Reshaping Medical Practice and Care with Health Information Systems

Ashish Dwivedi
University of Hull, UK

A volume in the Advances in Healthcare Information Systems and Administration (AHISA) Book Series

Medical Information Science Reference
An Imprint of IGI Global

Published in the United States of America by
Medical Information Science Reference (an imprint of IGI Global)
701 E. Chocolate Avenue
Hershey PA 17033
Tel: 717-533-8845
Fax: 717-533-8661
E-mail: cust@igi-global.com
Web site: http://www.igi-global.com

Library of Congress Cataloging-in-Publication Data

Names: Dwivedi, Ashish N., editor.
Title: Reshaping medical practice and care with health information systems / Ashish Dwivedi, editor.
Description: Hershey, PA : Medical Information Science Reference, [2016] | Includes bibliographical references and index.
Identifiers: LCCN 2015046928| ISBN 9781466698703 (hardcover) | ISBN 9781466698710 (ebook)
Subjects: LCSH: Medical informatics. | Medicine--Information technology.
Classification: LCC R858 .R47 2016 | DDC 610.285--dc23 LC record available at http://lccn.loc.gov/2015046928

This book is published in the IGI Global book series Advances in Healthcare Information Systems and Administration (AHISA) (ISSN: 2328-1243; eISSN: 2328-126X)

British Cataloguing in Publication Data
A Cataloguing in Publication record for this book is available from the British Library.

Advances in Healthcare Information Systems and Administration (AHISA) Book Series

ISSN: 2328-1243
EISSN: 2328-126X

Mission

The **Advances in Healthcare Information Systems and Administration (AHISA) Book Series** aims to provide a channel for international researchers to progress the field of study on technology and its implications on healthcare and health information systems. With the growing focus on healthcare and the importance of enhancing this industry to tend to the expanding population, the book series seeks to accelerate the awareness of technological advancements of health information systems and expand awareness and implementation.

Driven by advancing technologies and their clinical applications, the emerging field of health information systems and informatics is still searching for coherent directing frameworks to advance health care and clinical practices and research. Conducting research in these areas is both promising and challenging due to a host of factors, including rapidly evolving technologies and their application complexity. At the same time, organizational issues, including technology adoption, diffusion and acceptance as well as cost benefits and cost effectiveness of advancing health information systems and informatics applications as innovative forms of investment in healthcare are gaining attention as well. **AHISA** addresses these concepts and critical issues.

Coverage

- Measurements and Impact of HISA on Public and Social Policy
- Nursing Expert Systems
- E-Health and M-Health
- Clinical Decision Support Design, Development and Implementation
- Management of Emerging Health Care Technologies
- Decision Support Systems
- Virtual Health Technologies
- Rehabilitative Technologies
- Pharmaceutical and Home Healthcare Informatics
- IT Applications in Health Organizations and Practices

IGI Global is currently accepting manuscripts for publication within this series. To submit a proposal for a volume in this series, please contact our Acquisition Editors at Acquisitions@igi-global.com or visit: http://www.igi-global.com/publish/.

The Advances in Healthcare Information Systems and Administration (AHISA) Book Series (ISSN 2328-1243) is published by IGI Global, 701 E. Chocolate Avenue, Hershey, PA 17033-1240, USA, www.igi-global.com. This series is composed of titles available for purchase individually; each title is edited to be contextually exclusive from any other title within the series. For pricing and ordering information please visit http://www.igi-global.com/book-series/advances-healthcare-information-systems-administration/37156. Postmaster: Send all address changes to above address.

Titles in this Series

For a list of additional titles in this series, please visit: www.igi-global.com

Improving Health Management through Clinical Decision Support Systems
Jane D. Moon (The University of Melbourne, Australia) and Mary P. Galea (The University of Melbourne, Australia)
Medical Information Science Reference • copyright 2016 • 425pp • H/C (ISBN: 9781466694323) • US $225.00 (our price)

Maximizing Healthcare Delivery and Management through Technology Integration
Tiko Iyamu (Cape Peninsula University of Technology, South Africa) and Arthur Tatnall (Victoria University, Australia)
Medical Information Science Reference • copyright 2016 • 378pp • H/C (ISBN: 9781466694460) • US $235.00 (our price)

Flipping Health Care through Retail Clinics and Convenient Care Models
Amer Kaissi (Trinity University, USA)
Medical Information Science Reference • copyright 2015 • 306pp • H/C (ISBN: 9781466663558) • US $245.00 (our price)

Healthcare Informatics and Analytics Emerging Issues and Trends
Madjid Tavana (La Salle University, USA) Amir Hossein Ghapanchi (Griffith University, Australia) and Amir Talaei-Khoei (University of Technology, Sydney, Australia)
Medical Information Science Reference • copyright 2015 • 414pp • H/C (ISBN: 9781466663169) • US $235.00 (our price)

Laboratory Management Information Systems Current Requirements and Future Perspectives
Anastasius Moumtzoglou (Hellenic Society for Quality and Safety in Healthcare, Greece & P. & A. Kyriakou Children's Hospital, Greece) Anastasia Kastania (Athens University of Economics and Business, Greece) and Stavros Archondakis (Military Hospital of Athens, Greece)
Medical Information Science Reference • copyright 2015 • 354pp • H/C (ISBN: 9781466663206) • US $245.00 (our price)

Cloud Computing Applications for Quality Health Care Delivery
Anastasius Moumtzoglou (Hellenic Society for Quality and Safety in Healthcare, Greece & P. & A. Kyriakou Children's Hospital, Greece) and Anastasia N. Kastania (Athens University of Economics and Business, Greece)
Medical Information Science Reference • copyright 2014 • 342pp • H/C (ISBN: 9781466661189) • US $245.00 (our price)

In memory of Dr. S. N. Dwivedi and Mrs. Basanti Dwivedi

Editorial Advisory Board

List of Reviewers

Table of Contents

Preface xv

Chapter 1
The Benefits and Challenges of Using Mobile-Based Tools in Self-Management and Care 1
Rupananda Misra, Drexel University, USA

Chapter 2
A Transaction Cost Economics Perspective for Pervasive Technology 14
Nilmini Wickramasinghe, Epworth HealthCare, Australia & Deakin University, Australia
Indrit Troshani, University of Adelaide, Australia
Steve Goldberg, INET International Inc., Canada

Chapter 3
Constructive eHealth Evaluation: Involving the End-User 44
Anna Marie Balling Høstgaard, Aalborg University, Denmark

Chapter 4
Expanding Role of Telephone Systems in Healthcare: Developments and Opportunities 87
Jing Shi, North Dakota State University, USA
Ergin Erdem, North Dakota State University, USA
Heping Liu, North Dakota State University, USA

Chapter 5
Evaluating and Managing Electronic Commerce and Outsourcing Projects in Hospitals 132
Chad Lin, Curtin University, Australia
Geoffrey Jalleh, Curtin University, Australia
Yu-An Huang, National Chi Nan University, Taiwan

Chapter 6
Waseda University's E-School: 10 Years of E-Education in Japan 173
Shoji Nishimura, Waseda University, Japan
Douglass J. Scott, Waseda University, Japan

Chapter 7
From Healthcare Services to E-Health Applications: A Delivery System-Based Taxonomy 205
Riccardo Spinelli, University of Genoa, Italy
Clara Benevolo, University of Genoa, Italy

Chapter 8
Semantic Interoperability-Enabled Architecture for Connected Health Services 246
Adel Taweel, King's College London, UK & Birzeit University, Palestine

Chapter 9
SOA Governance in Healthcare: Beyond Early Ideas to a Structured Framework 266
Konstantinos Koumaditis, University of Piraeus, Greece, & Aarhus University, Denmark
Marinos Themistocleous, University of Piraeus, Greece & University of Coimbra, Portugal

Chapter 10
Healthy 3.0: Healthcare Digital Dimensions 287
Maria Teresa Borges Tiago, University of Azores, Portugal
Flávio Tiago, UAC, Portugal
Francisco Emanuel Batista Amaral, University of Azores, Portugal
Sandra Silva, Unidade de Saúde de Ilha de S. Miguel Azores, Portugal

Conclusion 323

Compilation of References 330

About the Contributors 394

Index 397

Detailed Table of Contents

Preface xv

Chapter 1
The Benefits and Challenges of Using Mobile-Based Tools in Self-Management and Care 1
Rupananda Misra, Drexel University, USA

An effective intervention tool in self-management and care is the patients' use of mobile-based devices. This tool reflects a paradigm shift in many areas of health management from healthcare professionals to the patients themselves. These mobile devices contribute to a growing public interest in self-care. This new use will save patients not only expensive hospitalization costs and doctor visits but will also save the US treasury millions of dollars. To successfully empower the patients who use these mobile-based tools to manage their own health as well as to see positive health outcomes, Mobile app developers need to consider many things when developing these mobile apps such as an engaging and easy-to-use interface, relevant content, and more. In addition, the developers must secure patient data and ensure user privacy.

Chapter 2
A Transaction Cost Economics Perspective for Pervasive Technology 14
Nilmini Wickramasinghe, Epworth HealthCare, Australia & Deakin University, Australia
Indrit Troshani, University of Adelaide, Australia
Steve Goldberg, INET International Inc., Canada

Numerous mobile technology solutions are being developed and implemented today to address a myriad of healthcare problems. However, it remains unclear what the true cost/benefit of these solutions is and who benefits from them. To investigate this we apply a transaction cost economics framework to a pervasive mobile solution that has been designed and developed to enhance diabetes self-care. Diabetes is one of the leading chronic diseases and its prevalence continues to rise. The solution examined in this paper relies on pervasive wireless technology and is designed to facilitate the effective management of diabetes in the context of gestational diabetes, a conditions that affects up to 8% of pregnant women. A transactions cost assessment of this solution is provided.

Chapter 3
Constructive eHealth Evaluation: Involving the End-User 44
Anna Marie Balling Høstgaard, Aalborg University, Denmark

Despite the existence of an extensive body of knowledge about best practices and factors that contribute to the successful development and adoption of eHealth, many eHealth development-projects still face a number of problems - many of them of an organizational nature. This chapter presents a new method: "The Constructive eHealth evaluation method" aimed at supporting real end-user participation - a well-known success factor in eHealth development. It provides an analytical framework for achieving real end-user participation during the different phases in the eHealth lifecycle. The method was developed and used for the first time during the evaluation of an EHR planning process in a Danish region. It has proven effective for providing management at more levels on-going information and feedback from end-users, allowing management to change direction during eHealth development in order to achieve the most successful adoption and implementation of eHealth in healthcare environments.

Chapter 4
Expanding Role of Telephone Systems in Healthcare: Developments and Opportunities 87
Jing Shi, North Dakota State University, USA
Ergin Erdem, North Dakota State University, USA
Heping Liu, North Dakota State University, USA

The telephone systems in healthcare settings serve as a viable tool for improving the quality of service provided to patients, decreasing the cost, and improving the patient satisfaction. It can play a pivotal role for transformation of the healthcare delivery for embracing personalized and patient centered care. This chapter presents a systematic review of new developments of healthcare telephone system operations in various areas such as tele-health. Current research on topics such as tele-diagnosis, tele-nursing, tele-consultation is outlined. Specific issues associated with the emerging applications such as underreferral, legal issues, patient acceptance, on-call physician are discussed. Meanwhile, the architecture and underlying technologies for healthcare telephone systems are introduced, and the performance metrics for measuring the system operations are provided. In addition, challenges and opportunities related with improving the healthcare telephone systems are identified, and the potential opportunities of optimizing these systems are pointed out.

Chapter 5
Evaluating and Managing Electronic Commerce and Outsourcing Projects in Hospitals 132
Chad Lin, Curtin University, Australia
Geoffrey Jalleh, Curtin University, Australia
Yu-An Huang, National Chi Nan University, Taiwan

Despite the huge popularity of outsourcing in electronic commerce/IT in the past two decades, many hospitals have failed to realize the expected benefits from their outsourcing projects. Not surprisingly, the management of electronic commerce/IT outsourcing contracts has become one of the top management issues for hospitals executives in recent years. Hence, the purpose of this study was to provide an overview of outsourcing in electronic commerce/IT investment evaluation and benefits realization processes and practices in Australian and Taiwanese hospitals. Inherent in this study was the opportunity to compare such practices between a developed economy (Australia) and a newly industrialized economy (Taiwan). Several key electronic commerce/IT investment evaluation and outsourcing issues and challenges faced by Australian and Taiwanese hospitals will be presented. The results will assist hospital executives to develop their own approaches and strategies to better manage the opportunities and threats that exist in undertaking electronic commerce/IT outsourcing projects in Australian and Taiwanese hospitals.

Chapter 6
Waseda University's E-School: 10 Years of E-Education in Japan 173
Shoji Nishimura, Waseda University, Japan
Douglass J. Scott, Waseda University, Japan

In 2003, the School of Human Sciences, Waseda University (Japan), established the e-School, Japan's first complete undergraduate program enabling students to earn their bachelor degrees solely through e-learning. Supported by the availability of high-speed Internet connections, it has become possible to economically transmit high-quality videotaped lectures across Japan and throughout the world. Waseda's e-School has many features that contribute to its success, among these are that lecture contents are transmitted with an image quality that allows students to easily read what is written on the blackboard. In addition, online classes are relatively small—21 students on average—and new classes are created to respond to students' needs and interests. This chapter outlines the e-School's first 10 years of operation: Its history, curriculum, administration, and management learning system. Data are also presented for student engagement with the e-School system for the first ten years of operation (2003-2012).

Chapter 7
From Healthcare Services to E-Health Applications: A Delivery System-Based Taxonomy 205
Riccardo Spinelli, University of Genoa, Italy
Clara Benevolo, University of Genoa, Italy

The increasing adoption of ICT – and especially Internet-based technologies – in healthcare has been very fruitful and has led to the innovative approach to healthcare practice commonly known as e-health. However, the boundaries of this new approach to healthcare are not clear, as it is reflected by the various properties and taxonomies of e-health applications which have been proposed. In this chapter, we first review the definition of e-health and the main taxonomies for its constituents. Then we propose an original taxonomy for e-health applications, based on the structural features of the delivery system of the services which are digitalized: the need for a physical interaction between the subjects involved in the service provisioning and the possibility of delivering the services through Internet-based technology.

Chapter 8
Semantic Interoperability-Enabled Architecture for Connected Health Services 246
Adel Taweel, King's College London, UK & Birzeit University, Palestine

With the increasing availability of connected health organisations, key medical information is expected to be accessible at the point of care. However, the high sensitivity of the clinical data and the large heterogeneity in health information systems pose a great interoperability challenge, including solutions that rely solely on the use of data exchange standards. Due to low adoption of these standards, such solutions will not sufficiently scale to achieve this objective. This chapter presents a service-based approach that utilises domain models combined with extensible problem models, enriched with domain terminology and knowledge services to enable autonomous data governance and semantic interoperability. The chapter addresses the resulting requirements, describes the proposed a solution and reports the results from the prototype of the approach.

Chapter 9
SOA Governance in Healthcare: Beyond Early Ideas to a Structured Framework 266
Konstantinos Koumaditis, University of Piraeus, Greece, & Aarhus University, Denmark
Marinos Themistocleous, University of Piraeus, Greece & University of Coimbra, Portugal

This chapter depicts the gradual development of a conceptual SOA Governance Framework tailored for healthcare organisations. The proposed framework presented herein is based on the authors' previous research and includes nine SOA Governance elements that need to be considered during the SOA process. The identification and conceptualisation of the elements were grounded in the normative literature and further developed to include healthcare specific aspects. This comes as a method to overcome the limitations identified in normative literature and enhance the elements' conceptualisation. Besides, the authors propose a unique design combining nine elements of SOA Governance with SOA Critical Success Factors (CSFs) and Healthcare Information Systems (HIS) challenges. This proposal aims to pinpoint attributes and guidelines for each element, required to successfully govern SOA and tackle longstanding HIS challenges. The framework is intended to be used as a decision supporting tool for SOA Governance in a healthcare setting.

Chapter 10
Healthy 3.0: Healthcare Digital Dimensions 287
Maria Teresa Borges Tiago, University of Azores, Portugal
Flávio Tiago, UAC, Portugal
Francisco Emanuel Batista Amaral, University of Azores, Portugal
Sandra Silva, Unidade de Saúde de Ilha de S. Miguel Azores, Portugal

Over the past few years, healthcare practice has evolved to include new forms of information and communication technologies, and healthcare providers have begun to leverage IT solutions and the internet to reach consumers in transformative ways. There is a common thought both in business and academia that the technology adoption process is a key component of success and allows firms to achieve and sustain competitive advantages. Therefore, this research attempts to reinforce the assessment of ICT impacts on healthcare, analyzing it from two different perspectives: 1) firm performance, which is measured as a combination of induced and intangible benefits beyond the traditional financial benefits; and 2) healthcare providers' acceptance and adoption of ICT tools. To assess the first perspective, a structural equation model was applied to a large database sample covering firms from 17 European countries. The results reinforce the importance of induced and structural benefits in firms' overall performance. The second perspective was analyzed only for the Portuguese healthcare providers sample. These results can be a starting point for rethinking the healthcare models emphasizing the perspectives of Healthy 2.0 and considering that patients' technological pattern evolution will lead to Healthy 3.0 in the short term. Nevertheless, some questions remain unanswered regarding the impacts of the ICT acceptance process on overall benefits; therefore, future research will focus on this domain.

Conclusion 323

Compilation of References 330

About the Contributors 394

Index 397

Preface

This edited book argues that new innovative practices from domains relating to Knowledge Management (KM) paradigm can offer solutions to healthcare institutions allowing them to face the challenge of transforming large amounts of medical data into relevant clinical information. This can be achieved by integrating information using workflow, context management and collaboration tools to provide a mechanism for effectively transferring the acquired knowledge as and when required.

This edited book establishes the interrelationship between KM and the healthcare sector by stating that both have been redefined by the ICT revolution and that both are bringing about fundamental changes which are redefining the work place of these organisations. Another common point is that both KM and the healthcare industry are concerned with dissemination of information in a manner which ensures that information is available when required. The contemporary focus is only on how best to disseminate the information, which could be fatal for the future of the healthcare applications (i.e. current use is static). Rather than creating or disseminating contextual knowledge, healthcare applications are being used to disseminate data and information. Future healthcare industry applications would have to support the transfer of information with context (i.e. such schemes would have to become dynamic in nature).

Such a scenario is likely to lead to a situation where healthcare institutions would be flooded with large amounts of clinical data. The introduction of the KM paradigm would enable these institutions to face the challenge of transforming large amounts of medical data into relevant clinical information. Future healthcare systems would have to shift their emphasis to deal with the intangibles of knowledge, institutions and culture. Healthcare institutions require a framework which would help to assess how best to identify and create knowledge from internal and external organisational experiences and how best to disseminate it on an organisation-wide basis in a manner which ensures that the acquired knowledge is available for preventive and operative medical diagnosis and treatment when required.

This would call for the contextual recycling of knowledge which has been acquired from the adoption of healthcare industry trials. KM can assist the healthcare industry to become viable by giving healthcare information context, so that other healthcare providers can use the healthcare industry to extract knowledge and not information.

ORGANISATION OF THIS BOOK

Chapter 1, titled "A Review of the Use of Mobile-Based Tools in Self-Management and Care," by Misra notes that evidence suggests that self management program is an effective intervention tool that can improve health status, reduce hospitalization costs, and reduce the providers workload. The terms "self-care" and "self-management" have been used interchangeably to imply the actions and decisions that people make in dealing with their health and illnesses. Self care in this context refers to the activities that the patients' undertake without the help of professionals in promoting their own health, preventing their own diseases, limiting their own illness, and restoring their own health. Increasingly, health experts agree that self-management is a strong determinant of positive health outcomes in illnesses such as chronic diseases. There is also a growing public interest in self-care because of epidemiological factors, personal responsibility for health, availability of self-care information and technology, etc. It is concluded that in order for self-management programs to be successful, patients have to achieve the skills and confidence to manage their own health, which means a shift from management by their healthcare provider to management by the patient themselves.

Chapter 2, titled "A Transaction Cost Economics Perspective for Pervasive Technology" by Wickramasinghe, Troshani, and Goldberg, observes that numerous mobile technology solutions are being developed and implemented today to address a myriad of healthcare problems. However, it remains unclear what the true cost/benefit of these solutions is and who benefits from them. To investigate this we apply a transaction cost economics framework to a pervasive mobile solution that has been designed and developed to enhance diabetes self-care. Diabetes is one of the leading chronic diseases and its prevalence continues to rise. The solution examined in this paper relies on pervasive wireless technology and is designed to facilitate the effective management of diabetes in the context of gestational diabetes, a conditions that affects up to 8% of pregnant women. A transactions cost assessment of this solution is provided.

Chapter 3, titled "Constructive eHealth Evaluation: Involving the End-User" by Høstgaard, notes that despite the existence of an extensive body of knowledge about best practices and factors that contribute to the successful development and adoption of eHealth, many eHealth development-projects still face a number of problems - many of them of an organizational nature. This chapter presents a new method: "The Constructive eHealth evaluation method" aimed at supporting real end-user participation - a well-known success factor in eHealth development. It provides an analytical framework for achieving real end-user participation during the different phases in the eHealth lifecycle. The method was developed and used for the first time during the evaluation of an EHR planning process in a Danish region. It has proven effective for providing management at more levels on-going information and feedback from end-users, allowing management to change direction during eHealth development in order to achieve the most successful adoption and implementation of eHealth in healthcare environments.

Chapter 4, titled "Expanding Role of Telephone Systems in Healthcare: Developments and Opportunities" by Shi, Erdem, and Liu, observes that the telephone systems in healthcare settings serve as a viable tool for improving the quality of service provided to patients, decreasing the cost, and improving the patient satisfaction. It can play a pivotal role for transformation of the healthcare delivery for embracing personalized and patient centered care. This chapter presents a systematic review of new developments of healthcare telephone system operations in various areas such as tele-health. Current research on topics such as tele-diagnosis, tele-nursing, tele-consultation is outlined. Specific issues associated with the emerging applications such as underreferral, legal issues, patient acceptance, on-call physician are discussed. Meanwhile, the architecture and underlying technologies for healthcare telephone systems are introduced, and the performance metrics for measuring the system operations are provided. In addition, challenges and opportunities related with improving the healthcare telephone systems are identified, and the potential opportunities of optimizing these systems are pointed out.

Chapter 5, titled "Evaluating and Managing Electronic Commerce and Outsourcing Projects in Hospitals" by Lin, Jalleh, and Huang, notes that despite the huge popularity of outsourcing in electronic commerce/IT in the past two decades, many hospitals have failed to realize the expected benefits from their outsourcing projects. Not surprisingly, the management of electronic commerce/IT outsourcing contracts has become one of the top management issues for hospitals executives in recent years. Hence, the purpose of this study was to provide an overview of outsourcing in electronic commerce/IT investment evaluation and benefits realization processes and practices in Australian and Taiwanese hospitals. Inherent in this study was the opportunity to compare such practices between a developed economy (Australia) and a newly industrialized economy (Taiwan). Several key electronic commerce/IT investment evaluation and outsourcing issues and challenges faced by Australian and Taiwanese hospitals will be presented. The results will assist hospital executives to develop their own approaches and strategies to better manage the opportunities and threats that exist in undertaking electronic commerce/IT outsourcing projects in Australian and Taiwanese hospitals.

Chapter 6, titled "Waseda University's E-School: 10 Years of E-Education in Japan" by Nishimura and Scott, comments that in 2003, the School of Human Sciences, Waseda University (Japan), established the e-School, Japan's first complete undergraduate program enabling students to earn their bachelor degrees solely through e-learning. Supported by the availability of high-speed Internet connections, it has become possible to economically transmit high-quality videotaped lectures across Japan and throughout the world. Waseda's e-School has many features that contribute to its success, among these are that lecture contents are transmitted with an image quality that allows students to easily read what is written on the blackboard. In addition, online classes are relatively small—21 students on average—and new classes are created to respond to students' needs and interests. This chapter outlines the e-School's first 10 years of operation: Its history, curriculum, administration, and management learning system. Data are also presented for student engagement with the e-School system for the first ten years of operation from 2003 to 2012.

Chapter 7, titled "From Healthcare Services to E-Health Applications: A Delivery System-Based Taxonomy" by Spinelli and Benevolo, estimates that the increasing adoption of ICT – and especially Internet-based technologies – in healthcare has been very fruitful and has led to the innovative approach to healthcare practice commonly known as e-health. However, the boundaries of this new approach to healthcare are not clear, as it is reflected by the various properties and taxonomies of e-health applications which have been proposed. In this chapter, we first review the definition of e-health and the main taxonomies for its constituents. Then we propose an original taxonomy for e-health applications, based on the structural features of the delivery system of the services which are digitalized: the need for a physical interaction between the subjects involved in the service provisioning and the possibility of delivering the services through Internet-based technology.

Chapter 8, titled "Semantic Interoperability Enabled Architecture For Connected Health Services" by Taweel, argues that with the increasing availability of connected health organisations, key medical information is expected to be accessible at the point of care. However, the high sensitivity of the clinical data and the large heterogeneity in health information systems pose a great interoperability challenge, including solutions that rely solely on the use of data exchange standards. Due to low adoption of these standards, such solutions will not sufficiently scale to achieve this objective. This chapter presents a service-based approach that utilises domain models combined with extensible problem models, enriched with domain terminology and knowledge services to enable autonomous data governance and semantic interoperability. The chapter addresses the resulting requirements, describes the proposed a solution and reports the results from the prototype of the approach.

Chapter 9, titled "SOA Governance in Healthcare: Beyond Early Ideas to a Structured Framework" by Koumaditis and Themistocleous, depicts the gradual development of a conceptual SOA Governance Framework tailored for healthcare organisations. The proposed framework presented herein is based on the authors' previous research and includes nine SOA Governance elements that need to be considered during the SOA process. The identification and conceptualisation of the elements were grounded in the normative literature and further developed to include healthcare specific aspects. This comes as a method to overcome the limitations identified in normative literature and enhance the elements' conceptualisation. Besides, the authors propose a unique design combining nine elements of SOA Governance with SOA Critical Success Factors (CSFs) and Healthcare Information Systems (HIS) challenges. This proposal aims to pinpoint attributes and guidelines for each element, required to successfully govern SOA and tackle longstanding HIS challenges. The framework is intended to be used as a decision supporting tool for SOA Governance in a healthcare setting.

Chapter 10, titled "Healthy 3.0: Healthcare Digital Dimensions" by Tiago, observes that over the past few years, healthcare practice has evolved to include new forms of information and communication technologies, and healthcare providers have begun to leverage IT solutions and the internet to reach consumers in transformative ways. There is a common thought both in business and academia that the technology adoption process is a key component of success and allows firms to achieve and sustain competitive advantages. Therefore, this research attempts to reinforce the assessment of ICT impacts on healthcare, analyzing it from two different perspectives: 1) firm performance, which is measured as a combination of induced and intangible benefits beyond the traditional financial benefits; and 2) healthcare providers' acceptance and adoption of ICT tools. To assess the first perspective, a structural equation model was applied to a large database sample covering firms from 17 European countries. The results reinforce the importance of induced and structural benefits in firms' overall performance. The second perspective was analyzed only for the Portuguese healthcare providers sample. These results can be a starting point for rethinking the healthcare models emphasizing the perspectives of Healthy 2.0 and considering that patients' technological pattern evolution will lead to Healthy 3.0 in the short term. Nevertheless, some questions remain unanswered regarding the impacts of the ICT acceptance process on overall benefits; therefore, future research will focus on this domain.

I hope that academics, clinical and non-clinical practitioners, managers, and students will find some issues of interest and value in the ensuing pages.

Ashish N. Dwivedi
Hull University, UK
May 2015

Chapter 1
The Benefits and Challenges of Using Mobile-Based Tools in Self-Management and Care

Rupananda Misra
Drexel University, USA

ABSTRACT

An effective intervention tool in self-management and care is the patients' use of mobile-based devices. This tool reflects a paradigm shift in many areas of health management from healthcare professionals to the patients themselves. These mobile devices contribute to a growing public interest in self-care. This new use will save patients not only expensive hospitalization costs and doctor visits but will also save the US treasury millions of dollars. To successfully empower the patients who use these mobile-based tools to manage their own health as well as to see positive health outcomes, Mobile app developers need to consider many things when developing these mobile apps such as an engaging and easy-to-use interface, relevant content, and more. In addition, the developers must secure patient data and ensure user privacy.

DOI: 10.4018/978-1-4666-9870-3.ch001

BACKGROUND

Evidence suggests that a self-management program is an effective intervention tool that can improve health status, reduce hospitalization costs (Effing, et al., 2007; Lorig, et al., 1999), and reduce the provider's workload (Nazareth & Murray, 2010). The terms "self-care" and "self-management" are interchangeable and imply the actions and decisions people make in dealing with their health and illnesses (Wagner & McCorkle, 2010). Self-care in this context refers to the activities the patients undertake, without the help of professionals, in promoting their own health, preventing their own diseases, limiting their own illnesses, and restoring their own health (Levin & Idler, 1983). Increasingly, health experts agree that self-management is a strong determinant of positive health outcomes in illnesses such as chronic diseases (Janson, McGrath, Covington, Cheng, & Boushey, 2009), diabetes (Funnell, et al., 2009), asthma (Krishna, et al., 2003), mental illness (Cook, et al., 2009), arthritis (Lorig, Ritter, Laurent, & Plant, 2008), eating habits (Irvine, Ary, Grove, & Gilfillan-Morton, 2004), and other illnesses. There's also a growing public interest in self-care because of epidemiological factors, personal responsibility for health, availability of self-care information and technology, and more (Levin & Idler, 1983). In order for self-management programs to succeed, patients have to achieve the skills and confidence to manage their own health, which means a shift from management by their healthcare provider to management by the patients themselves (Bourbeau & van der Palen, 2009).

Self-management entails learning about the illnesses, treatment options, and understanding medical terminologies, which means the patients need the skills and the tools to empower themselves to manage their health (Alpay, Verhoef, Xie, Te'eni, & Zwetsloot-Schonk, 2009). Self-management also means that in designing applications for consumers, developers need a deep understanding of the consumer's background, needs, and preferences because today's consumers are a lot more involved in their own healthcare and more technology-minded (Alpay, et al., 2009). Therefore, self-management programs are much more than patient education; they must also include assessments of progress and problems, goal-setting, and problem-solving (Bourbeau & van der Palen, 2009). Although modern technologies hold tremendous potential in developing effective health communication interventions, there are a few challenges to reach its full potential such as the design must (1) maximize interactive communication with users to encourage their active involvement, (2) work effectively across communication platforms, (3) personally engage the users, and (4) have broad reach across diverse populations (Kreps & Neuhauser, 2010).

Much evidence exists to suggest that mobile phone technology can support behavior change (Whittaker, Merry, Dorey, & Maddison, 2012). So, the question becomes what is the best way to deliver self-management and care using mobile phone technology or mobile health technologies? The use of mobile health technologies in healthcare can become a major digital health revolution. In today's world, the concept of mobile health (or mHealth) broadly describes the use of mobile telecommunication technologies to deliver or communicate healthcare to support wellness (Steinhubl, Muse, & Topol, 2013). Use of mobile IT devices such as personal digital assistants (PDAs) and cellular phones in healthcare is increasing (Mitseva, Kyriazakos, Litke, Papadakis, & Prasad, 2009).

Cell phones are the most ubiquitous of the mobile devices in the world (Kahn, Yang, & Kahn, 2010). According to Pew Internet Research, as of December 2009, 83 percent of adults own a cell phone whether it is a Blackberry or iPhone or any other device that is also called a cell phone (Lenhart, Purcell, Smith, & Zickuhr, 2010). The technologies that underlie mobile phones are not just cheaper but are also getting powerful, a circumstance already recognized in the delivery of healthcare services and the promotion of personal health (Patrick, Griswold, Raab, & Intille, 2008). In the developed world, its penetration is almost 90 percent and in the developing world, it is around 33 percent. Other than easily accessing health website information on mobile devices, consumers can access around 30,000 to 90,000 health-related apps for download (Steinhubl, et al., 2013). Therefore, since mobile technologies are widely available, it can play a critical role in healthcare at the regional, community, and the individual level (Kahn, et al., 2010).

Already research studies show that learners prefer mobile devices to carrying a lot of pieces of paper. Also, learning through mobile devices supports lifelong learning because they allow access any time and from anyplace; allow greater engagement with learning and assessment (Taylor, et al., 2010); and allow remote patient data capture (Mitseva, et al., 2009). From an economic perspective, using mobile phones as a means of delivery of healthcare makes sense because US expenditure on healthcare is projected to reach $4 trillion per year (Patrick, et al., 2008). Also, because mobile phone users can use text-based communication along with accessing the Internet, it is a great resource for doctors and patients to keep in touch (Peirce & Bakke, 2010).

A recent study focusing on patients diagnosed with Type 1 insulin-dependent diabetes to manage their disease using mobile phones suggests the application was successful, and the overall patient satisfaction level was positive (Preuveneers & Berbers, 2008). The findings of another study to examine the feasibility of using cell phone technology to assist with diabetes self-care in a clinic population indicate that the intervention using a cell phone had a positive impact on clinical outcome and self-efficacy (Faridi, et al., 2008). A recent systematic review of behavior change interventions delivered by mobile telephone short-message services indicates that 13 out of 14 reviewed articles reported positive behavior change outcomes. Tailoring of SMS along with interactivity was the important feature (Fjeldsoe, Marshall, & Miller, 2009). Other parts of the world such as Uganda (Chang, et al., 2008) have successfully implemented mobile phone intervention in healthcare.

In another recent systematic review for all controlled trials of mobile technology-based health interventions to assess the effectiveness of mobile technology interventions delivered to healthcare consumers between Jan. 1990 and Sept. 2010, the authors found that text messaging interventions increased adherence to antiretroviral adherence and smoking cessation and providers should include these interventions in their services (Free, et al., 2013).

Although there is a strong perception among the general public about the side effects from the exposure to mobile phones, it is still inconclusive whether cell phone radiation causes electronsensitivity (Rubin, Cleare, & Wessely, 2008). Health communication has used telephone-based technology for more than a decade, but what is significant now is that computer technology is behind much of the innovation in telephone technology in health communication (Suggs, 2006). For health information to stay effective, the health message designers should pay attention to the inherent strength of the medium as well as to the principles of the effective message design in enhancing knowledge (Maibach & Parrott, 1995). With the proliferation of new health information technologies comes the daunting responsibility to design health applications that are interoperable, easy to use, and engaging and communicates the right information to diverse audiences (Kreps & Neuhauser, 2010; Mitseva, et al., 2009).

Bridging the gap between access to the information and understanding the information can lead to empowering the patients (Alpay, et al., 2009). These new communication technologies such as mobile phones also bring in new challenges in empowering the patients and transitioning the patient's role from a passive to an active one in which the patient stays informed, has choices, and becomes involved in the decision-making process (Mitseva, et al., 2009). While mobile phones are primarily communication devices, the newer smartphones can mimic what a personal computer can do with the transmission of a variety of data, including a multimedia learning environment such as text, graphics, audio, and video (Patrick, et al., 2008). Although several commercial applications run on mobile phones, a recent usability study on the design of mobile dietary and nutritional support for individuals living with diabetes indicates that these commercial applications still have opportunities to enhance their design (Arsand, Tufano, Ralston, & Hjortdahl, 2008). Studies suggest that patients with limited health literacy may require an improved communication mechanism to support their self-management strategies (Sarkar, et al., 2008).

MHealth can potentially help patients in several ways. For instance, it can allow patients to diagnose their acute symptoms and enhance monitoring, tracking, and communication of various biometric information for the patients to send to their healthcare providers to rapidly diagnose and treat their conditions (Steinhubl, et al., 2013). One of the important objectives of self-management programs is to bring about change in a patient's behavior, but there are challenges, as well. A lot of self-management programs failed because of a failure of knowing how to intervene (Bourbeau & van der Palen, 2009).

Even though mobile devices with their ubiquitous presence can help disease prevention and management around-the-clock with lots of locations and in real time (Chen, et al., 2012), there are a number of obstacles and complexities in the use of mHealth technologies, especially reimbursement, patient-physician relationship, possible increase in the workload of healthcare providers, lack of oversight by governments, and other factors (Steinhubl, et al., 2013). Also, health apps are overloading medical professionals and regular citizens, and it is challenging to find the right app for their needs. On top of that, health information fragments across too many apps (van Velsen, Beaujean, & van Gemert-Pijnen, 2013).

Here are few important points about the use of mobile devices in self-care that can potentially help an effective health intervention tool and transform health.

Interoperabilty with Other Clinical Systems

One of the great things that mobile apps circumvent is the unnecessary paper work and technical challenges that come with using electronic health systems (Logan, 2013). One of the important points to keep in mind is how compatible or interoperable the mobile apps are with other clinical systems in terms of communicating and exchanging data. Interoperability is a critical issue in mHealth because many of the patient's mobile apps may not be compatible with the patient's other health systems. Many mobile apps such as text messages may seem simple to the patients when reminding them of their next appointment, but other apps may need to exchange information, such as microscopy images taken with a mobile phone, with other health systems, and it's important it can securely import into the patient's electronic health record (Editors, 2013).

For example, a diabetic patient may record her insulin use, nutrition intake, exercise, blood sugar values, and other data in several different mobile apps, but without a shared architecture for data analysis, the patient and clinician may have a difficult time to correlate the blood sugar values with corresponding exercise or diet (Chen, et al., 2012).

Information Design of the Mobile Health Apps and the Application of Health Theories

While mobile technologies rapidly evolve as a method for delivering health behavior interventions, the content and the timing of those interventions were not consistently grounded in health behavior theories (Riley, et al., 2011). While most of the smoking and weight loss studies reviewed had a theoretical basis for the intervention, most of the adherence and disease management studies did not (Riley, et al., 2011).

The health researchers in mobile app development may be primarily interested about how the application would contain traditional theory-based behavioral strategies such as self-regulation theory, but the app developers primarily care about the user interface and how to keep the users engaged (Azar, et al., 2013).

There are several theory-based behavioral modification strategies used in the clinical field for weight loss, changes in diet, and so on, but many of those traditional theories may not work in the mobile-based interventions because these interventions are often more responsive, interactive, and dynamic (Azar, et al., 2013). For example, theories such as persuasive technology theory and the Fogg Behavioral Model (FBM) may seem more appropriate for a digital medium to increase motivation and trigger changes in the patient's behavior (Azar, et al., 2013).

Management of Acute Conditions

Now approximately 34 percent of all physician office visits relate to acute care. Many of these patients can potentially forgo such visits and manage their health using effective and informed management from home (Steinhubl, et al., 2013). Even though there are rich sources of passive and actively collected data from mHealth applications, they lack in three essential areas for improving health outcomes (Chen, et al., 2012)

(1) patient-facing feedback to guide patients' self-care (e.g., how does taking the medication topiramate affect my pain?), (2) clinician-directed summary data to guide clinical decision-making for individual patients (e.g., how do the side effects and therapeutic benefits of topiramate balance for my patient?), and (3) research evidence to improve clinical care for groups of patients (populations) (e.g., in patients with neuropathic pain, does topiramate reduce pain intensity and improve quality of life?)

Lack of visualization tools, absence of analysis tools as well as biases in the data make it difficult for patients to make sense of the data to improve health outcomes (Chen, et al., 2012).

Decision-Making and Scalability

Traditional forms of interventions such as 1-to-1 doctor or pharmacy visits are either too costly or do not engage patients in decision-making (Logan, 2013). Mobile app use, however, can help to overcome those limitations. By using mobile technologies, health professionals can monitor a large number of patients passively to ensure patients maintain their health and minimize or reduce office visits of most common acute and chronic issues (Steinhubl, et al., 2013).

Traditionally, physicians were the gatekeepers of the patients' health information, and the patients and their families did not participate in the important decision-making process. But the Internet technologies have changed that. Nowadays, the focus has changed toward patient-centered care, which actively engages the patients in the decision-making process (Barry & Edgman-Levitan, 2012).

One aspect of the decision-making process is providing proper feedback from the mobile app. Feedback can help in various things such as providing cues or reinforcement to learners, reducing discrepancies, performing tasks, clarifying the goals, making progress toward the goal, and giving activities to the patient to achieve the goal. It is advisable not to think of extrinsic rewards as feedback since it is possible it is not that effective in enhancing achievement (Hattie & Timperley, 2007). Research studies suggest that feedback is more effective if provided on information on correct responses instead of incorrect responses (Hattie & Timperley, 2007).

Security of Data

In today's world, every single day, some company launches a new mobile health app. The protection of patient data is critical, but with the emerging complex mobile technologies, communication capabilities and user expectations, they require sophisticated technological safeguards to protect unauthorized access and threats to data integrity (Luxton, Kayl, & Mishkind, 2012). Even though it is important to safeguard the patients' personal health information, app developers do not follow appropriate and stringent methods to do this, and the apps go on the market without proper security and privacy mechanisms to protect the users' data and users' consent collection (Martínez-Pérez, de la Torre-Díez, & López-Coronado, 2014). The laws about privacy and security both in the EU and USA are based on obsolete technology and are not up-to-date; they are too open and too old. The regulators need to create more specific rules to solve security problems (Martínez-Pérez, et al., 2014).

Many researchers propose many different security schemes for the use of wireless sensors with smartphone applications. Many mobile applications use wireless sensors to monitor the wellbeing of critical patients who have chronic conditions such as cardiac problems, Parkinson's disease, or epilepsy. In such cases where confidentially of the patient data is highly essential, some researchers propose the use of a three-tier security architecture for the mobile application (Sahoo, 2012). Given the use of disparate mobile technologies, it is apparent that the different stakeholders must collaborate and find a solution to create or follow "standardized policies, technologies, administrative practices to assure data security." (Luxton, et al., 2012)"

Use of Open Standards

The current use of close standards in eHealth and mHealth can potentially lead to knowledge barriers for IT professionals in different countries because of the lack of access to the standards (Editors, 2013). In that case, IT professionals cannot make appropriate decisions in designing health systems. For example, Health Level Seven (HL7), which is a comprehensive framework and related standards in terms of the exchange, integration, sharing, and retrieval of electronic health information, and SNOMED CT are comprehensive clinical terminologies, which define healthcare concepts relating to diseases, findings, procedures, and so forth. Both are nonprofit organizations, but neither is yet freely available for use (Editors, 2013).

Other than that, there are other platforms such as the Open mHealth project, which is supposed to make it easier in data sharing across platforms and thereby integrating disparate health data. It is creating a repository of shared, open-source, and interoperable modules for mHealth data interpretation and presentation (Kumar, et al., 2013). By using open standards, it will also facilitate the use of common metrics and standards for mHealth research as well as in the creation of databases to make data aggregation possible (Kumar, et al., 2013).

Authenticity and Evaluation of Data

Even though there are many mobile apps that help patients to quit smoking, improve HIV medication adherence, there is not just a need to better evaluate but also to challenge the understanding of how to evaluate (Editors, 2013). In two systematic reviews of randomized trials relating to interventions to improve health behaviors, improve disease self-management, and facilitate healthcare delivery, the authors suggest that just focusing exclusively on the randomized trials as the gold standards may be too restrictive in evaluating the mHealth interventions (Editors, 2013).

Summary

In this chapter, we reviewed some of the critical issues regarding the effectiveness of mobile device-based intervention in health self-management and care. The aim of this chapter is to better understand the benefits and challenges of using mobile device-based tools to aid in self-management and care.

By using mobile health apps to monitor patient self-management, physicians can now spend extra time with critical patients who need them most (Steinhubl, et al., 2013). This can also increase physician satisfaction. So from that perspective, mobile health technologies can potentially transform healthcare. But, with that comes many challenges such as the lack of standardized data security for patient data privacy and interoperability, among other things. Consequently, health practitioners cannot harness the full potential of mobile apps, which presents a significant barrier to self-care and management of health. Although, key components of traditional behavior theory are the basis of many of the mobile-based health apps, but the user interface of mobile health is critical to engage the user and support long-term maintenance of that behavior change (Azar, et al., 2013).

REFERENCES

Alpay, L., Verhoef, J., Xie, B., Te'eni, D., & Zwetsloot-Schonk, J. (2009). Current challenge in consumer health informatics: Bridging the gap between access to information and information understanding. *Biomedical Informatics Insights*, *2*(1), 1. PMID:20419038

Arsand, E., Tufano, J., Ralston, J., & Hjortdahl, P. (2008). Designing mobile dietary management support technologies for people with diabetes. *Journal of Telemedicine and Telecare*, *14*(7), 329–332. doi:10.1258/jtt.2008.007001 PMID:18852310

Azar, K. M., Lesser, L. I., Laing, B. Y., Stephens, J., Aurora, M. S., Burke, L. E., & Palaniapan, L. (2013). Mobile applications for weight management: Theory-based content analysis. *American Journal of Preventive Medicine*, *45*(5), 583–589. doi:10.1016/j.amepre.2013.07.005 PMID:24139771

Barry, M. J., & Edgman-Levitan, S. (2012). Shared decision making—the pinnacle of patient-centered care. *The New England Journal of Medicine*, *366*(9), 780–781. doi:10.1056/NEJMp1109283 PMID:22375967

Bourbeau, J., & van der Palen, J. (2009). Promoting effective self-management programmes to improve COPD. *The European Respiratory Journal*, *33*(3), 461–463. doi:10.1183/09031936.00001309 PMID:19251792

Chang, L., Kagaayi, J., Nakigozi, G., Packer, A., Serwadda, D., Quinn, T., & Reynolds, S. J. et al. (2008). Responding to the human resource crisis: Peer health workers, mobile phones, and HIV care in Rakai, Uganda. *AIDS Patient Care and STDs*, *22*(3), 173–174. doi:10.1089/apc.2007.0234 PMID:18290750

Chen, C., Haddad, D., Selsky, J., Hoffman, J. E., Kravitz, R. L., Estrin, D. E., & Sim, I. (2012). Making sense of mobile health data: An open architecture to improve individual-and population-level health. *Journal of Medical Internet Research*, *14*(4), e112. doi:10.2196/jmir.2152 PMID:22875563

Cook, J., Copeland, M., Hamilton, M., Jonikas, J., Razzano, L., Floyd, C., & Gray, D. D. et al. (2009). Initial outcomes of a mental illness self-management program based on wellness recovery action planning. *Psychiatric Services (Washington, D.C.)*, *60*(2), 246–249. doi:10.1176/ps.2009.60.2.246 PMID:19176420

Editors, P. M. (2013). A reality checkpoint for mobile health: Three challenges to overcome. *PLoS Medicine*, *10*(2), e1001395. doi:10.1371/journal.pmed.1001395 PMID:23468597

Effing, T., Monninkhof, E., van der Valk, P., Zielhuis, G., Walters, E., van der Palen, J., & Zwerink, M. (2007). *Self-management education for patients with chronic obstructive pulmonary disease*. Academic Press.

Faridi, Z., Liberti, L., Shuval, K., Northrup, V., Ali, A., & Katz, D. (2008). Evaluating the impact of mobile telephone technology on type 2 diabetic patients' self-management: The NICHE pilot study. *Journal of Evaluation in Clinical Practice*, *14*(3), 465–469. doi:10.1111/j.1365-2753.2007.00881.x PMID:18373577

Fjeldsoe, B., Marshall, A., & Miller, Y. (2009). Behavior change interventions delivered by mobile telephone short-message service. *American Journal of Preventive Medicine*, *36*(2), 165–173. doi:10.1016/j.amepre.2008.09.040 PMID:19135907

Free, C., Phillips, G., Galli, L., Watson, L., Felix, L., Edwards, P., & Haines, A. et al. (2013). The effectiveness of mobile-health technology-based health behaviour change or disease management interventions for health care consumers: A systematic review. *PLoS Medicine*, *10*(1), e1001362. doi:10.1371/journal.pmed.1001362 PMID:23349621

Funnell, M., Brown, T., Childs, B., Haas, L., Hosey, G., Jensen, B., & Weiss, M. et al. (2009). National standards for diabetes self-management education. *Diabetes Care*, *32*(Supplement 1), S87–S94. doi:10.2337/dc09-S087 PMID:19118294

Hattie, J., & Timperley, H. (2007). The power of feedback. *Review of Educational Research*, *77*(1), 81–112. doi:10.3102/003465430298487

Irvine, A. B., Ary, D. V., Grove, D. A., & Gilfillan-Morton, L. (2004). The effectiveness of an interactive multimedia program to influence eating habits. *Health Education Research, 19*(3), 290–305. doi:10.1093/her/cyg027 PMID:15140849

Janson, S. L., McGrath, K. W., Covington, J. K., Cheng, S. C., & Boushey, H. A. (2009). Individualized asthma self-management improves medication adherence and markers of asthma control. *The Journal of Allergy and Clinical Immunology, 123*(4), 840–846. doi:10.1016/j.jaci.2009.01.053 PMID:19348923

Kahn, J. G., Yang, J., & Kahn, J. S. (2010). 'Mobile' health needs and opportunities in developing countries. *Health Affairs, 29*(2), 252–258. doi:10.1377/hlthaff.2009.0965 PMID:20348069

Kreps, G. L., & Neuhauser, L. (2010). New directions in eHealth communication: Opportunities and challenges. *Patient Education and Counseling, 78*(3), 329–336. doi:10.1016/j.pec.2010.01.013 PMID:20202779

Krishna, S., Balas, E. A., Francisco, B. D., Konig, P., Graff, G. R., & Madsen, R. W. (2003). Internet-enabled interactive multimedia asthma education program: A randomized trial. *Pediatrics, 111*(3), 503–510. doi:10.1542/peds.111.3.503 PMID:12612228

Kumar, S., Nilsen, W. J., Abernethy, A., Atienza, A., Patrick, K., Pavel, M., & Swendeman, D. et al. (2013). Mobile health technology evaluation: The mHealth evidence workshop. *American Journal of Preventive Medicine, 45*(2), 228–236. doi:10.1016/j.amepre.2013.03.017 PMID:23867031

Lenhart, A., Purcell, K., Smith, A., & Zickuhr, K. (2010). *Social media & mobile Internet use among teens and young adults*. Pew Internet and American Life Project.

Levin, L. S., & Idler, E. L. (1983). Self-care in health. *Annual Review of Public Health, 4*(1), 181–201. doi:10.1146/annurev.pu.04.050183.001145 PMID:6860437

Logan, A. G. (2013). Transforming hypertension management using mobile health technology for telemonitoring and self-care support. *The Canadian Journal of Cardiology, 29*(5), 579–585. doi:10.1016/j.cjca.2013.02.024 PMID:23618506

Lorig, K., Ritter, P., Laurent, D., & Plant, K. (2008). The Internet-based arthritis self-management program: A one-year randomized trial for patients with arthritis or fibromyalgia. *Arthritis Care and Research, 59*(7), 1009–1017. doi:10.1002/art.23817 PMID:18576310

Lorig, K., Sobel, D., Stewart, A., Brown, B. Jr, Bandura, A., Ritter, P., & Halstead, R. et al. (1999). Evidence suggesting that a chronic disease self-management program can improve health status while reducing hospitalization: A randomized trial. *Medical Care, 37*(1), 5–14. doi:10.1097/00005650-199901000-00003 PMID:10413387

Luxton, D. D., Kayl, R. A., & Mishkind, M. C. (2012). mHealth data security: The need for HIPAA-compliant standardization. *Telemedicine Journal and e-Health, 18*(4), 284–288. doi:10.1089/tmj.2011.0180 PMID:22400974

Maibach, E., & Parrott, R. (1995). *Designing health messages: approaches from communication theory and public health practice*. Thousand Oaks, CA: Sage Publications.

Martínez-Pérez, B., de la Torre-Díez, I., & López-Coronado, M. (2014). Privacy and security in mobile health apps: A review and recommendations. *Journal of Medical Systems, 39*(1). PMID:25486895

Mitseva, A., Kyriazakos, S., Litke, A., Papadakis, N., & Prasad, N. (2009). ISISEMD: Intelligent System for Independent living and self-care of SEniors with mild cognitive impairment or Mild Dementia. *The Journal on Information Technology in Healthcare, 7*(6), 383–399.

Nazareth, I., & Murray, E. (2010). Promoting self care for minor illness. *British Medical Journal, 340*, c2913.

Patrick, K., Griswold, W., Raab, F., & Intille, S. (2008). Health and the mobile phone. *American Journal of Preventive Medicine, 35*(2), 177–181. doi:10.1016/j.amepre.2008.05.001 PMID:18550322

Peirce, L., & Bakke, E. (2010, June 21). Healthcare perceptions and mobile phone use: a predictive model of text-based health communication. *Annual meeting of the International Communication Association, Suntec,* Singapore.

Preuveneers, D., & Berbers, Y. (2008). Mobile phones assisting with health self-care: a diabetes case study. *10th Annual Conference on Human Computer Interaction with Mobile Devices and Services.*

Riley, W. T., Rivera, D. E., Atienza, A. A., Nilsen, W., Allison, S. M., & Mermelstein, R. (2011). Health behavior models in the age of mobile interventions: Are our theories up to the task? *Translational Behavioral Medicine, 1*(1), 53–71. doi:10.1007/s13142-011-0021-7 PMID:21796270

Rubin, G., Cleare, A., & Wessely, S. (2008). Psychological factors associated with self-reported sensitivity to mobile phones. *Journal of Psychosomatic Research, 64*(1), 1–9. doi:10.1016/j.jpsychores.2007.05.006 PMID:18157992

Sahoo, P. K. (2012). Efficient security mechanisms for mHealth applications using wireless body sensor networks. *Sensors (Basel, Switzerland), 12*(9), 12606–12633. doi:10.3390/s120912606 PMID:23112734

Sarkar, U., Piette, J. D., Gonzales, R., Lessler, D., Chew, L. D., Reilly, B., & Schillin.ger, D. et al. (2008). Prefere.nces for self-management support: Findings from a survey of diabetes patients in safety-net health systems. *Patient Education and Counseling, 70*(1), 102–110. doi:10.1016/j.pec.2007.09.008 PMID:17997264

Steinhubl, S. R., Muse, E. D., & Topol, E. J. (2013). Can mobile health technologies transform health care? *Journal of the American Medical Association, 310*(22), 2395–2396. doi:10.1001/jama.2013.281078 PMID:24158428

Suggs, L. (2006). A 10-year retrospective of research in new technologies for health communication. *Journal of Health Communication, 11*(1), 61–74. doi:10.1080/10810730500461083 PMID:16546919

Taylor, J., Dearnley, C., Laxton, J., Coates, C., Treasure-Jones, T., Campbell, R., & Hall, I. (2010). Developing a mobile learning solution for health and social care practice. *Distance Education, 31*(2), 175–192. doi:10.1080/01587919.2010.503343

van Velsen, L., Beaujean, D. J., & van Gemert-Pijnen, J. E. (2013). Why mobile health app overload drives us crazy, and how to restore the sanity. *BMC Medical Informatics and Decision Making, 13*(1), 23. doi:10.1186/1472-6947-13-23 PMID:23399513

Wagner, E., & McCorkle, R. (2010). Self-management support. In *Psycho-Oncology*. London: Oxford University Press. doi:10.1093/med/9780195367430.003.0063

Whittaker, R., Merry, S., Dorey, E., & Maddison, R. (2012). A development and evaluation process for mHealth interventions: examples from New Zealand. *Journal of Health Communication, 17*(sup1), 11-21.

Chapter 2
A Transaction Cost Economics Perspective for Pervasive Technology

Nilmini Wickramasinghe
Epworth HealthCare, Australia & Deakin University, Australia

Indrit Troshani
University of Adelaide, Australia

Steve Goldberg
INET International Inc., Canada

ABSTRACT

Numerous mobile technology solutions are being developed and implemented today to address a myriad of healthcare problems. However, it remains unclear what the true cost/benefit of these solutions is and who benefits from them. To investigate this we apply a transaction cost economics framework to a pervasive mobile solution that has been designed and developed to enhance diabetes self-care. Diabetes is one of the leading chronic diseases and its prevalence continues to rise. The solution examined in this paper relies on pervasive wireless technology and is designed to facilitate the effective management of diabetes in the context of gestational diabetes, a conditions that affects up to 8% of pregnant women. A transactions cost assessment of this solution is provided.

DOI: 10.4018/978-1-4666-9870-3.ch002

INTRODUCTION

Mobile technology has created many opportunities for a plethora of new applications to emerge. More recently, many of these new applications are focused on addressing health and wellness issues such as obesity, diabetes, and wellness aspects including nutritional intake, and exercise. Many believe that these applications will assist in addressing the current health concerns including diabetes and obesity; however it is still unclear how cost effective these solutions really are and who benefits from them. In an attempt to shed light on these issues and guide existing and future research, we examine a specific pervasive mobile solution that is designed to enable diabetes self-care. We assess this solution the transaction economics cost perspective to assess its key cost and benefit aspects. The study contributes to both theory and practice.

BACKGROUND

Diabetes mellitus is one of the leading chronic diseases affecting Australians and its prevalence continues to rise expontially. The total number of diabetes patients worldwide is estimated to rise to 366 million in 2030 from 171 million in 2000 (Wild, Roglic, Green, Sicree, & King, 2004). With increasingly growing prevalence which includes an estimated 275 Australians developing diabetes daily (DiabetesAustralia, 2008), Australia is expected to be a significant contributor to this projected trend. An estimated 700,000 Australians, representing approximately 3.6% of the population, were diagnosed with diabetes in 2004-05. Between 1989-90 and 2004-05 the proportion of Australians diagnosed with this disease more than doubled from 1.3% to 3.3%. Additionally, between 2000-01 and 2004-05, Australian diabetes hospitalizations increased by 35% from 1,932 to 2,608 hospitalizations per 100,000 people (AIHW, 2007, 2008). For every person diagnosed with diabetes, it is estimated that there is another who has yet to be diagnosed, which doubles the number of diabetes sufferers (DiabetesAustralia, 2008). Diabetes is, thus, one of the fastest growing chronic diseases in Australia (AIHW, 2008; Catanzariti, Faulks, & Waters, 2007; Chittleborough, Grant, Phillips, & Taylor, 2007). Diabetes and its complications incur significant costs for the health system in Australia, including costs incurred by carers, government, and the entire health system (DiabCostAustralia, 2002). In 2004-05 direct healthcare expenditure on diabetes was A$907 million, which constituted approximately 2% of the allocatable recurrent health expenditure in that year (AIHW, 2007, 2008). Further costs include societal costs that represent productivity losses for both patients and their carers (DiabCostAustralia, 2002).

Gestational diabetes mellitus (GDM) is a common form of diabetes that presents in pregnancy, sometimes with symptoms but often diagnosed in otherwise normal women on routine screening tests. Some women, particularly those in whom the diagnosis of GDM is made early in pregnancy, may have pre-existing undiagnosed diabetes. In Australia and New Zealand, universal screening for GDM is recommended by the Australasian Diabetes in Pregnancy Society (ADIPS) (Hoffman, Nola, Wilson, Oats, & Simmons, 1998), although the uptake of this recommendation is variable (Rumbold & Crowther, 2001). It is estimated that in Australia, 3-6% of pregnant women will develop GDM at around 24-28 weeks gestation, with a smaller number earlier and later in pregnancy. An Australian study of 210 pregnant women found that screening for GDM had an adverse impact on women's perceptions of their own health (Rumbold & Crowther, 2001, 2002). GDM is more common in older women, in those with a family history of diabetes, in those who are overweight, and in those of non-Caucasian heritage (Carolan, Steele, & Margetts, 2010). Maternal complications of GDM can be serious and include polyhydramnios and premature labour, maternal hypertension, low birth weights and stillbirth (Fan, Yang, Gao, Lintu, & Sun, 2006; Hoffman et al., 1998). It recurs in subsequent pregnancy in 30-80% of women, the incidence varying with ethnicity, being lower in Caucasian women (Kim, Berger, & Chamany, 2007).

Treatment of women with GDM aims to control maternal, and therefore fetal, hyperglycaemia and the associated tendency of fetal hyperinsulinaemia which is at the root of the fetal complications (Metzger & al-others), 2008). After many years of uncertainty as to the value of such treatment in GDM, two trials have now shown benefit for both mother and offspring for antenatal initiation of lifestyle modification and glucose monitoring, coupled with insulin therapy as necessary (Crowther et al., 2005; Landon & al(others), 2009). Antenatal treatment of detected mild GDM was also associated with improved health status for women during the antenatal period and at 3 months after birth, with less postnatal depression (Crowther et al., 2005). Specifically, there is agreement in the literature that specific self-management activities including glucose monitoring, dietary restrictions, and exercise regimes can result in good outcomes for mothers and babies suggesting that self-management behaviors can be critical (Crowther et al., 2005; Fan et al., 2006).

Recognizing the need to have a solution that can enable the ubiquitous monitoring of GDM patients while also continuously educating them, the goal of this paper is to investigate the development and application of DiaMonD – a diabetes monitoring device. Powered by pervasive technology software developed by INET, DiaMonD is a wireless enabled mobile phone that can facilitate superior diabetes self-management for GDM patients. The realization of this goal can contribute by establishing a benchmark for theoretical and empirical testing. We examine DiaMonD in the context of GDM. Critical to the GDM and to successful pregnancy outcomes is careful and systematic monitoring of maternal glycaemia and appropriate adjustment of lifestyle, dietary and pharmacological therapy in the light of the results. The end results of GDM are similar to other types of diabetes (e.g. Types 1 and 2). However, unlike other types of diabetes GDM is generally transient which can have implications on awareness of impacts and self-management attitudes (Carolan et al., 2010; Crowther et al., 2005; Fan et al., 2006). To achieve our goal, first we provide a general background on the Australian health scene and critically review existing research and then, we elaborate the proposed pervasive mobile technology solution and assess it using a preliminary transaction cost economics framework.

Current Australian Health Scene

Both healthcare professionals and diabetes patients require quality information if disease conditions are to be effectively managed. There are several deficiencies in the information provided by the existing system for monitoring diabetes in Australia (Dixon & Webbie, 2006; Sprivulis et al., 2007; Swerissen & Taylor, 2008). First, data collected in hospitals are episode-based rather than patient-based, making it difficult to determine statistics concerning individual admissions, re-admissions, and treatment patterns. Second, there is a lack of data on incidence and prevalence by diabetes type, so as to assess reliably the magnitude of the problem. Third, the accuracy of recording data in administrative data sets, such as hospital morbidity, mortality and general practice is uncertain. Finally, clinical management information is derived from uncoordinated and fragmented data collections that are not representative of the entire population of diabetes patients, making comparisons, analysis and trend identification difficult. These deficiencies are the result of the current health system set-up. Based on fee-for-service episodic doctor-patient consultation, the current Australian healthcare system is well placed to handle short-term illnesses involving a limited range of interventions including their diagnosis and treatment (Hunt, 2007). However, this system is comprised of a mixture of fragmented private and public healthcare subsystems that provide both healthcare funding and delivery. Largely uncoordinated, these subsystems are deemed to be unsuitable for the treatment of long-term chronic diseases, including diabetes more generally and GDM in particular (Dixon & Webbie, 2006; Sprivulis et al., 2007). In particular, the chronic and multisystem nature of diabetes and its complications requires teams of various health professionals and long-term support to help sufferers make effective healthy lifestyle changes and constantly maintain them (Hunt, 2007).

Current Diabetes Self-Management Research

As there is no cure for diabetes, non-medical approaches are used jointly with medical ones, so that patients with the disease can have a life which is as normal as possible. Such non-medical approaches require effective and ongoing lifestyle management, together with meticulous attention and monitoring by both patients and healthcare professionals (Britt et al., 2007). Particularly, to be successful, patients need to be both informed and active in their treatment regimen (AIHW, 2007, 2008). These aims can be achieved by effective self-management, which is a non-medical approach and which constitutes the focus of this paper.

Self-management is important as it empowers diabetes patients while acknowledging their central role and responsibility for managing their healthcare (ICIC, 2008). Active participation of diabetes patients in self-management is a key strategy for managing their condition and reaching improved treatment outcomes (Colagiuri, Colagiuri, & Ward, 1998; Poulton, 1999; Rasmussen, Wellard, & Nankervis, 2001; Wellard, Rennie, & King, 2008). However, self-management is constantly time-consuming and requires significant self-discipline (Russell, Churl Suh, & Safford, 2005) and support strategies including assessment, goal-setting, action-planning, problem-solving and follow-up (ICIC, 2008). Moreover, because effective self-management may require patient interaction with various healthcare professionals, including diabetes physicians, general practitioners, diabetes educators, dieticians, and community nurses (Knuiman, Welborn, & Bartholomew, 1996), difficulties can arise when diabetes patients encounter problems ranging from making appointments to needing to travel to many locations (Van Eyk & Baum, 2002; Wellard et al., 2008; Zigbor & Songer, 2001). Given both the importance and complexity of applying self-management effectively for both prevention and early detection of diabetes, there are increasing calls for further research to facilitate self-management (Wellard et al., 2008).

Although current research has provided solutions for supporting self-management (Chau & Turner, 2006; Rudi & Celler, 2006) these have not always been effective due to the reality that "patients did not learn how to do it [apply the solutions] or they did not understand the rules which were explained to them, or they are not sure enough of their knowledge, uncertainty entailing indecision" (Reach, Zerrouki, Leclercq, & d'Ivernois, 2005). Additionally, a number of recent attempts at implementing diabetes self-management monitoring systems found them to be either impractical or costly. For example, a system implemented in France uses a combination of personal digital assistants (PDAs) and mobile phones, but downloads glucose readings data weekly or bi-weekly potentially resulting in feedback delays and quality for patients and, thus, questionable effectiveness (Farmer et al., 2005). A telephone support system was trialed in the UK with nurse facilitators.

While this system was shown to improve glucose readings overtime, it did not use systematic transmission of glucose results, again, potentially adversely impacting on effectiveness while also being costly to run and maintain (Farmer et al., 2005). Nevertheless, research shows that computer-assisted telemedicine generally can help people with diabetes improve both self-management (Balas et al., 2004) and their relationship with healthcare professionals (Bodenheimer, Lorig, Holman, & Grumbach, 2002; Downer, Meara, Da Costa, & Sethuraman, 2006). Therefore, in this paper, we investigate the application of a pervasive mobile technology solution to facilitate superior self-management of GDM.

A Transaction Cost Economics Assessment Framework

Transaction cost economics (TCE) theory represents a natural and logical theoretical setting for guiding the evaluation of actor interactions in a diabetes monitoring healthcare setting (Hesterly, Liebeskind, & Zenger, 1990; Hesterly & Zenger, 1993; Jones, Hesterly, & Borgatti, 1997; Troshani & Rao, 2007a; Williamson, 1991). That is, TCE focuses on economic exchange relations amongst organizational actors, including diabetes patients and healthcare providers that are typically involved in interactions. Using the TCE extensions proposed by Jones, Hesterly, and Borgatti (1997) as a basis, the interactions of these actors are comprised of economic exchanges the efficiency of which is jointly determined by four conditions, namely, 1) demand uncertainty, 2) complexity, 3) asset specificity, and 4) frequency. We explain these in turn.

Demand uncertainty is defined as the inability of an actor to predict future events concerning the success or failure of new product offerings, such as a diabetes monitoring solution (Milliken, 1987; Troshani & Rao, 2007a). It can be caused by many sources including rapid changes in knowledge and technology or even by the actors themselves. Understanding potential sources of demand uncertainty is important because it helps control it and reduce the impact of associated risks. *Task complexity* refers to the number of different specialized behavioral inputs that are required to fully develop and distribute a product or service (Jones et al., 1997; Troshani & Rao, 2007a). Task complexity creates behavioral interdependencies while increasing the need for coordinating actors involved in related processes (Pfeffer & Salancik, 1978; Troshani & Rao, 2007a).

Asset-specific exchanges can be based on both unique human (e.g. unique processes and knowledge developed by various actors) and non-human assets (e.g. unique equipment) which actors can use to enable economic exchanges. Asset-specific exchanges create dependencies which can in turn require enhanced cooperation, coordination, and proximity for the effective transfer of both assets or their deliverables amongst actors (Jones et al., 1997; Troshani & Rao, 2007a; Williamson, 1991). *Frequency* concerns how often actors are involved in exchanges with each another (Jones et al., 1997; Williamson, 1985). Jones, Hesterly, and Borgatti (1997) argue that "frequency allows human asset specificity to develop from learning-by-doing and to "deepen" through continued interaction; this creates exchanges where the "identity" of the other [actors] matters and enhances the transfer of tacit knowledge…" (p. 922) while also maximizing the cost efficiencies of existing interaction structures (Troshani & Rao, 2007a; Williamson, 1985).

THE DEVELOPMENT OF A PERVASIVE MOBILE TECHNOLOGY SOLUTION

We propose DiaMonD – a diabetes monitoring device – as a solution which incorporates software that facilitates the ubiquitous monitoring of an individual's GSM, thereby, contributing to diabetes self-management. The solution is grounded in trying to support key components of a chronic disease care model (Table 1).

Table 1. Components of a Chronic Care Model (Rachlis, 2006)

Component	Description
Organisation of Health System	• Leadership in chronic disease management (CDM) • Goals for CDM • Improvement strategy for CDM • Incentives and regulations for CDM • Benefits
Self-management support	• Assessment and documentation of needs and activities • Addressing concerns of patients • Effective behaviour change interventions
Decision Support	• Evidence-based guidelines • Involvement of specialists in improving primary care • Providing education for CDM • Informing patients about guidelines
Delivery System design	• Practice team functioning • Practice team leadership • Appointment system • Follow-up • Planned visits for CDM • Continuity of Care
Clinical Information Systems	• Registry • Reminders to providers • Feedback • Information about relevant subgroups of patients needing services • Patient treatment plans
Community	• Linkages for patients to resources • Partnerships with community organizations • Policy and plan development

INET International Inc.'s research (S. Goldberg, 2009; S. e. a. Goldberg, 2002a, 2002b, 2002c, 2002d, 2002e; Wickramasinghe & Goldberg, 2003, 2004) starts with a 30-day e-business acceleration project in collaboration with many key players in hospitals, such as clinicians, medical units, administration, and IT departments. Together, they follow a rigorous procedure that refocuses the traditional 1-5-year system development lifecycle (SDLC) into concurrent 30-day projects to accelerate healthcare delivery improvements. At completion, an e-business acceleration project delivers a scope document to develop a handheld technology application (HTA) proof-of-concept specific to the unique needs of a particular environment. The proof-of-concept is a virtual lab case scenario which operates within a mobile Internet (wireless) environment by working with hospitals and technology vendors. The final step is the collection of additional data with clinical HTA trials consisting of two-week hospital evaluations.

The INET web-based model (figure 1) provides the necessary components to enable the delivery framework to be positioned in the best possible manner so it can indeed facilitate enacting the key components of the chronic disease model successfully (table 1). The model is positioned to suit the complex nature of healthcare environments by iteratively, systematically, and rigorously incorporating lessons

Figure 1. INET web-based model

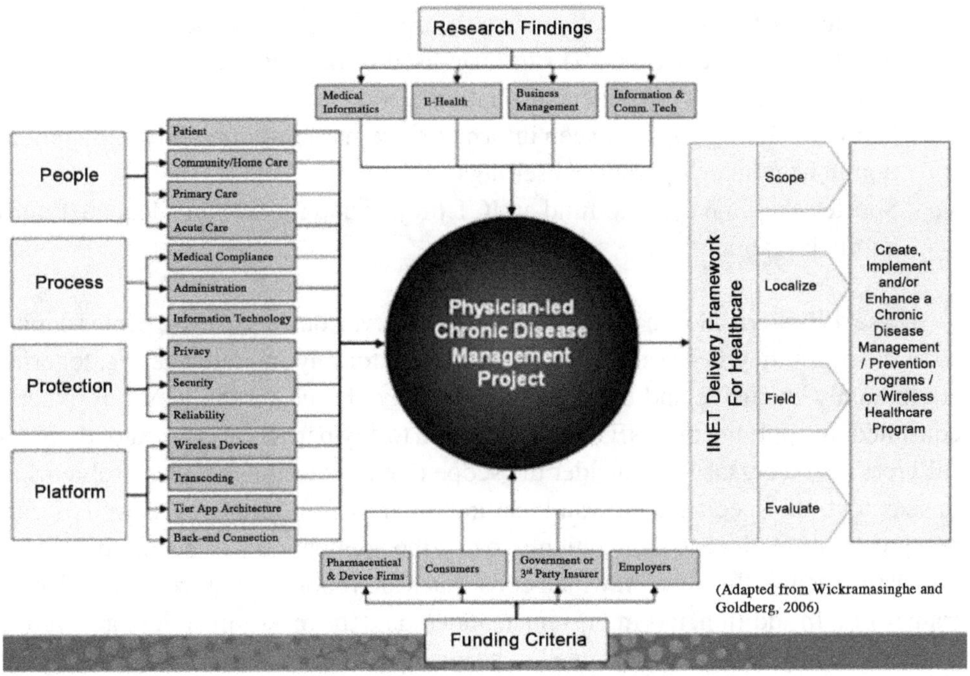

(Adapted from Wickramasinghe and Goldberg, 2006)

learnt data to healthcare processes for ensuring superior healthcare delivery. This manner not only maximizes the value of past data and organizational learning, but it also makes processes amendable as complex needs and requirements evolve.

It is important to note that in the INET web-based model the three key areas of risk, namely, people, processes and technology, are minimized through the use of pervasive technology, which we believe is a unique benefit of the INET solution. Specifically, since the proposed solution is an application that is compatible with any mobile phone or wireless device (e.g. a PDA), data transfers occur between patients and providers on a well-vetted model. Therefore, the learning curve for patients may be minimal as they are likely to be in possession of mobile devices.

What makes this model unique and most beneficial is its focus on enabling and supporting all areas necessary for the actualization of ICT initiatives in healthcare. By design, the model identifies the inputs necessary to bring an innovative chronic disease management solution to market. These solutions are developed and implemented through a physician-led mobile e-health project. This project is the heart of the model that bridges the needs and requirements of many different players into a final (output) deliverable, a "Wireless Healthcare Program".

To accomplish this, the model is continually updated to identify, select and prioritize the ICT project inputs that will:

- Accelerate healthcare system enhancements and achieve rapid healthcare benefits. The model identifies key healthcare system inputs with the four Ps, namely, 1) ***People*** that deliver healthcare, 2) ***Process*** to define the current healthcare delivery tasks, 3) ***Platform*** used in the healthcare technology infrastructure, and 4) ***Protection*** of patient data.
- Close the timing gaps between information research studies and their application in healthcare operational settings.
- Shorten the time cycle to fund an ICT project and receive an adequate return on the investment.

These 4 Ps were chosen after discussions with various healthcare professionals as to the areas they believed were critical inputs for any model. These categories are mutually exclusive and collectively exhaustive based on the views of experts consulted. In applying the INET-based solution to any particular context of diabetes sufferers it is necessary to consider the scope or extent of the diabetes problems in this context, the specific contextual features such as demographics as well as current processes in place to treat patients so that the application will be tailored to this population hence "localize" it which constitutes an important aspect in the delivery framework. In addition, it is important to understand the make-up of the care team or field and finally the results that need to be evaluated. Thus, the delivery framework helps making the solution applicable to any context of diabetes patients which is an essential consideration given that diabetes cuts across all areas of the community. Together the components of the model will help in actualizing physician-led solution for the management of chronic diseases in general and of diabetes in particular. To successfully implement the INET web-based model described above, it was necessary to have an appropriate methodology. Based on this need, the adaptive mapping to realization methodology (AMR) was developed (figure 2). The idea of the methodology was to apply a systematic rigorous set of predetermined protocols to each business case and then to map the post-prior results back to the model. In this way, it was possible to compare and contrast both a priori and post priori findings. From such a comparison, first a diagnosis of the current state was made then prescriptions were derived for the next business case. Hence, each pilot study incorporated the lessons learnt from the previous one and the model was adapted in real time.

By applying the tools and techniques of today's knowledge economy as presented in an intelligence continuum (IC), it is possible to make the AMR methodology into a very powerful knowledge-based systems development model. The IC was developed by Wickramasinghe and Schaffer (2006) to enable the application of tools and technologies of the knowledge economy to be applied to healthcare

Figure 2. AMR Methodology

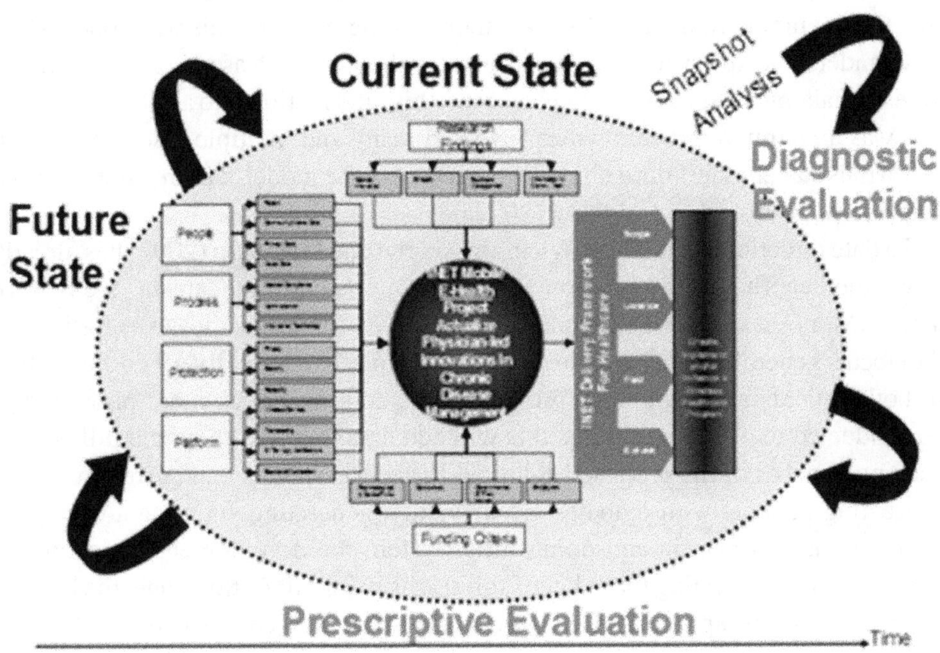

processes in a systematic and rigorous fashion, thereby ensuring superior healthcare delivery. The collection of key tools, techniques and processes that make up the IC include, but are not limited to, data mining, business intelligence/analytics and knowledge management (Wickramasinghe & Schaffer, 2006).

Taken together, they represent a very powerful system for refining the raw data stored in data marts and/or data warehouses, thereby maximizing the value and utility of these data assets for any organization. To maximize the value of the data generated through specific healthcare processes and then to use this to improve processes, IC techniques and tools must be applied in a systematic manner. Once applied, the results become part of the data set that are subsequently reintroduced into the system and combined with other inputs of people, processes, and technology to develop an improvement continuum. Thus, the IC includes the generation of data, the analysis of these data to provide a “diagnosis”, and their reintroduction into the cycle as a “prescriptive” solution. In this way, the IC is well suited to the dynamic and complex nature of healthcare environments and ensures that the future state is always built upon the extant knowledge-base of the preceding state. Through the incorporation of the IC with the AMR methodology we then have a knowledge-based systems development model that can be applied to any setting, not necessarily to chronic disease management. The power of this model is that it brings best practices and the best available germane knowledge to each iteration and is both flexible and robust.

Given the uniqueness of this approach it was necessary to develop this model from the beginning rather than look at other existing models. This was done by trying to understand key criteria from various stakeholders such as patients, healthcare professionals and hospital personnel and sort this information into a coherent whole. This was an iterative process which involved many and multiple discussions with the various stakeholders until all parties agreed that the model captured the essential elements as discussed in Goldberg (2002a-e)

To date directional data from Wickramasinghe and Goldberg (2007) has already shown the benefits of this solution in various pilot studies in Canada. We believe that DiaMonD is a most beneficial solution given the huge and growing impact of diabetes generally and GDM in particular. In particular, it is very cost effective for both patients and healthcare providers. We believe that as more pilot studies are conducted in different settings this will add data that will show the full and far reaching benefits of the proposed solution. What is certain is that current methods for treating patients with diabetes are unwieldy, generating significant costs, not especially patient-centric and doing little to stem the development of secondary complications, suggesting that a better solution is required. At this stage, the INET’s solution looks to be appropriate as it offers a real-time user-centric solution. It offers an innovative approach to transmit blood glucose readings for GDM patients while providing support and instant feedback to patients and clinicians on both mobile devices and web-browsers, significantly enhancing accessibility and patient care. Additionally, the solution has the potential to establish critical self-management behaviors for GDM patients or, where they already exist, enhance them. It also addresses issues of existing solutions which either do not systematically capture glucose readings data or when they do, do not provide the data to clinicians in a timely manner (Farmer et al., 2005; Young et al., 2005).

Thus, DiaMonD represents a pervasive ICT enabled solution, which, while not exorbitantly expensive, can facilitate the superior monitoring of GDM (figure 3). DiaMonD also enables patient empowerment by way of enhancing self-management. This is a desirable objective because it allows patients to become more like partners with their clinicians in the management of their own healthcare (Opie, 1998; Radin, 2006) by enhancing the traditional clinical-patient interactions (Mirza, Norris, & Stockdale, 2008; Wickramasinghe, Troshani, & Goldberg, 2009, 2010).

Figure 3. ICT Support for Diabetes

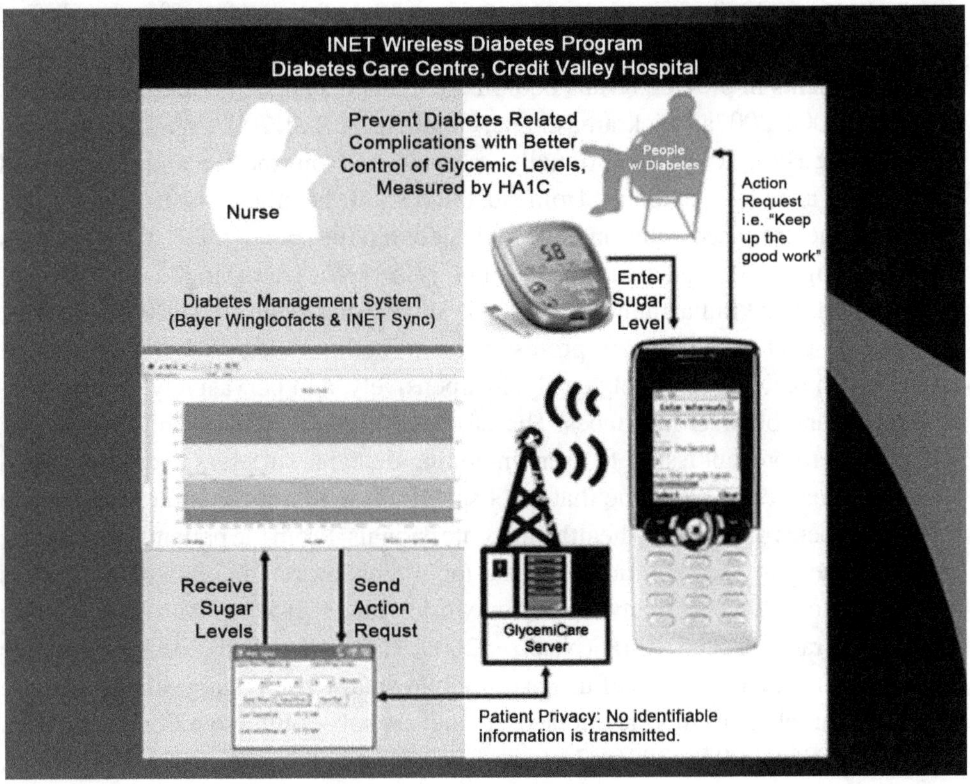

A PRELIMINARY ASSESMENT OF THE SOLUTION

Demand Uncertainty: Given the growing incidences of diabetes and GDM sufferers and the relative ineffectiveness of existing non-medical approaches (Reach et al., 2005), it is anticipated that upon being made available there will be demand for the proposed solution, i.e. DiaMonD. Additionally, costs incurred by diabetes patients to operate the solution, that is, to systematically send glucose readings to their diabetes healthcare professionals (Figure 3), are likely to be negligible since data transfer charges have recently become inexpensive. It is, therefore, expected that uncertainty is not likely to adversely affect demand for DiaMonD as a solution for self-management for diabetes patients generally and GDM patients in particular.

Complexity: We argue that the proposed solution is easy to use and useful for both diabetes patients and healthcare professionals. As shown in Figure 3, DiaMonD requires diabetes sufferers to input their glucose readings systematically via a simple user interface before sending them for processing. In fact, the solution is very similar to Short Message Service (SMS) applications which are renowned for their popularity (Mackay & Weidlich, 2007; O'Doherty, Rao Hill, Mackay, & McPherson, 2010; Oh et al., 2008). It is, therefore, anticipated that diabetes sufferers will find the solution intuitive, easy to use and useful as also supported in preliminary studies and assessments in previous trials both in the US and Canada (Wickramasinghe & Goldberg, 2004, 2007a; Wickramasinghe, Goldberg, & Bali, 2007; Wickramasinghe, Goldberg, & Bali, 2008). Additionally, as evidence from the US and Canada and preliminary anecdotal evidence from Australia show, healthcare professionals that have used the proposed solution have indicated that the functionality that concerns them (see Figure 3) is also easy to use and useful (Wickramasinghe & Goldberg, 2004, 2007a; Wickramasinghe et al., 2007; Wickramasinghe et al., 2008). That is, the solution enables healthcare professionals to both monitor diabetes trends and interact with patients relatively easily, inexpensively, and pervasively on both mobile device and browser interfaces. Therefore, we argue that DiaMonD complexity is not likely to present issues to users including diabetes sufferers and clinicians.

Asset Specificity: We argue that asset specificity will not constitute an obstacle for both diabetes patients and healthcare professionals. From the patients' viewpoint, operating the proposed solution entails a mobile handset and a data plan. Current evidence shows that in many countries worldwide, including Australia, mobile penetration rates exceed 100% (Netsize, 2009; Rao & Troshani, 2006). Evidence also shows increasing trends of usage of mobile data services suggesting that there is growing numbers of mobile phone users that are subscribing to mobile data plans (Informa, 2005a, 2005b, 2006a; Netsize, 2009; Rao & Troshani, 2006). Therefore, as a mobile diabetes self-management solution DiaMonD can be run on assets, i.e. mobile handset, which diabetes patients are likely to already own. Similar arguments can be made for healthcare professionals and their organization. Additionally, healthcare professionals may also access DiaMonD reporting functions (Figure 3) using web browser interfaces which only require internet computers and are not expected to require specific expensive assets. Thus, aside from software upgrades in existing servers and corresponding license fees, upgrades to new assets including computer hardware, are not necessary.

Frequency: We argue that interaction frequency between diabetes patients and healthcare providers using the proposed mobile solution will be high, though dictated by the treatment regimen that healthcare professionals prescribe to patients. For example, some patients may be required send their glucose readings to their healthcare professional six times daily, i.e. three times daily before and after each meal, while other patients may be required to fulfill different patterns. We argue that interaction frequency is only a means of maximizing cost efficiencies, but also as a way of strengthening and complementing long term patient-healthcare professional relationships thereby improving the overall quality of healthcare services offered.

CONCLUSION

We set out to assess the cost/benefit issues pertaining to a pervasive mobile solution. We focused on a particular mobile solution–DiaMonD–a diabetes self-care solution used in the context of gestational diabetes patients. We assessed this solution using the transaction economic cost framework to assess key cost and benefit aspects. The study contributes to both theory and practice in many significant ways. In particular, it highlights the need to assess both qualitative and quantitative issues when assessing benefits. Moreover, it also serves to underscore the need to examine the web of players not just the direct users such as patient and clinicians. In particular these types of solutions also enable compliance with Meaningful Use and The Affordable Care Act (which is especially important in the United States), as well as other key regulations for compliance in other countries.

Given the general global consensus that effective and efficient healthcare delivery will only occur through the judicious application of ICTs (FS, 2004; Kulkarni & Nathanson, 2005; Lacroix, 1999; Porter & Tiesberg, 2006; Wickramasinghe, 2007), it is inevitable that, as we move into the second decade of the 21st century, the prevalence of ICTs to facilitate the delivery of value-driven healthcare will increase. In such a climate, DiaMonD will be even more appropriate, not only because it utilizes ICTs to provide superior healthcare delivery in the case of GDM patients, but also because it is both simple to implement and use, and also cost effective both at the micro and macro levels. These levels include individual patients, clinicians and organizations, including public and private healthcare providers.

While still only initial assessments, we believe that mobile solutions might hold the key to addressing many current challenges playing healthcare delivery today including escalating costs and the rise in chronic diseases. Consequently, we call for more research in this area.

REFERENCES

AIHW. (2007). *National Indicators for Monitoring Diabetes: Report of the Diabetes Indicators Review Subcommittee of the National Diabetes Data Working Group: AIHW cat. no. CVD 38*. Canberra: AIHW.

AIHW. (2008). *Diabetes: Australian Facts 2008*. Canberra: Australian Institute of Health and Welfare.

Balas, E. A., Krishna, S., Kretschmer, R. A., Cheek, T. R., Lobach, D. F., & Boren, S. A. (2004). Computerized knowledge management in diabetes care. *Medical Care, 42*(6), 610–621. doi:10.1097/01.mlr.0000128008.12117.f8 PMID:15167329

Bodenheimer, T., Lorig, K., Holman, H., & Grumbach, K. (2002). Patient self-management of chronic disease in primary care. [JAMA]. *Journal of the American Medical Association, 288*(19), 2469–2475. doi:10.1001/jama.288.19.2469 PMID:12435261

Britt, H., Miller, G. C., Charles, J., Pan, Y., Valenti, L., Henderson, J., …Knox, S. (2007). General Practice Activity in Australia 2005-06, Cat. no. GEP 16. Canberra: AIHW.

Carolan, M. C., Steele, C., & Margetts, H. (2010). Attitudes towards Gestational Diabetes among a multi-ethnic cohort in Australia. *Journal of Clinical Nursing, 19*(17/18), 2446–2453. doi:10.1111/j.1365-2702.2010.03305.x PMID:20920072

Catanzariti, L., Faulks, K., & Waters, A.-M. (2007). *National Diabetes Register: Statistical Profile 1999-2005, AIHW cat. no. CVD 39*. Canberra: AIHW.

Chau, S., & Turner, P. (2006). Utilisation of mobile handheld devices for care management at an Australian aged care facility. *Electronic Commerce Research and Applications, 5*(4), 305–312. doi:10.1016/j.elerap.2006.04.005

Chittleborough, C. R., Grant, J. F., Phillips, P. J., & Taylor, A. W. (2007). The increasing prevalence of diabetes in South Australia: The relationship with population ageing and obesity. *Public Health, 121*(2), 92–99. doi:10.1016/j.puhe.2006.09.017 PMID:17166533

Colagiuri, S., Colagiuri, R., & Ward, J. (1998). *National Diabetes Strategy and Implementation Plan*. Canberra: Diabetes Australia.

Crowther, C. A., Hiller, J. E., Moss, J. R., McPhee, A. J., Jeffries, W. S., & Robinson, J. S. (2005). The effect of treatment of gestational diabetes mellitus on pregnancy outcomes. *The New England Journal of Medicine*, *352*(24), 2477–2486. doi:10.1056/NEJMoa042973 PMID:15951574

DiabCostAustralia. (2002). *Assessing the Burden of Type 2 Diabetes in Australia*. Adelaide: DiabCost Australia.

DiabetesAustralia. (2008). *Diabetes in Australia*. Retrieved from http://www.diabetesaustralia.com.au/Understanding-Diabetes/Diabetes-in-Australia/

Dixon, T., & Webbie, K. (2006). *The National System for Monitoring Diabetes in Australia (AIHW Cat. No. CVD 32)*. Canberra: Australian Institute of Health and Wealfare.

Downer, S. R., Meara, J. G., Da Costa, A. C., & Sethuraman, K. (2006). SMS text messaging improves outpatient attendance. *Australian Health Review*, *30*(3), 389–396. doi:10.1071/AH060389 PMID:16879098

Fan, Z., Yang, H., Gao, H., Lintu, H., & Sun, W. (2006). Pregnancy outcome in gestational diabetes. *International Journal of Gynaecology and Obstetrics: the Official Organ of the International Federation of Gynaecology and Obstetrics*, *94*(1), 12–16. doi:10.1016/j.ijgo.2006.03.021 PMID:16733056

Farmer, A., Gibson, O., Hayton, P., Bryden, K., Dudley, C., Neil, C., & Tarrassenko, L. (2005). A real-time, mobile phone-based telemedicine system to support young adults with type 1 diabetes. *Informatics in Primary Care*, *13*(3), 171–177. PMID:16259856

FS. (2004). *Frost and Sullivan Country Industry Forecast*. Retrieved from http://www.news-medical.net/print_article.asp?id=1405

Goldberg, S. a. (2002a). *Building the Evidence for a standardized Mobile Internet (wireless) Environment in Ontario, Canada, January Update, Internal INET Documentation*. Ontario, Canada: INET.

Goldberg, S. a. (2002b). *HTA Presentational Selection and Aggregation Component Summary. Internal INET Documentation*. Ontario, Canada: INET.

Goldberg, S. a. (2002c). *Wireless POC Device Component Summary, Internal INET documentation*. Ontario, Canada: INET.

Goldberg, S. a. (2002d). *HTA Presentation Rendering Component Summary, Internal INET documentation*. Ontario, Canada: INET.

Goldberg, S. a. (2002e). *HTA Quality Assurance Component Summary, Internal INET documentation*. Ontario, Canada: INET.

Goldberg, S. (2009). *An Evolution of using social networks in chronic disease management.* Paper presented at the 22nd Bled eConference: Facilitating an Open, Effective and Representative Society, Bled, Slovenia.

Hesterly, W. S., Liebeskind, J., & Zenger, T. R. (1990). Organizational economics: An impeding revolution in organizational theory. *Academy of Management Review*, *15*(3), 402–420. doi:10.2307/258016

Hesterly, W. S., & Zenger, T. R. (1993). The myth of a monolithic economics: Fundamental assumptions and the use of economic models in policy and strategy research. *Organization Science*, *4*(3), 496–510. doi:10.1287/orsc.4.3.496

Hoffman, L., Nola, C., Wilson, J. D., Oats, J. J. N., & Simmons, D. (1998). Gestational diabetes mellitus -- management guidelines. *The Medical Journal of Australia*, *169*, 93–97. PMID:9700346

Hunt, D. (2007). *Urgent health system reform needed to tackle disease epidemic, says head of new University of Melbourne centre*. Retrieved 25 November, 2008, from http://uninews.unimelb.edu.au/view.php?articleID=4615

ICIC. (2008). *Improving Chronic Illness Care: The Chronic Care Model*. Retrieved from http://www.improvingchroniccare.org/indix.php?p=The_Chronic_Care_Model&s=2

Informa. (2005a). *Mobile Content and Services: Worldwide Market Analysis & Strategic Outlook*. London: Informa Telecoms & Media.

Informa. (2005b). *Global Mobile Forecasts to 2010: Worldwide Market Analysis & Strategic Outlook 2005-2010* (5th ed.). London: Informa Telecoms & Media.

Jones, C., Hesterly, W. S., & Borgatti, S. P. (1997). A general theory of network governance: Exchange conditions and social mechanisms. *Academy of Management Review*, *22*(4), 911–945.

Kim, C., Berger, D. K., & Chamany, S. (2007). Recurrence of gestational diabetes mellitus: A systematic review. *Diabetes Care*, *30*(5), 1314–1319. doi:10.2337/dc06-2517 PMID:17290037

Knuiman, M. W., Welborn, T. A., & Bartholomew, H. C. (1996). Self-reported health and use of health services: A comparison of diabetic and nondiabetic persons from a national sample. *Australian and New Zealand Journal of Public Health, 20*(3), 241–247. doi:10.1111/j.1467-842X.1996.tb01023.x PMID:8768412

Kulkarni, R., & Nathanson, L. A. (2005). *Medicine Informatics in Medicine.* Retrieved from http://www.emedicine.com/emerg/topic879.htm

Lacroix, A. (1999). International concerted action on collaboration in telemedicine: G8sub-project 4. *Studies in Health Technology and Informatics, 64*, 12–19. PMID:10747530

Landon, M. B., Spong, C. Y., Thom, E., Carpenter, M. W., Ramin, S. M., Casey, B., & Anderson, G. B. et al. (2009). A multicenter, randomized trial of treatment for mild gestational diabetes. *The New England Journal of Medicine, 361*(14), 1339–1348. doi:10.1056/NEJMoa0902430 PMID:19797280

Mackay, M. M., & Weidlich, O. (2007, March). *Australian Mobile Phone Lifestyle Index* (3rd ed.). Australian Interactive Media Industry Association (AIMIA), Mobile Content Industry Development Group (MCIDG). Retrieved 8 April, 2007, from http://www.aimia.com.au/mobile

Metzger, B. E. (2008). Hyperglycemia and adverse pregnancy outcomes. *The New England Journal of Medicine, 358*(19), 1191–2002. PMID:18463375

Milliken, F. J. (1987). Three types of perceived uncertainty about the environment: State, effect, and response uncertainty. *Academy of Management Review, 12*(1), 133–143.

Mirza, F., Norris, T., & Stockdale, R. (2008). Mobile technologies and the holistic management of chronic diseases. *Health Informatics Journal, 14*(4), 309–321. doi:10.1177/1460458208096559 PMID:19008280

Netsize. (2009). *Netsize Guide 2009 Edition: Mobile Society and Me: When worlds combine*. Levallois-Perret: Netsize.

O'Doherty, K., Rao Hill, S., Mackay, M. M., & McPherson, J. (2010). Mobile Data Service usage and preference: An investigation of Australian consumers. *International Journal ofMobile Communications, 8*(1), 106–127. doi:10.1504/IJMC.2010.030523

Oh, S., Yang, S., Kurnia, S., Lee, H., Mackay, M. M., & O'Doherty, K. (2008). The characteristics of mobile data users in Australia. *International Journal of Mobile Communications, 8*(2), 217–230. doi:10.1504/IJMC.2008.016578

Opie, A. (1998). Nobody's asked me for my view: Users' empowerment by multidisciplinary health teams. *Qualitative Health Research, 18*(2), 188–206. doi:10.1177/104973239800800204

Pfeffer, J., & Salancik, G. R. (1978). *The external control of organizations: a resource dependence perspective*. New York: Harper & Row.

Porter, M., & Tiesberg, E. (2006). *Re-defining health care delivery*. Boston: Harvard Business Press.

Poulton, B. C. (1999). User involvement in identifying health needs and shaping and evaluating services: Is it being raised? *Journal of Advanced Nursing, 30*(6), 1289–1296. doi:10.1046/j.1365-2648.1999.01224.x PMID:10583638

Rachlis, M. (2006). *Key to sustainable healthcare system*. Retrieved 21 June, 2008, from http://www.improveinchroniccare.org

Radin, P. (2006). To me, it's my life: Medical communication, trust, and activism in cyberspace. *Social Science & Medicine, 6*(3), 591–601. doi:10.1016/j.socscimed.2005.06.022 PMID:16039031

Rao, S., & Troshani, I. (2006). AMC-ER Preliminary Research Report: Understanding Market and Mobile Content Selection for Distribution. Adelaide, South Australia: Australian Mobile Content – Export Research Initiative, m.Net Corporation Ltd.

Rasmussen, B., Wellard, S., & Nankervis, A. (2001). Consumer issues in navigating health care services for type I diabetes. *Journal of Clinical Nursing, 10*(5), 628–634. doi:10.1046/j.1365-2702.2001.00550.x PMID:11822513

Reach, G., Zerrouki, D., Leclercq, D., & d'Ivernois, J. F. (2005). Adjusting insulin doses: From knowledge to decision. *Patient Education and Counseling, 56*(1), 98–103. doi:10.1016/j.pec.2004.01.001 PMID:15590229

Rudi, R., & Celler, B. G. (2006). *Design and implementation of expert-telemedicine system for diabetes management at home*. Paper presented at the International Conference on Biomedical and Pharmaceutical Enginering 2006 (ICBPE2006), Singapore.

Rumbold, A. R., & Crowther, C. A. (2001). Guideline use for gestational diabetes mellitus and current screening, diagnostic and management practices in Australian hospitals. *Australian and New Zealand Journal of Obstetrics and Gynaecology, 41*(1), 86–90. doi:10.1111/j.1479-828X.2001.tb01301.x PMID:11284655

Rumbold, A. R., & Crowther, C. A. (2002). Women's experiences of being screened for gestational diabetes mellitus. *Australian and New Zealand Journal of Obstetrics and Gynaecology, 42*(2), 131–137. doi:10.1111/j.0004-8666.2002.00131.x PMID:12069138

Russell, L. B., Churl Suh, D., & Safford, M. M. (2005). Time requirements for diabetes management: Too much for many? *The Journal of Family Practice*, *54*(1), 52–56. PMID:15623407

Sprivulis, P., Walker, J., Johnston, D., Pan, E., Adler-Milstein, J., Middleton, B., & Bates, D. W. (2007). The economic benefits of health information exchange interoperability. *Australian Health Review*, *31*(4), 531–539. doi:10.1071/AH070531 PMID:17973611

Swerissen, H., & Taylor, M. J. (2008). Reforming funding for chronic illness: Medicare-CDM. *Australian Health Review*, *32*(1), 76–84. doi:10.1071/AH080076 PMID:18241151

Troshani, I. & Rao, S. (2007a). The diffusion of mobile services in Australia: an evaluation using stakeholder and transaction cost economics theories. *IADIS International Journal of WWW/Internet,* *5*(2), 40-57.

Van Eyk, H., & Baum, F. (2002). Learning about interagency collaboration: Trialling collaborative projects between hospitals and community health services. *Health & Social Care in the Community*, *10*(4), 262–269. doi:10.1046/j.1365-2524.2002.00369.x PMID:12193170

Wellard, S. J., Rennie, S., & King, R. (2008). Perceptions of people with type 2 diabetes about self-management and the efficiency of community based services. *Contemporary Nurse*, *29*(2), 218–226. doi:10.5172/conu.673.29.2.218 PMID:18844535

Wickramasinghe, N. (2007). Fostering knowledge assets in healthcare with the KMI model. *International Journal of Management and Enterprise Development*, *4*(1), 52–65. doi:10.1504/IJMED.2007.011455

Wickramasinghe, N., & Goldberg, S. (2003). *The wireless panacea for healthcare.* Paper presented at the 36th Hawaii International Conference on System Sciences, Hawaii, HI.

Wickramasinghe, N., & Goldberg, S. (2004). How M=EC2 in healthcare. *International Journal of Mobile Communications*, *2*(2), 140–156. doi:10.1504/IJMC.2004.004664

Wickramasinghe, N., & Goldberg, S. (2006). M-health: A New Paradigm for Mobilizing Healthcare Delivery. IGI Global.

Wickramasinghe, N., & Goldberg, S. (2007). Adaptive mapping to realisation methodology (AMR) to facilitate mobile initiatives in healthcare. *International Journal of Mobile Communications*, *5*(3), 300–318. doi:10.1504/IJMC.2007.012396

Wickramasinghe, N., Goldberg, S., & Bali, R. (2007). Enabling superior m-health project success: A tri-country validation. *International Journal of Services and Standards*, *4*(1), 97–117. doi:10.1504/IJSS.2008.016087

Wickramasinghe, N., & Schaffer, J. (2006). Creating knowledge driven healthcare processes with the intelligence continuum. *International Journal of Electronic Healthcare*, *2*(2), 164–174. doi:10.1504/IJEH.2006.008830 PMID:18048242

Wickramasinghe, N., Troshani, I., & Goldberg, S. (2009). Supporting diabetes self-management with pervasive wireless technology solutions. *International Journal of Healthcare Delivery Reform Initiatives*, *1*(4), 17–31. doi:10.4018/jhdri.2009100102

Wickramasinghe, N., Troshani, I., & Goldberg, S. (2010). An investigation into the use of pervasive wireless technologies to support diabetes healthcare. In A. Coronato & G. De Pietro (Eds.), *Pervasive and Smart Technologies for Healthcare: Ubiquitous Methodologies and Tools* (Vol. 114-129). New York: IGI Global. doi:10.4018/978-1-61520-765-7.ch006

Wild, S., Roglic, G., Green, A., Sicree, R., & King, H. (2004). Global prevalence of diabetes: Estimates for the year 2000 and projections for 2030. *Diabetes Care*, *27*(5), 1047–1053. doi:10.2337/diacare.27.5.1047 PMID:15111519

Williamson, O. E. (1985). *The Economic Institutions of Capitalism: Firms, Markets, and Relational Contracting*. New York: Free Press.

Williamson, O. E. (1991). Comparative economic organization: The analysis of discrete structural alternatives. *Administrative Science Quarterly*, *36*(2), 269–296. doi:10.2307/2393356

Young, R. J., Taylor, J., Friede, T., Hollis, S., Mason, J. M., Lee, P., & Gibson, J. M. et al. (2005). Pro-active call centre treatment support (PACCTS) to improve glucose control in type 2 diabetes: A randomized controlled trial. *Diabetes Care*, *28*(2), 278–282. doi:10.2337/diacare.28.2.278 PMID:15677779

Zigbor, J. C., & Songer, T. J. (2001). External barriers to diabetes care: Addressing personal and health systems issues. *Diabetes Spectrum*, *14*(1), 23–28. doi:10.2337/diaspect.14.1.23

ADDITIONAL READING

AIHW. (2007). *National Indicators for Monitoring Diabetes: Report of the Diabetes Indicators Review Subcommittee of the National Diabetes Data Working Group: AIHW cat. no. CVD 38*. Canberra: AIHW.

AIHW. (2008). *Diabetes: Australian Facts 2008*. Canberra: Australian Institute of Health and Welfare.

Balas, E. A., Krishna, S., Kretschmer, R. A., Cheek, T. R., Lobach, D. F., & Boren, S. A. (2004). Computerized knowledge management in diabetes care. *Medical Care*, *42*(6), 610–621. doi:10.1097/01.mlr.0000128008.12117.f8 PMID:15167329

Bodenheimer, T., Lorig, K., Holman, H., & Grumbach, K. (2002). Patient self-management of chronic disease in primary care. [JAMA]. *Journal of the American Medical Association*, *288*(19), 2469–2475. doi:10.1001/jama.288.19.2469 PMID:12435261

Britt, H., Miller, G. C., Charles, J., Pan, Y., Valenti, L., Henderson, J., & Knox, S. (2007). *General Practice Activity in Australia 2005-06, Cat. no. GEP 16*. Canberra: AIHW.

Carolan, M. C., Steele, C., & Margetts, H. (2010). Attitudes towards Gestational Diabetes among a multi-ethnic cohort in Australia. *Journal of Clinical Nursing*, *19*(17/18), 2446–2453. doi:10.1111/j.1365-2702.2010.03305.x PMID:20920072

Catanzariti, L., Faulks, K., & Waters, A.-M. (2007). *National Diabetes Register: Statistical Profile 1999-2005, AIHW cat. no. CVD 39*. Canberra: AIHW.

Chau, S., & Turner, P. (2006). Utilisation of mobile handheld devices for care management at an Australian aged care facility. *Electronic Commerce Research and Applications*, *5*(4), 305–312. doi:10.1016/j.elerap.2006.04.005

Chittleborough, C. R., Grant, J. F., Phillips, P. J., & Taylor, A. W. (2007). The increasing prevalence of diabetes in South Australia: The relationship with population ageing and obesity. *Public Health*, *121*(2), 92–99. doi:10.1016/j.puhe.2006.09.017 PMID:17166533

Colagiuri, S., Colagiuri, R., & Ward, J. (1998). *National Diabetes Strategy and Implementation Plan*. Canberra: Diabetes Australia.

Crowther, C. A., Hiller, J. E., Moss, J. R., McPhee, A. J., Jeffries, W. S., & Robinson, J. S. (2005). The effect of treatment of gestational diabetes mellitus on pregnancy outcomes. *The New England Journal of Medicine*, *352*(24), 2477–2486. doi:10.1056/NEJMoa042973 PMID:15951574

DiabCostAustralia. (2002). *Assessing the Burden of Type 2 Diabetes in Australia*. Adelaide: DiabCost Australia.

DiabetesAustralia. (2008). Diabetes in Australia. http://www.diabetesaustralia.com.au/Understanding-Diabetes/Diabetes-in-Australia/ Retrieved from http://www.diabetesaustralia.com.au/Understanding-Diabetes/Diabetes-in-Australia/

Dixon, T., & Webbie, K. (2006). *The National System for Monitoring Diabetes in Australia (AIHW Cat. No. CVD 32)*. Canberra: Australian Institute of Health and Wealfare.

Downer, S. R., Meara, J. G., Da Costa, A. C., & Sethuraman, K. (2006). SMS text messaging improves outpatient attendance. *Australian Health Review*, *30*(3), 389–396. doi:10.1071/AH060389 PMID:16879098

Fan, Z., Yang, H., Gao, H., Lintu, H., & Sun, W. (2006). Pregnancy outcome in gestational diabetes. *International Journal of Gynaecology and Obstetrics: the Official Organ of the International Federation of Gynaecology and Obstetrics*, *94*(1), 12–16. doi:10.1016/j.ijgo.2006.03.021 PMID:16733056

Farmer, A., Gibson, O., Hayton, P., Bryden, K., Dudley, C., Neil, C., & Tarassenko, L. (2005). A real-time, mobile phone-based telemedicine system to support young adults with type 1 diabetes. *Informatics in Primary Care*, *13*(3), 171–177. PMID:16259856

Fischhoff, B. “Setting standards: a systematic approach to managing public health and safety risks,” Management Science (30:7) 1984, pp 823-843.

FS. (2004). *Frost and Sullivan Country Industry Forecast, May 11, 2004, Available:* http://www.news-medical.net/print_article.asp?id=1405: European Union Healthcare Industry.

Gazmararian, J., Curran, J., Parker, R., Bernhardt, J., and DeBuono, B. “Public health literacy in America: an ethical imperative,” American Journal of Preventative Medicine (28:3) 2005, pp 317-322.

Goldberg, S. a. (2002a). *Building the Evidence for a standardized Mobile Internet (wireless) Environment in Ontario, Canada, January Update, Internal INET Documentation*. Ontario, Canada: INET.

Goldberg, S. a. (2002b). *HTA Presentational Selection and Aggregation Component Summary. Internal INET Documentation*. Ontario, Canada: INET.

Goldberg, S. a. (2002c). *Wireless POC Device Component Summary, Internal INET documentation*. Ontario, Canada: INET.

Goldberg, S. a. (2002d). *HTA Presentation Rendering Component Summary, Internal INET documentation*. Ontario, Canada: INET.

Goldberg, S. a. (2002e). *HTA Quality Assurance Component Summary, Internal INET documentation*. Ontario, Canada: INET.

Goldberg, S. (2009). *An Evolution of using social networks in chronic disease management*. Paper presented at the 22nd Bled eConference: Facilitating an Open, Effective and Representative Society, Bled, Slovenia.

Gururajan, R., & Murugesan, S. "Wireless solutions developed for the Australian healthcare: A review," *4th International Conference on Mobile Business*, IEEE, Sydney, Australia, 2005. doi:10.1109/ICMB.2005.116

Halkias, D., Harkiolakis, N., and Thurman, P. "Internet use for health-related purposes among Greek consumers," Telemedicine and e-Health (14:3) 2008, pp 255-260.

Harvey, P. W., Petkov, J. N., Misan, G., Fuller, J., Battersby, M. W., Cayetano, T. N., Warren, K., and Holmes, P. "Self-management support and training for patients with chronic and complex conditions improves health-related behaviour and health outcomes," Australian Health Review (32:2) 2008, pp 330-338.

Hesterly, W. S., Liebeskind, J., & Zenger, T. R. (1990). Organizational economics: An impeding revolution in organizational theory. *Academy of Management Review*, *15*(3), 402–420. doi:10.2307/258016

Hesterly, W. S., & Zenger, T. R. (1993). The myth of a monolithic economics: Fundamental assumptions and the use of economic models in policy and strategy research. *Organization Science*, *4*(3), 496–510. doi:10.1287/orsc.4.3.496

Hoffman, L., Nola, C., Wilson, J. D., Oats, J. J. N., & Simmons, D. (1998). Gestational diabetes mellitus -- management guidelines. *The Medical Journal of Australia*, *169*, 93–97. PMID:9700346

Holliday, I., and Tam, W.-K. "E-health in the East Asian tigers," International Journal of Medical Informatics (73:11-12) 2004, pp 759-769.

Hunt, D. (2007). Urgent health system reform needed to tackle disease epidemic, says head of new University of Melbourne centre. Retrieved from http://uninews.unimelb.edu.au/view.php?articleID=4615

ICIC. (2008). Improving Chronic Illness Care: The Chronic Care Model. http://www.improvingchroniccare.org/indix.php?p=The_Chronic_Care_Model&s=2 Retrieved from http://www.improvingchroniccare.org/indix.php?p=The_Chronic_Care_Model&s=2

Informa. (2005a). *Mobile Content and Services: Worldwide Market Analysis & Strategic Outlook*. London: Informa Telecoms & Media.

Informa. (2005b). *Global Mobile Forecasts to 2010: Worldwide Market Analysis & Strategic Outlook 2005-2010* (5th ed.). London: Informa Telecoms & Media.

Informa. (2006a). Global Mobile: The International Business Newsletter of Mobile Communications Markets. *13*(6).

Jones, C., Hesterly, W. S., & Borgatti, S. P. (1997). A general theory of network governance: Exchange conditions and social mechanisms. *Academy of Management Review*, *22*(4), 911–945.

Kim, C., Berger, D. K., & Chamany, S. (2007). Recurrence of gestational diabetes mellitus: A systematic review. *Diabetes Care*, *30*(5), 1314–1319. doi:10.2337/dc06-2517 PMID:17290037

Knuiman, M. W., Welborn, T. A., & Bartholomew, H. C. (1996). Self-reported health and use of health services: A comparison of diabetic and nondiabetic persons from a national sample. *Australian and New Zealand Journal of Public Health*, *20*(3), 241–247. doi:10.1111/j.1467-842X.1996.tb01023.x PMID:8768412

Kulkarni, R., & Nathanson, L. A. (2005). *Medicine Informatics in Medicine. Available:* http://www.emedicine.com/emerg/topic879.htm

Lacroix, A. (1999). International concerted action on collaboration in telemedicine: G8sub-project 4. *Studies in Health Technology and Informatics*, *64*, 12–19. PMID:10747530

Landon, M. B., Spong, C. Y., Thom, E., Carpenter, M. W., Ramin, S. M., Casey, B., & Anderson, G. B. et al. (2009). A multicenter, randomized trial of treatment for mild gestational diabetes. *The New England Journal of Medicine*, *361*(14), 1339–1348. doi:10.1056/NEJMoa0902430 PMID:19797280

Liang, H., Xue, Y., Laosethakul, K., and Lloyd, S. J. "Information systems and healthcare-I: trust, uncertainty, and online prescription filling," Communications of the Association for Information Systems (15) 2005, pp 41-60.

Mackay, M. M., & Weidlich, O. (2007, March 2007). Australian Mobile Phone Lifestyle Index, 3rd Edition, Australian Interactive Media Industry Association (AIMIA), Mobile Content Industry Development Group (MCIDG). Retrieved from http://www.aimia.com.au/mobile

Metzger, B. E., & al-others), e. (2008). Hyperglycemia and adverse pregnancy outcomes. *The New England Journal of Medicine*, *358*(19), 1191–2002. PMID:18463375

Milliken, F. J. (1987). Three types of perceived uncertainty about the environment: State, effect, and response uncertainty. *Academy of Management Review*, *12*(1), 133–143.

Min, S. D., Lee, B. W., Yoon, S. W., Lee, Y. B., Kim, J. K., Lee, M., & Park, C. O. "Actual condition of Korean e-health: What do enterprisers want for developing e-health industry?" in: 9th International Conference on e-Health Networking, Application and Services, IEEE, Taipei, Taiwan, 19-22 June, 2007, pp. 304-307. doi:10.1109/HEALTH.2007.381658

Mirza, F., Norris, T., & Stockdale, R. (2008). Mobile technologies and the holistic management of chronic diseases. *Health Informatics Journal*, *14*(4), 309–321. doi:10.1177/1460458208096559 PMID:19008280

Netsize. (2009). *Netsize Guide 2009 Edition: Mobile Society and Me: When worlds combine*. Levallois-Perret: Netsize.

O'Doherty, K., Rao Hill, S., Mackay, M. M., & McPherson, J. (2010). Mobile Data Service usage and preference: An investigation of Australian consumers. *International Journal of Mobile Communications*, *8*(1), 106–127. doi:10.1504/IJMC.2010.030523

Oh, S., Yang, S., Kurnia, S., Lee, H., Mackay, M. M., & O'Doherty, K. (2008). The characteristics of mobile data users in Australia. *International Journal of Mobile Communications*, *8*(2), 217–230. doi:10.1504/IJMC.2008.016578

Opie, A. (1998). Nobody's asked me for my view: Users' empowerment by multidisciplinary health teams. *Qualitative Health Research*, *18*(2), 188–206. doi:10.1177/104973239800800204

Pfeffer, J., & Salancik, G. R. (1978). *The external control of organizations: a resource dependence perspective*. New York: Harper & Row.

Porter, M., & Tiesberg, E. (2006). *Re-defining health care delivery*. Boston: Harvard Business Press.

Poulton, B. C. (1999). User involvement in identifying health needs and shaping and evaluating services: Is it being raised? *Journal of Advanced Nursing*, *30*(6), 1289–1296. doi:10.1046/j.1365-2648.1999.01224.x PMID:10583638

Rachlis, M. (2006). *Key to sustainable healthcare system. Available:* http://www.improveinchroniccare.org, *21 June 2006* (Vol. 2008).

Radin, P. (2006). To me, it's my life: Medical communication, trust, and activism in cyberspace. *Social Science & Medicine*, *6*(3), 591–601. doi:10.1016/j.socscimed.2005.06.022 PMID:16039031

Rao, S., & Troshani, I. (2006). AMC-ER Preliminary Research Report: Understanding Market and Mobile Content Selection for Distribution. Adelaide, South Australia: Australian Mobile Content – Export Research Initiative, m.Net Corporation Ltd.

Rasmussen, B., Wellard, S., & Nankervis, A. (2001). Consumer issues in navigating health care services for type I diabetes. *Journal of Clinical Nursing*, *10*(5), 628–634. doi:10.1046/j.1365-2702.2001.00550.x PMID:11822513

Reach, G., Zerrouki, D., Leclercq, D., & d'Ivernois, J. F. (2005). Adjusting insulin doses: From knowledge to decision. *Patient Education and Counseling*, *56*(1), 98–103. doi:10.1016/j.pec.2004.01.001 PMID:15590229

Rudi, R., & Celler, B. G. (2006). *Design and implementation of expert-telemedicine system for diabetes management at home*. Paper presented at the International Conference on Biomedical and Pharmaceutical Enginering 2006 (ICBPE2006), IEEE, 11-14 December 2006, Singapore.

Rumbold, A. R., & Crowther, C. A. (2001). Guideline use for gestational diabetes mellitus and current screening, diagnostic and management practices in Australian hospitals. *Australian and New Zealand Journal of Obstetrics and Gynaecology*, *41*(1), 86–90. doi:10.1111/j.1479-828X.2001.tb01301.x PMID:11284655

Rumbold, A. R., & Crowther, C. A. (2002). Women's experiences of being screened for gestational diabetes mellitus. *Australian and New Zealand Journal of Obstetrics and Gynaecology*, *42*(2), 131–137. doi:10.1111/j.0004-8666.2002.00131.x PMID:12069138

Russell, L. B., Churl Suh, D., & Safford, M. M. (2005). Time requirements for diabetes management: Too much for many? *The Journal of Family Practice*, *54*(1), 52–56. PMID:15623407

Sprivulis, P., Walker, J., Johnston, D., Pan, E., Adler-Milstein, J., Middleton, B., & Bates, D. W. (2007). The economic benefits of health information exchange interoperability. *Australian Health Review*, *31*(4), 531–539. doi:10.1071/AH070531 PMID:17973611

Swerissen, H., & Taylor, M. J. (2008). Reforming funding for chronic illness: Medicare-CDM. *Australian Health Review*, *32*(1), 76–84. doi:10.1071/AH080076 PMID:18241151

Troshani, I., & Rao, S. (2007a). The diffusion of mobile services in Australia: an evaluation using stakeholder and transaction cost economics theories. *IADIS International Journal of WWW/Internet*, *5*(2), 40-57.

Van Eyk, H., & Baum, F. (2002). Learning about interagency collaboration: Trialling collaborative projects between hospitals and community health services. *Health & Social Care in the Community*, *10*(4), 262–269. doi:10.1046/j.1365-2524.2002.00369.x PMID:12193170

Wellard, S. J., Rennie, S., & King, R. (2008). Perceptions of people with type 2 diabetes about self-management and the efficiency of community based services. *Contemporary Nurse*, *29*(2), 218–226. doi:10.5172/conu.673.29.2.218 PMID:18844535

Wickramasinghe, N. (2007). Fostering knowledge assets in healthcare with the KMI model. *International Journal of Management and Enterprise Development*, *4*(1), 52–65. doi:10.1504/IJMED.2007.011455

Wickramasinghe, N., & Goldberg, S. (2003). *The wireless panacea for healthcare.* Paper presented at the 36th Hawaii International Conference on System Sciences, Hawaii, 6-10 January, IEEE.

Wickramasinghe, N., & Goldberg, S. (2004). How M=EC2 in healthcare. *International Journal of Mobile Communications*, *2*(2), 140–156. doi:10.1504/IJMC.2004.004664

Wickramasinghe, N., & Goldberg, S. (2007a). Adaptive mapping to realisation methodology (AMR) to facilitate mobile initiatives in healthcare. *International Journal of Mobile Communications*, *5*(3), 300–318. doi:10.1504/IJMC.2007.012396

Wickramasinghe, N., Goldberg, S., & Bali, R. (2007). Enabling superior m-health project success: A tri-country validation. *International Journal of Services and Standards*, *4*(1), 97–117. doi:10.1504/IJSS.2008.016087

Wickramasinghe, N., Goldberg, S., & Bali, S. (2008). Enabling superior m-health project success: A tri-country validation. *International Journal of Services and Standards*, *4*(1), 97–117. doi:10.1504/IJSS.2008.016087

Wickramasinghe, N., & Schaffer, J. (2006). Creating knowledge driven healthcare processes with the intelligence continuum. *International Journal of Electronic Healthcare*, *2*(2), 164–174. doi:10.1504/IJEH.2006.008830 PMID:18048242

Wickramasinghe, N., Troshani, I., & Goldberg, S. (2009). Supporting diabetes self-management with pervasive wireless technology solutions. *International Journal of Healthcare Delivery Reform Initiatives*, *1*(4), 17–31. doi:10.4018/jhdri.2009100102

Wickramasinghe, N., Troshani, I., & Goldberg, S. (2010). An investigation into the use of pervasive wireless technologies to support diabetes healthcare. In A. Coronato & G. De Pietro (Eds.), *Pervasive and Smart Technologies for Healthcare: Ubiquitous Methodologies and Tools* (Vol. 114-129). New York: IGI Global. doi:10.4018/978-1-61520-765-7.ch006

Wild, S., Roglic, G., Green, A., Sicree, R., & King, H. (2004). Global prevalence of diabetes: Estimates for the year 2000 and projections for 2030. *Diabetes Care*, *27*(5), 1047–1053. doi:10.2337/diacare.27.5.1047 PMID:15111519

Williamson, O. E. (1985). *The Economic Institutions of Capitalism: Firms, Markets, and Relational Contracting*. New York: Free Press.

Williamson, O. E. (1991). Comparative economic organization: The analysis of discrete structural alternatives. *Administrative Science Quarterly*, *36*(2), 269–296. doi:10.2307/2393356

Young, R. J., Taylor, J., Friede, T., Hollis, S., Mason, J. M., Lee, P., & Gibson, J. M. et al. (2005). Pro-active call centre treatment support (PACCTS) to improve glucose control in type 2 diabetes: A randomized controlled trial. *Diabetes Care*, *28*(2), 278–282. doi:10.2337/diacare.28.2.278 PMID:15677779

Zigbor, J. C., & Songer, T. J. (2001). External barriers to diabetes care: Addressing personal and health systems issues. *Diabetes Spectrum*, *14*(1), 23–28. doi:10.2337/diaspect.14.1.23

KEY TERMS AND DEFINITIONS

Asset-Specific Exchanges: Create dependencies which can in turn require enhanced cooperation, coordination, and proximity for the effective transfer of both assets or their deliverables amongst actors.

Data Protection: Ensuring appropriate privacy and security of medical data ensues at all times.

Demand Uncertainty: Is defined as the inability of an actor to predict future events concerning the success or failure of new product offerings.

Diabetes Self-Management: The combination of medical and non-medical approaches so that patients with the disease can have a life which is as normal as possible.

Frequency: Concerns how often actors are involved in exchanges with each another.

GDM: Gestational diabetes mellitus (GDM) is a common form of diabetes that presents in pregnancy.

Pervasive Technology Solution: A technology solution that can be used and is as useful anywhere and anytime to the user.

Platform Independent: Not being restricted to one or another technology platform.

Task Complexity: Refers to the number of different specialized behavioral inputs that are required to fully develop and distribute a product or service.

Transaction Cost Economics (TCE) Theory: Represents a natural and logical theoretical setting for guiding the evaluation of actor interactions. TCE focuses on economic exchange relations amongst organizational actors, including diabetes patients and healthcare providers that are typically involved in interactions.

Chapter 3
Constructive eHealth Evaluation:
Involving the End-User

Anna Marie Balling Høstgaard
Aalborg University, Denmark

ABSTRACT

Despite the existence of an extensive body of knowledge about best practices and factors that contribute to the successful development and adoption of eHealth, many eHealth development-projects still face a number of problems - many of them of an organizational nature. This chapter presents a new method: "The Constructive eHealth evaluation method" aimed at supporting real end-user participation - a well-known success factor in eHealth development. It provides an analytical framework for achieving real end-user participation during the different phases in the eHealth lifecycle. The method was developed and used for the first time during the evaluation of an EHR planning process in a Danish region. It has proven effective for providing management at more levels on-going information and feedback from end-users, allowing management to change direction during eHealth development in order to achieve the most successful adoption and implementation of eHealth in healthcare environments.

DOI: 10.4018/978-1-4666-9870-3.ch003

INTRODUCTION

During the past decades an extensive body of knowledge and many research experiences about factors that contribute to successful development and implementation of eHealth technologies have been obtained (Ash, Stavre, & Kuperman, 2003; Berg, 2001; Kaplan & Harris-Salamone, 2009; Kaye, Kokia, Shalev, Idar, & Chinitz, 2010; Van der Meijden, Tange, Troost, & Hasman, 2003). Yet, lessons are still to be learned as many eHealth implementations still face a number of problems, many of them of an organizational nature (Ash, Stavre, & Kuperman, 2003; Cresswell, Bates, & Sheikh, 2013; Edmondson, 2003a; Høstgaard & Nøhr, 2004b; Pagliari, 2007; Van der Meijden, Tange, Troost, & Hasman, 2001; van Gemert-Pijnen et al., 2011). One of the most crucial organizational success factors in eHealth development is *end-user participation,* which has been increasingly recognized during the past decades (Berg & Winthereik, 2004; Cresswell, Bates, & Sheikh, 2013; Høstgaard, 2009; Kensing, Simonsen, & Bødker, 1996; Kensing & Blomberg, 1998; Kushniruk & Turner, 2011; Pagliari, 2007). However, the concept of "end-user participation" has a broad range of meanings, ranging from end-users as consultants (e.g.to test technologies before they are being implemented) to involving end-users during all the phases in the full technological development process (Arnstein, 2007).

In this chapter the concept is used in the sense of enabling end-users to exert influence in decision-making throughout the full eHealth life cycle. That is, *real* influence by participating in decision-making during all phases in the eHealth development process. Most methods developed to support and facilitate end-user participation so far have been developed for organizations in general and have focused on the design stage (Bødker, Kensing, & Simonsen, 2004; Kensing, Simonsen, & Bødker, 1996; Mumford & Weir, 1979). Methods designed for the full eHealth life cycle – formative evaluation methods - have been proposed by Catwell & Sheikh, Clarke et al. and van Gemert-Pijnen (Catwell & Sheikh, 2009; Clarke et al., 1994; van Gemert-Pijnen et al., 2011). However, none of these methods have end-user involvement as a fulcrum. Thus, so far, no methods have been developed with a specific focus on supporting end-user participation during the full eHealth lifecycle, i.e. during all the different phases in the eHealth development process.

A new formative evaluation method aiming at supporting end-user participation during the full eHealth lifecycle is presented in this chapter: "*Constructive eHealth evaluation*". It is meant for eHealth management at all levels – and others working in the field of eHealth technology. The method provides tools for learning during the eHealth development process by involving end-users throughout the eHealth lifecycle. This allows eHealth management to benefit from the unique knowledge on the clinical work practices that end-users possess. Thus, based on feedback from the end-users, management is provided the opportunity to make adjustments in project plans accordingly, hence to solve problems as they arise. In contrast, when using summative evaluation methods, problems are often first identified when the technology is completed, which means that only minor changes can be made, as major changes often can only be made with great difficulty and at great expenses.

The Constructive eHealth evaluation method was used for the first time in a research study of an EHR planning process in a Danish region. Thus, it was developed within and specifically for the healthcare sector.

Initially, the chapter will provide the background for developing the method. Next, the Constructive eHealth evaluation method will be described - including the theoretical framework on which it is based, its target groups, and when and how to use it. Then a more detailed review of the method will be provided through a thorough description of its different phases, where examples from using the method in practice will be provided. Finally, the strengths and the limitations of the method will be discussed as well as its relation to other approaches.

BACKGROUND

During recent years the type, the extent and especially the introduction rate of new eHealth technologies (e.g. telemedicine technologies, technologies for self management of health and electronic health records) aimed at improving patient health, patient safety and / or the quality of treatment and care has increased significantly. However, studies show that the introduction of new eHealth technologies, besides offering new solutions and solving some problems, often brings with it a number of new problems, often of an organizational nature (Ash, Stavre, & Kuperman, 2003; Cresswell, Bates, & Sheikh, 2013; Edmondson, 2003b; Høstgaard & Nøhr, 2004a; Pagliari, 2007; Seemann, 2013; Van der Meijden, Tange, Troost, & Hasman A., 2001; van Gemert-Pijnen et al., 2011). Research has also revealed not only pitfalls to be aware of but also success factors to be met in order for eHealth implementation to be successful (Ash, Stavre, & Kuperman, 2003; Berg, 2001; Kaplan & Harris-Salamone, 2009; Kaye, Kokia, Shalev, Idar, & Chinitz, 2010; Seemann, 2013; Van der Meijden, Tange, Troost, & Hasman, 2003). Some crucial – and well-known – organizational success factors are that the clinicians must obtain *positive clinical benefits* (Ash, Stavre, & Kuperman, 2003; Robertson et al., 2010; Simonsen & Hertzum, 2006) as a result of eHealth implementation and *joint ownership* (Cresswell, Bates, & Sheikh, 2013) of the decisions made during the development process. A prerequisite for both is *real* participation in the development process – not pretended or symbolic – enabling clinicians to exert real influence in decision-making (Berg, 2001; Bødker, Kensing, & Simonsen, 2004; Cresswell, Bates, & Sheikh, 2013; Høstgaard, 2009; Pagliari, 2007; Pare, Sicotte, & Jacques, 2006). Experience and research have shown the following prerequisites for achieving real end-user participation:

Early Involvement

Mumford classifies end-user participation in information technology (IT) development into three different types according to depth: consultative, representative and consensus participation. According to Mumford, real influence in IT-development is best achieved by using the consensus type of participation, where end-users are involved *throughout* the technological development process (Mumford E. & Weir M., 1979; Mumford E., 1983). In line with this, Johnson, Lorentzen, Müller et al. and Protti state that early involvement of clinicians (end-users) in eHealth development is essential because, as the technological development process proceeds, the scope of influence of the clinicians and the possibility of changing the decisions already made are progressively limited. Therefore, by involving the clinicians already in the planning stage, their influence on decision-making increases considerably (Johnson C.W., 2006; Lorentzen A., 1994; Müller, Kjaer-Rasmussen, & Nohr, 1989; Protti D., 2002).

Representation

Representation of all groups of clinicians is important in order to achieve joint ownership from all relevant participant-groups (Avison.D.E. & Fitzgerald G., 1995; Kensing F. & Blomberg J., 1998; Mumford E., 1983). Avison et al. argue that in order to achieve real participation of the end-users, "all major interests should be represented, including each section and function, grade, age group and so on" (Avison.D.E. & Fitzgerald G., 1995)p.357). However, Berg describes how trying to accommodate "everybody's" requests and "needs" can result in an EHR process losing direction and momentum (Berg M., 2001) p.149. Thus, for eHealth working groups to be able to reach agreements, not *all* wards and *all* medical specialties can be represented. The goal is for upper management to set frames allowing end-users the *best possible* representation.

Workload Reduction

Kensing et al. have found that *workload reduction* – meaning that colleagues take over part/all of the clinical duties for the clinicians involved (it does not involve extra payment) - is a precondition for *real* end-user participation at certain stages in eHealth development. The authors argue that "it is the responsibility of the management to provide users with the time and possibilities to participate in this process" (Kensing F., Simonsen J., & Bødker K., 1996) p.132. Also Høstgaard found workload reduction to be essential for obtaining real end-user participation in eHealth development (A. M. Høstgaard, 2009).

Involving End-Users through Formative Evaluation Methods

Despite the existence of an extensive body of knowledge about best practices and success factors, eHealth development and implementation *still* faces a number of organizational problems (Black A.D. et al., 2011; Robertson A. et al., 2010; Sheikh, Cornford, & Barber, 2011; Wears R.L. & Berg M., 2005). This is supported by Kaplan et al. who - based on a literature review and the results of an AMIA workshop - report that many eHealth systems are not successful "despite an accumulation of best practices research identifying success factors" (Kaplan B. & Harris-Salamone K, 2009) p. 291). These authors therefore call for further research into the development of new methods to support successful eHealth development. In line with this, Black et al. have found, in a recently published study, that the empirical evidence for the beneficial impact on the quality and safety of healthcare of most eHealth technologies is often absent or modest, and the authors state that if the expected benefits of eHealth are to be realized, substantial future research resources will be required (Black A.D. et al., 2011). Also the results of the final evaluation of the implementation and adoption of nationwide electronic health records in secondary care in England in "early adopter" hospitals showed that the benefits for clinicians and patients were limited or even missing, mainly because of problems of an organizational nature. One of the main findings was that the systems had difficulties in fulfilling organizational and user needs because of a lack of organizational and user involvement in decision making (Sheikh, Cornford, & Barber, 2011). All these findings call for further research into how the existing knowledge within the health informatics research field on the importance of supporting well known success factors can be applied in practice.

Formative evaluation methods offer a basis for the development of new methods to support successful eHealth development while building on one of the most well-known success factors: the involvement of end-users in the eHealth development process. The aim of formative evaluation methods is to improve eHealth system development by providing feedback and learning from all relevant actor-groups involved – including end-users - to e.g. management and it-professionals during all phases in the eHealth lifecycle (Nykänen et al., 2011; Yusof, Papazafeiropoulou, Paul, & Stergioulas, 2008). Formative evaluation methods have been proposed by Catwell & Sheikh, Clarke et al. and van Gemert-Pijnen (Catwell & Sheikh, 2009; Clarke et al., 1994; van Gemert-Pijnen et al., 2011)However, the focus in these formative methods is on monitoring the eHealth development process by setting up various evaluation measures and checkpoints during the different phases in the technological lifecycle (Nykänen et al., 2011; Yusof, Papazafeiropoulou, Paul, & Stergioulas, 2008). They do not have a specific focus on end-users. Besides, they do not provide any guidance on how activities are undertaken during the development process as an independent activity separated from other project activities (Nykänen et al., 2011).

Constructive eHealth Evaluation

Within recent years researchers at the Danish Centre for Health Informatics (DaCHI) at Aalborg University (AAU) in Aalborg, Denmark have developed a new formative evaluation method with a specific focus on end-user involvement: the Constructive eHealth evaluation method. This method is a further development of formative evaluation methods developed in the 1980s and forward by researchers within the early science-technology-society (STS) movements in the Netherlands, Scandinavia, the UK and USA respectively: Constructive Technology Assessment (CTA) methods. CTA methods were aimed at evaluation of technology in general (Bijker, 2009; Müller, Kjaer-Rasmussen, & Nohr, 1989; Schot & Rip, 1997). These researchers set up a new research agenda aiming at challenging the limitations to summative technology evaluation, which generally is conducted, when the technology is fully developed. This means that only minor changes can be made, as major changes can only be made with great difficulty and at great expenses. Thus, with CTA the focus shifted from only assessing the various impacts of fully developed technologies to also paying attention to the technological development process as a learning and feedback process, when new technologies are developed and implemented (Müller, Kjaer-Rasmussen, & Nohr, 1989).

During the late 1980s researchers at Aalborg University further developed the CTA for the evaluation of eHealth specifically (Müller, Kjaer-Rasmussen, & Nohr, 1989; Müller, Kjaer-Rasmussen, & Nøhr, 1988). The objective was to deliver a constructive evaluation of both intended and unintended consequences of eHealth implementation. Besides, it was to involve the end-users at an early stage in the process, as they were seen as the most important knowledge capacity with respect to the work practices into which the technology was to be integrated (Müller, 1990). However, this CTA method did not gain ground in eHealth development at that time – possibly because end-user involvement was not yet recognised by management as an important success factor.

During the past decades, the importance of end-user involvement in eHealth development has been increasingly recognised (Bødker K., Kensing F., & Simonsen J., 2004; Cresswell, Bates, & Sheikh, 2013; A. M. Høstgaard, 2009; Kushniruk A. & Turner P., 2011; Pagliari, 2007; Pare G., Sicotte C., & Jacques H., 2006), and in the newly published eHealth Task Force Report: "Redesigning Health in Europe in 2020" by the European Union, end-user involvement is mentioned as a key recommendation (The European Union, 2012). Thus, in this perspective, the present Constructive eHealth evaluation method will fill a void in the current body of knowledge about success factors and best practices in eHealth development and implementation and, not least of all, on how to apply these in practice. The method is based on Müller et al.'s method from the 1980s and further developed on the basis of a number of recent evaluation studies within the healthcare sector (A. M. Høstgaard, 2009; A. M. Høstgaard, 2010; A. M. Høstgaard, Bertelsen, & Nøhr, 2010a; Nøhr, Høstgaard,

Botin, & Kjær-Andersen, 2004; Pape-Haugaard, Haugaard, Carøe, & Høstgaard, 2013). The Constructive eHealth evaluation method offers an analytical framework for involving end-users during the different phases in the full eHealth lifecycle. It also offers specific methods for achieving this in each of the phases in the lifecycle. Besides, it offers an eHealth evaluation method as an independent activity during the technological development process (A. M. Høstgaard, Bertelsen, Petersen, & Nøhr, 2013).

THEORETICAL FRAMEWORK

The Constructive eHealth evaluation method is based on the combination of the following two theories:

- The Socio-Technical theory
- The Social-Carrier-of-Technology theory

The combination of the two theories is called the Socio-Technical-Carrier-of-Technology theory (STCT). It was developed by researchers at Aalborg University in the 1990s (Müller, 1990; Müller, Kjaer-Rasmussen, & Nøhr, 1988)

The Socio-Technical Theory

The Socio-Technical theory provides a broad concept of technology, focusing on the micro level and the actor as opposed to the macro level. This concept is open-ended to enable an understanding of the relation between technological- and social change. According to the concept, technology embraces a combination of four constituents: technique (meaning the technological object in question), knowledge, organization and product. These four constituents are inseparable components of any technology. A qualitative change in any one of the components will eventually result in supplementary, compensatory, and/or retaliatory change in the other components. For a technology to be considered as such, it has to be applied and result in a product, and for this to happen, actors have to be active within each of the four components. The Socio-Technical theory is process-oriented and focuses on the technological development process. It can be described in five stages. Within each of these stages, the actors make their selections based on possibilities and interests. This means that at every stage a selection takes place (black circles) which leaves out many potential actions not chosen (grey circles) (figure 1) (Kuanda J., 2003; Müller J., 1991; Müller, Kjaer-Rasmussen, & Nøhr, 1988).

Figure 1. The five stages in the technological development process (Müller, Kjaer-Rasmussen, & Nøhr, 1988)

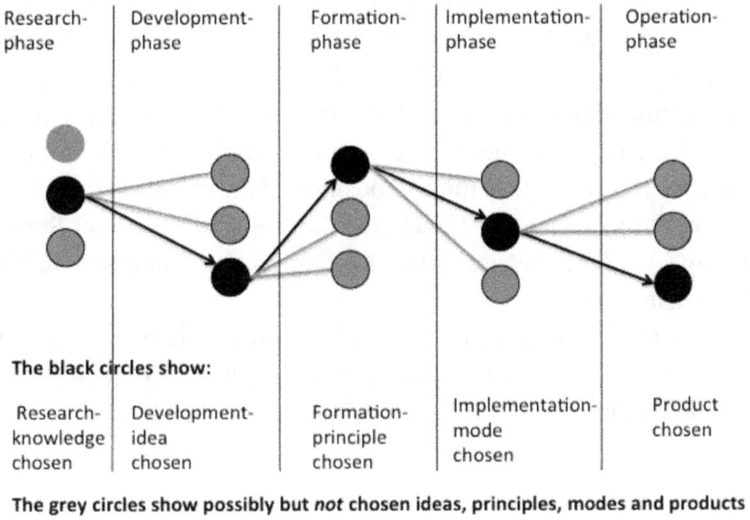

The Social-Carrier-of-Technology Theory

The focus in the Social-Carrier-of-Technology theory is the actors. It was developed to identify and study the relevant "Social-Carriers-of-Technology" involved in the development of new technology. The concept refers to a group of actors, or a social entity, which chooses a new technology and carries it forward towards the next stage in the technological development process. According to this theory, this will happen only if the "Social-Carriers-of-Technology" have the necessary resources (interest, power, organization, information, access and knowledge) to change their status from *potential* to *actual* carriers of the technology in question. All actors who have interest in a new technology are potential carriers, but only if all the six conditions mentioned above are fulfilled, they will become actual carriers. However, interest and power are the two most important conditions of the six (Edquist C. & Edquist O., 1979).

Often two or more Social-Carrier-of-Technology groups choose and implement the technology together. These groups are named *combined* Social-Carriers-of-Technology. When, on the other hand, the social groups involved carry the technology in different stages of the development process and, in this way, are sequentially linked to each other, they are named *linked* Social-Carriers-of-Technology. In reality the combined and linked Social-Carriers-of-Technology are most often intertwined (Edquist C. & Edquist O., 1979).

The Socio-Technical-Carrier-of-Technology Theory (STCT)

According to the STCT theory - developed by combining and further developing the two above theories - the choices made by the actors include not only the technique but *all* four components in the socio-technological technology concept: technique, knowledge, organization and product. The STCT theory states that every qualitative change – and the final outcome/product – in a technological development process can be traced back to a change in the composition of the social carriers of technology and in the conditions necessary to achieve the status of an actual Social-Carrier-of-Technology (A. M. Høstgaard, 2009; Müller, Kjaer-Rasmussen, & Nøhr, 1988; Nøhr & Bernstein, 1992).

The STCT theory provides a framework for understanding the interactions that occur between the relevant social groups in eHealth development, hence during Constructive eHealth evaluation, which comprises the full technological lifecycle.

OBJECTIVE

The objective of the Constructive eHealth evaluation method is to support successful eHealth development and implementation by providing an analytical framework for achieving the best possibly end-user participation during all the phases in the eHealth technological lifecycle, which is a well-known success factor in eHealth development. Hence, it is to improve the adoption of eHealth in healthcare environments. Besides it is to offer specific methods for achieving this in each single phase. Finally, it is to offer an eHealth evaluation method as an independent evaluation activity, which takes place parallel to the tasks of the overall project management in contrast to being an intrinsic part of these. The Constructive eHealth evaluation method thus fills a void in the current body of knowledge on how to apply knowledge about success factors and best practices in eHealth development in practice.

Preconditions for Using the Constructive eHealth Evaluation Method

It is important to stress the following preconditions for using the Constructive eHealth evaluation method. The first two apply for the Constructive eHealth evaluation method specifically, the last for evaluation in general:

- Management at all levels must recognize end-user participation as a crucial success factor in achieving the key objectives in healthcare: patient safety and quality of treatment and care. Hence, end-users are considered indispensable knowledge capacities, when it comes to eHealth development

- The evaluation must be an independent activity running in parallel to the tasks of the project management. This means that the manager/members of the evaluation team cannot be identical to the project manager/project management, as conflicts of interests might occur during the process (this is further dealt with later on in this chapter)
- Guidelines for good evaluation practice has to be followed throughout the evaluation process (Nykänen et al., 2011)

When to Use the Method

eHealth development can be divided into different stages within the technological lifecycle (figure 2). The technological lifecycle is an on going process in any technological development. This means that when a technology has been designed, developed, implemented and taken into operation, i.e. the first so-called life-circle in eHealth development is completed, the next one starts. This is because all technologies – including eHealth technologies - will be subject to on-going redesign (of greater or lesser), until the technology might be permanently phased out.

As mentioned before in this chapter, early involvement of end-users in eHealth development is crucial for achieving eHealth technologies providing clinical benefits, as the end-users are considered the most important knowledge capacity with respect to the work practices into which the technology is to be integrated. Therefore, end-users should be involved as early in the technological lifecycle as possibly – i.e.

Figure 2. The technological lifecycle (own figure based on (Müller, Kjaer-Rasmussen, & Nøhr, 1988))

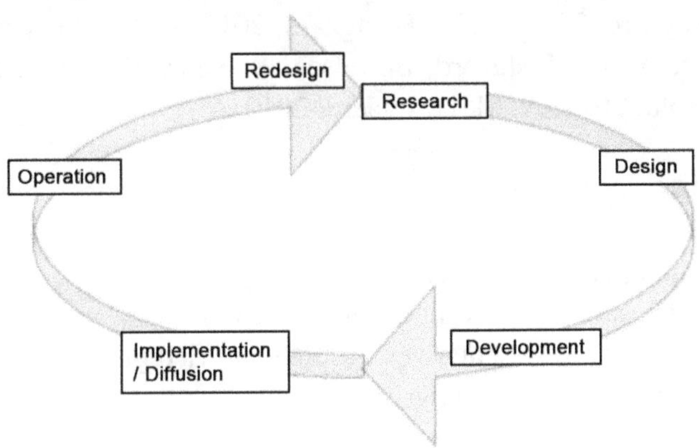

in the early phases in *first* technological lifecycle, because the possibility of changing the decisions already made are progressively limited as the technological development process proceeds (Johnson C.W., 2006; Lorentzen A., 1994; Protti D., 2002). However, end-user involvement in the early phases in the technological lifecycle requires thoughtfulness: according to Avison et al. and Berg, participation in the early stages of a technological development process requires more than *clinical* knowledge Thus, for end-users to make informed decisions in the early stages, they must possess both technical and clinical knowledge. Otherwise they will, according to Avison et al. be subject to the influence from other more powerful groups. Berg argues that end-users/clinicians generally are incompetent as regards speaking the language of "specifications" and "configurations" and of expressing their "needs" in the work situation. The skills needed for this can only be developed over time by taking them on board early in the process and - according to Avison et al. - by giving them the necessary skills *before* they enter into the process (Avison.D.E. & Fitzgerald G., 1995; Berg M., 2001). This is important to bear in mind for eHealth project management aiming at supporting real end-user involvement.

Thus, the optimal way to conduct Constructive eHealth evaluation is to involve the end-users already in the early phases of the *first* lifecycle while having the above considerations in mind. However, the method can also be used during forthcoming lifecycles – i.e. in later "lifecycle rounds" where redesign is on the agenda. Of course, the end-users degree of influence will be significantly diminished compared to participating during the first cycle.

ANALYTICAL FRAMEWORK

Based on a number of studies within the healthcare sector, an analytical framework for the Constructive eHealth evaluation method was developed by DaCHI researchers (A. M. Høstgaard, 2009; A. M. Høstgaard, 2010; A. M. Høstgaard, Bertelsen, & Nøhr, 2010a; A. M. Høstgaard, Bertelsen, & Nøhr, 2010b; A. M. Høstgaard, Bertelsen, & Nøhr, 2011; A. M. Høstgaard, 2012):

Pre Analysis

1. Research and planning phase:
    a. Identification of relevant groups of actors
    b. Selection of representatives for the identified groups
    c. Technology-carrier analysis

2. Design phase
    a. Identifying needs
    b. Requirement specifications
3. Development phase
4. Implementation and diffusion phase
5. Summative evaluation and reporting phase

It is important to notice that in practice, the phases are not distinct, but overlap.

Below general recommendations for each phase is first presented. Then the role of the manager of the evaluation process/ the evaluation team (referred to as "the evaluator" forward from this point) in the respective phases is described. The evaluator can be hired from outside as a consultant or be from inside the eHealth organization, but cannot be identical to the project manager/project management as mentioned before. This depends e.g. on the system being assessed and on the decisions taken by the upper management. The overall responsibility of the evaluator is to facilitate learning and feedback between the different groups involved with a specific focus on the end-users during the entire development process and to direct the summative evaluation in phase 5.

Pre Analysis

Any eHealth evaluations should be initiated with answering the following questions:

What is the problem?

1. *What* is going to be evaluated (the aspects or the focus for the evaluation)?
2. *Why* the planned evaluation (objective)?
3. *When* in the eHealth lifecycle is the evaluation going to take place (phase)?
4. *Who* are the relevant actors involved and whose perspective is to be followed (perspective)? (E.g. the end-users, the management, others?)
5. *How* are the results going to be used?

If it is not possible to answer these questions, the evaluation should not take place! (Brender J., 2006; Yusof, Papazafeiropoulou, Paul, & Stergioulas, 2008).

1. Research and Planning Phase
    1a) Identification of relevant groups of actors: The identification of the relevant groups of actors to be involved in the different eHealth development phases can be conducted by using e.g. partner analysis (Kørnøv, 2007; Mitchell, Agle, & Wood, 1997). Obvious groups in eHealth development are: various groups of clinicians, management, vendors and

it-professionals. The evaluator's role is to ensure that when e.g. steering committees and eHealth-working groups are assembled, all relevant actor groups are represented – and that focus is on the end-users.

1b) Selection of representatives for the identified groups: Experience show that it is important to make sure that the representatives from the various identified groups of actors are appointed by members of the respective groups themselves - and not handpicked by management. This is essential in order to achieve ownership to the decisions taken during the process (Kensing F. & Blomberg J., 1998; Pare G., Sicotte C., & Jacques H., 2006). At regional and hospital level it is recommended to ask the respective professional associations representing the different groups to identify their own representatives. At ward level a useful method is the "Participatory method" (Kanstrup & Bertelsen, 2006). The evaluator's role is to ensure that the selection of especially the end-user groups are performed according to the recommendations mentioned above.

1c) Technology-carrier analysis: An analysis of the interactions that occur between the identified relevant groups of actors in eHealth development in order to shed light on possibly conflicts of interests and power can be an important part of phase 1. The technology-carrier analysis is not always a necessary part of a Constructive eHealth evaluation. However, it is recommended to carry through, if former experiences or experiences gained through phase 1a) and 1b) have shown that more detailed information on and understanding of the interactions that occur between the relevant actor groups is needed in order to ensure the involvement of all groups – with a special focus on the end-users - in the forthcoming process. The analysis comprises examination, synthesis and conclusion on separate analysis of each of the six conditions for becoming an actual carrier of the new technology, hence for becoming involved in decision making during the eHealth development process (A. M. Høstgaard, 2009). The six separate analyses are:

- Interest-analysis of the vested interests of the different relevant social carrier groups (the identified actor groups) of technology in relation to the technology in question
- Power analysis of their options to carry through their interests
- Organizational-analysis of the possibly support from their professional association
- Access-analysis of their opportunities to see and test the system in practice and -
- Knowledge and information analysis of the amount of knowledge and information that they have acquired about technology in ques-

tion both in general and particularly regarding the different options available. The evaluator's role is to direct and to carry through the analysis and to discuss the results with the upper management if they show that some of the conditions mentioned above are not fulfilled – and with a special focus on the end-users. It is important to bear in mind that in order to benefit from using the Constructive eHealth evaluation method, upper management must recognize end-user participation as a crucial success factor for achieving the key objectives in healthcare. And, as a consequence that they are willing to take the necessary steps to support real end-user involvement, if the technology-carrier analysis shows that some of the conditions mentioned above are not fulfilled.

2. Design Phase

2a) Identifying needs: In order to identify the needs the new eHealth technology must fulfil, the following analysis should be carried through:

Needs and problem analysis - e.g. identification of:

- The kind of problems the new eHealth technology is meant to solve
- Internal and/or external communication needs
- The relationships between the different relevant user groups when it comes to supporting communication on the operational level
- Localization of where in the organization the communication needs are to be supported

Assessment of impact of existing technology - e.g. identification of:

- To which degree the existing technology has fulfilled and lived up to the functions and needs, it was meant to meet
- To which degree the existing technology has *not* fulfilled and lived up to the functions and needs, it was meant to meet
- The consequences of using the existing technology
- The assessment from the various relevant user groups in relation to using the existing technology

Assessment of operational experience from existing technology - e.g. identification of:

- Which aspects from using the existing technology – especially those of an organizational nature – should be preserved, and which should be changed

Assessment of design experience from existing technology - e.g. identification of:

- Which design characteristics of the existing technology should be preserved and which should be modified

Search for new research and development ideas - e.g. identification of:

- New knowledge relevant to be included in the design of the new technology
- The possible - perhaps long-term - development perspectives which seem most promising in relation to the needs and problem analysis

Outline of possible technical designs conceivably into possible operational contexts - e.g. identification of:

- A (limited) number of technical design options - outlined and incorporated one by one into concrete operational contexts and organizational patterns

Impact assessment of the outlined new technology - e.g. identification of:

- Which of the available proposals for design and operation for a new technology will best meet the stated needs and functional requirements
- The outcome of a comparison between the various impact assessments
- Which of the available proposals for design and operation for a new technology will best be accepted among the different user groups

This leads to:

2b) Requirement specifications: In 2005 the EU announced a new way to conduct a tender process: *The Competitive Dialogue Process* (CDP). The CDP is aimed at particularly complex contracts, where the provider (the eHealth project management) is not able to define technical, legal or financial matters related to the project (Falch & Jensen, 2005) (fig.3). The CDP can be applied in eHealth development (of e.g. a new EHR systems) when no off-the-shelf items meet the provider's needs and requirements. This way of conducting an eHealth development process is fully in line with the aim of the Constructive eHealth evaluation method, as the CDP supports end-user involvement in decision-making during the design phase.

During the design phase – including 2a) and 2b) - the evaluator's role is to ensure that the requirements for supporting end-users possibility for exerting real influence on the decisions making are accommodated (e.g. workload reduction). Besides, it is to facilitate learning between all groups involved. This must be done in close collaboration with the project management.

3. Development Phase: During the development phase, the project management in close collaboration with the end-users and the vendor/it professionals outline possible technical configurations thought into different clinical contexts. A useful method for this process is the "User Innovation Management" (UIM) method,

Figure 3. The different phases in the Competitive Dialogue Process method (Falch & Jensen, 2005)

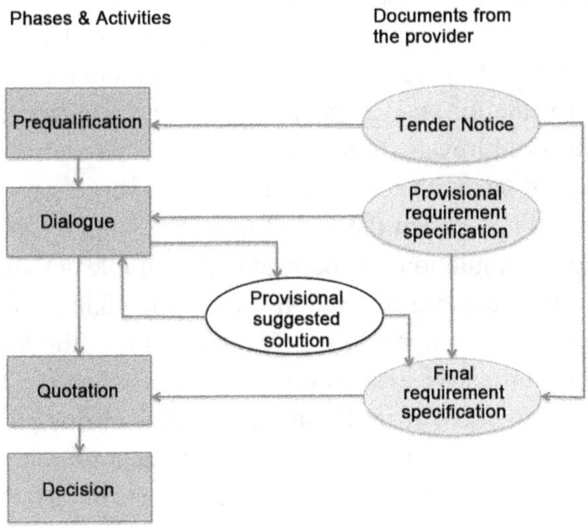

where the focus is on involving the end-users in designing the functionalities of the new technology (Kanstrup & Bertelsen, 2011). The outcome of this process is the development of an early prototype of the eHealth system (a so-called pre-proto type). This might first be tested in a usability laboratory or in clinical set-ups in order to assess e.g. user-friendliness and the consequences of using it in clinical word-practice. Jacob Nielsen's ten heuristics for usability studies could be useful to follow in this phase (Nielsen, 2005). When the usability/ laboratory testing is completed, the next step is to test a prototype in a real clinical setting. Experience show that no matter how realistic a usability study has been performed, unforeseen disruptions and communication challenges can be hard to imitate (Kaipio, 2011). The role of the evaluator in this phase is to ensure that the end-users are involved throughout the phase, and that they are working closely together with the vendor/it-professionals. Besides, it is – like in previous phases – to facilitate learning between all groups involved.

4. Implementation and Diffusion Phase: During this phase, prototypes of the new eHealth system are usually implemented at selected wards for pilot testing. At this point of time, working-groups at ward level are set up to provide feed-back on the system's functionalities and user friendliness in various clinical contexts. The evaluator's role in this phase is to: a) make sure that all relevant actor groups are represented in the new groups. It is especially important to ensure that the vendor/ it-professionals are an integrated part of the groups,

as they must work closely together with the end-user in order to ensure that the new system meets the requirements in order to be able to support clinical work practices. b) To provide feedback from observations and interviews at ward level between different professional groups in order to share experiences and knowledge, and to management for learning and management purposes.

5. Summative Evaluation and Reporting Phase: The summative evaluation in the Constructive eHealth evaluation method is different from traditional summative evaluations methods with outcomes decided on very early in the process and rigidly assessed up upon at the end of the process. In a Constructive eHealth evaluation, the formulation of precise and measurable outcomes is an on-going process, and the outcomes are reconsidered and changed during the process based on new insights gained during this – and with methodological reflections in mind. The summative evaluation takes place when the eHealth system is fully developed in line with traditional summative evaluation methods like e.g. health technology assessment (HTA). The evaluator's role is to direct and to carry through the evaluation process in order to ensure that the objective of the summative evaluation is fulfilled. Moreover, it is to ensure that all results of the evaluation are reported through the appropriate channels and to all relevant parties.

PRESENTATION OF THE CONSTRUCTIVE eHEALTH EVALUATION METHOD USED DURING AN EHR DEVELOPMENT PROCESS IN A DANISH REGION

The Constructive eHealth evaluation method was first used and further developed in a research and evaluation study of an EHR planning process in a Danish region. In the following section a presentation of how the method was used in practice during the different phases in the technological lifecycle will be provided.

Background

In Denmark, where the healthcare system is public and financed by taxation and the five regions govern the hospitals, there has been extensive discussion about the EHR in Danish hospitals. Since 1999, the Danish national strategy for IT in the healthcare sector has required all Danish counties (counties at that time, now regions, because the counties were reorganized into 5 regions in 2007) – to implement an EHR (The Ministry of Health1999). In Denmark, the concept of "EHR" is defined as a platform with different modules delivered by different vendors. This means that the EHR in the five Danish regions each have their own development strategy and different platforms. The national strategy for IT resulted in The North Denmark Region (NDR) (at that time named "the County of North Jutland") developed an overall IT-strategy for the EHR development process (Nordjyllands Amt (The County of North Jutland), 2000). In October 2003, the EHR planning process was initiated in NDR.

The evaluation of the EHR in NDR was conducted in different ways during the different phases in the Constructive eHealth evaluation method, hence during the EHR development process. From April 2004 until December 2009 the research- and planning- and the design phases (phase 1 and 2) were studied by this author as part of a Ph.d. study with a focus on end-user involvement. The objective of the Ph.d. study was to study to which degree the end-users (with a specific focus on physicians) were involved during these phases. Thus, this author was not conducting a formative evaluation in the proper sense, but rather observing the interactions going on between the different actor groups involved during the research- and the design phases in the EHR development process (A. M. Høstgaard, 2009). However, the experiences gained during the Ph.d. study helped to inform the recommendations provided for some of the phases in the Constructive eHealth evaluation method in combination with experiences gained from a number of other studies performed by the Danish Centre for Health Informatics (DaCHI) (A. M. Høstgaard, 2009; A. M. Høstgaard, 2010; A. M. Høstgaard, Bertelsen, & Nøhr, 2010a; A. M. Høstgaard, Bertelsen, & Nøhr, 2010b; A. M. Høstgaard, Bertelsen, & Nøhr, 2011; A. M. Høstgaard, 2012). Besides, the Ph.d. study resulted in the development of a new method aimed at collecting more detailed information on end-user participation in health information (HIT) development in order to support, facilitate and improve *real* end-user participation: the EUPHIT (**e**nd-**u**ser **p**articipation in **h**ealth **i**nformation **t**echnology development) method (A. M. Høstgaard, 2010; A. M. Høstgaard, 2012).

Between June 2008 and December 2010, the AAU evaluation team: "DaCHI" was hired as an external evaluator to carry through the evaluation of the development- and the first part of the implementation- and diffusion phases (phase 3 and 4 in the Constructive eHealth evaluation method) (A. M. Høstgaard, Bertelsen, & Nøhr, 2010a). Because of unforeseen circumstances the EHR development process in NDR has been significantly delayed, and the implementation is still not completed. Hence, the summative evaluation (phase 5) remains to be carried through once the implementation phase is completed.

It is important to notice that more of the phases mentioned above were not distinct, but overlapped.

Methods

Phase 1 (Research and Planning) and 2 (Design) in the Constructive eHealth Evaluation Method Used in NDR

This author undertook the evaluation of Phase 1 and 2 as part of a Ph.d. study. (A. M. Høstgaard, 2009; A. M. Høstgaard, 2010).

Design

The study was designed as a single case study of the EHR research- and planning phases in NDR.

The relevant groups of actors during this phase were:

- Clinicians: Nurses and Physicians (members of the EHR working group)
- Secretaries (members of the EHR working group)
- IT-professionals (members of the EHR working group)
- The EHR project management
- The executive board
- The vendors

For phase 1c (The technology-carrier analysis) some of these groups of actors were combined, resulting in the following three groups:

- Clinicians (nurses, physicians and secretaries)
- It-professionals (the it-professionals at NDR and the vendors)
- Administrators (the EHR project management and the executive board)

Data Collection

Data were collected through observations at the EHR working group meetings, interviews and insight gathered from documents.

Data Analysis

Empirical data were analysed using the software programme ATLAS (Muhr, 2004) with a focus on the six conditions to be a social carrier of EHR (interest, power, organization, information, access and knowledge) – and an “open mind” towards other themes.

Phase 3 (Development) in the Constructive eHealth Evaluation Method Used in NDR

The Constructive eHealth evaluation method was applied during this phase in a single case study aiming at evaluating the development and implementation of a pre-prototype - and the further development of this into a prototype based on the gained experiences - of the new EHR system for NDR. Evaluators from DaCHI conducted the evaluation during this phase. The evaluation took place at one hospital ward from June 2008 to January 2010 (A. M. Høstgaard, 2010).

Design

The design was a single case study with the participation of The Infectious Diseases ward at Aalborg Hospital, Aalborg, Denmark

The relevant groups of actors during this phase were:

- Clinicians: Nurses, Physicians and other clinical staff at the ward (members of the EHR working group at ward level)
- Secretaries (members of the EHR working group at ward level)
- The EHR project management
- The executive board
- The vendor

Data Collection

Data were collected through questionnaires, interviews (personal and focus-group), and personal observations and insight into documents

Data Analysis

Empirical data were analysed using the software programme ATLAS (Muhr, 2004)

Phase 4 (Implementation and Diffusion) in the Constructive eHealth Evaluation Method Used in NDR

Evaluators from DaCHI conducted the evaluation during this phase. The Constructive eHealth evaluation method was applied during this phase in a multiple case study with the objective of evaluating the implementation of the prototype of the new EHR system for NDR resulting from phase 3 in more different clinical contexts. The evaluation took place at different locations at four hospitals in NDR from January 2010 to December 2010 (A. M. Høstgaard, Bertelsen, & Nøhr, 2010a).

Design

The design was a multiple case study with the participation of the following wards:

Case 1: The Gynaecological /Obstetrical Department at Aalborg Hospital, Aalborg, Denmark
Case 2: The Orthopaedic, Surgery Department at Vendsyssel Hospital, Frederikshavn, Denmark
Case 3: The Medical department at Himmerland Hospital, Hobro, Denmark
Case 4: The Medical department at Himmerland Hospital, Farsø, Denmark
Case 5: The emergency room at Aalborg Hospital, Aalborg, Denmark

The relevant groups of actors during this phase were:

- Clinicians: Nurses, Physicians and other clinical staff at the wards (members of the EHR working group at ward level)
- Secretaries (members of the EHR working group at ward level)
- The EHR project management
- The executive board
- The vendor (CSC)

Data Collection

Data were collected through questionnaires, interviews (personal and focus-group), video- and personal observations and insight into documents for all five cases (A. M. Høstgaard, 2009; A. M. Høstgaard, 2010; A. M. Høstgaard, Bertelsen, & Nøhr, 2010a)

Data Analysis

Empirical data were analysed using the software programme ATLAS (Muhr, 2004)

Trustworthiness: All Phases

Trustworthiness was sought through data triangulation, approval of the transcripts by the interviewed persons and a thoroughly description of all activities throughout the process (transparency).

Results of the Constructive eHealth Evaluation in NDR

Below the results of the evaluation in the different phases during the EHR development in NDR will be provided. The EHR development process in NDR will be referred to as the "NDR case".

Pre Analysis

The first step in any eHealth evaluation is to answer the question: What is the problem? The answer to this question is given through the answers to the sub-questions below:

1. *What* is going to be evaluated (the aspects or focus for the evaluation)?
    a. *Answer:* The specific eHealth technology, which was the focus for the evaluation in question, was a future electronic health record (EHR) for NDR in Denmark.
2. Why should the evaluation take place (objective)?
    a. *Answer*: The objective of the evaluation was twofold:
        - To provide feedback between the end-users and the management on experiences and learning during the development process
        - To assess the clinical benefits of the EHR based on the clinicians' assessments
3. When in the eHealth lifecycle is the evaluation going to take place (phase)?
    a. *Answer:* The evaluation was carried through during the research-, design-, development- and the first part of the implementation phases and took place from 2004 until 2010.
4. Who are the relevant actors involved and whose perspective is to be followed (perspective)?
    a. *Answer:* A local EHR working group of physicians, nurses and secretaries, members of the EHR project management and the executive board, IT-professionals and the vendor were involved in the evaluation in phase 1 and 2. In phase 3 and 4, also local working groups of physicians, nurses and secretaries from the respective wards involved were included in the evaluation. The perspective was on the clinician's during all phases, as one of the main objectives was to assess the clinical benefits of the EHR based on the clinicians' assessments
5. How are the results to be used?
    a. *Answer:* The results of the evaluation were used in different ways according to the objectives:
        - As an important part of the learning process, the results from the formative evaluation should inform the on-going process through continuously feedback during all phases in the technological lifecycle, thereby making it possibly to change direction during the process if necessary. The feedback should be provided both through direct contact between the evaluator and the management (e.g. telephone or mail contact) for results important to pass on

quickly, and through sub-reports and presentations at meetings at all levels during the process.

- The results of the assessments of clinical benefits were provided in a final report at the end of the evaluation.

Phase 1: Research and Planning Phase and Phase 2a): Design Phase (Identifying Needs)

1a) Identification of relevant groups of actors and 1b) selection of representatives for the identified groups:

In the NDR case, an EHR working group was set up in March 2004 by the executive board to prepare requirement specifications and to choose between four different EHR systems. The members of the working group included physicians, nurses, secretaries and IT-professionals. No partner analysis or other participatory methods were used to identify and assemble the relevant groups of actors to participate in the working group. On the contrary, the executive board "handpicked" the members by choosing participants known from previous projects. Half way through phase1, this approach resulted in protests from physicians at ward level, because they found that their interests were not accommodated in the working group. Because of the critique, the executive board in collaboration with the EHR project management decided to expand the group with six more physicians. This time, a more democratic way to select members was used, as the professional association representing the physicians in NDR was asked to identify the six members, who were going to represent them in the working group. However, the fact that only two out of eight physicians in the EHR working group were members from the start, while the six newcomers joined the group, when the process had been going on for 18 months, made it impossibly for the newcomers to acquire the necessary knowledge to make informed decisions. As a consequence, the decisions made through this phase were taken primarily on the basis of advice from the it-professionals in the group; hence the physicians in the working group did not feel any ownership to the decisions taken (A. M. Høstgaard, 2009).

The – predominantly informal – planning strategy for the EHR planning process meant that there was no clinical workload reduction at all during the process, i.e. the full technologic lifecycle. Physicians were expected to handle their full-time clinical duties while, at the same time, participating in the planning process. As a result, seven out of the eight physicians in the working group were senior physicians from Aalborg Hospital (the largest hospital in NDR), whose work was characterized by the fact that they had more administrative- than clinical tasks. This meant that they could plan their daily work more flexible than younger colleagues, hence they had better possibilities to participate in meetings during day-time and to read the vast number of ICT- technical papers and reports that they were expected to gain insight into. Only one younger physician at ward level – and from a hospital outside Aalborg – joined the group. He participated in two meetings, whereupon he left the group due to a lack of time. It meant that junior physicians (more than half of the physicians in NDR) and physicians from hospitals outside Aalborg were not represented in the EHR working group at all (A. M. Høstgaard, 2009)

During the planning phase, the EHR-project management made no attempts to learn from the experiences from EHR planning-processes in the other Danish counties/regions – including experiences on the need for workload reductions in one form or another. The EHR-project management's main argument for not allowing workload reduction (paid by the county/region) was a general principle about leaving decisions about workload reduction to the individual hospitals in the county/region. From the executive boards point of view, the local hospital's incentive to pay for workload reduction was the fact that the individual hospitals were allowed to keep any rationalization gains from the EHR implementation process. This principle meant that the responsibility for prioritizing costs for workload reduction, e.g. within treatment and care, was moved from county-level to hospital-level. Based on experiences regarding the prerequisites for a successful implementation of EHR, a decision like this should be made at regional level to ensure the best possible implementation across regions (A. M. Høstgaard, 2009).

1c) Technology-carrier analysis and 2a) Identifying needs:

The results of the evaluation of phase 1c) will be presented together with the results of the evaluation of phase 2a) because in the NDR-case, the technology- carrier analysis, during which the interactions between the different relevant actor groups were studied, was performed while at the same time evaluating phase 2a): the process of "identifying needs". Thus, the technology-carrier analysis was not carried through during phase 1 - i.e. *before* identifying needs for the new eHealth technology - which it should according to the Constructive eHealth evaluation method. This issue will be dealt with in the Solutions and recommendations / Discussion section. Besides, phase 2b (requirement specifications) occasionally overlap with phase 1c) and 2a).

Three main actor/technology-carrier groups were identified for the technology-carrier analysis: clinicians (with a focus on physicians), it-professionals and administrators (the project management and the executive board).

Interest

The three technology-carrier groups had different interests in the implementation of the EHR. The physicians' main interest was to ensure positive clinical benefits. Hence, the physicians found it crucial that it was physicians, who formulated the clinical requirements for the requirement specification. The IT-professionals' main interests were concerned with optimizing administrative functions in the EHR, while the administrators had a major interest in complying with the national requirements about implementing EHR in all Danish counties.

A new way of conducting the planning process was used in the NDR case: *The Competitive Dialogue Process* (CDP). This method facilitated dialogue between the members of the working group and the four vendors, who participated in the bidding round, and it made it possible for each of the vendors to further develop different functionalities during the process based on the feedback from members in the working group. The physicians felt that by using this method, they were enabled to gain insight into more - including technical - functionalities of the systems and to better argue for their clinical requirements and interests in the EHR. However, the physicians did not have sufficient time (because of no workload reduction) to go through all documents related to the process. Neither did they have the time to participate in all meetings in the EHR working group or meetings and workshops in the sub-groups established in relation to the process. As a consequence, IT-professionals with past clinical background (non-physicians) developed most of the clinical requirements for the requirement specifications. This implies, according to Kensing et al., Brandt and Simonsen et al., a great risk; namely that the clinical requirements do not reflect clinical practice, because experience shows that professional knowledge has to be presented by professionals (Brandt E., 2006; Kensing F. & Blomberg J., 1998; Simonsen J. & Hertzum J., 2008). At the same time, it implies a great risk that the physicians' interests were not, or only partially, met during the process (A. M. Høstgaard, 2009).

All four EHR systems were at a very early stage of development at the time for phase 2a) (identifying needs). None of them were in operation in any hospital ward - they only existed as schematic diagrams and early prototypes. This fact taken together with the fact that all the vendors further developed and changed functionalities important to clinical work practices (e.g. configuration of the user interface, the number of mouse clicks and integration with other systems) during this phase, resulted in the four systems becoming almost alike. Therefore, clinical functionalities had to be abandoned as criteria for the selection of an EHR system at the time for finally choosing among the systems. Thus, only technical functionalities were used as a basis for choosing between the systems. Thus, the physicians made their choice according to feelings, sensations and advice from the IT-professionals, according to their own words. That is, the final choice of EHR system was primarily made on the basis of the interests of the IT-professionals and the administrators, namely according to technical and economic criteria (A. M. Høstgaard, 2009).

Power and Organization

The Danish Medical Association was not involved in the EHR development process in any way. The organizational support and encouragement that the physicians in the working group achieved during the process was from colleagues in the different professional associations at Aalborg Hospital.

Compared to the physicians, the IT-professionals had a much stronger organizational support and thereby more power. The fact that the head of their professional organization was a member of the project management, and that most of the documents prepared during the EHR process were prepared by members of their organization, gave them a significant amount of power.

The physicians and the IT-professionals used the power associated with professional knowledge to accommodate their own respective interests. However, the physicians' clinical knowledge turned out to be inadequate as a basis for choosing between systems. Technical knowledge was essential. The administrators had the power to make final decisions – which they did, when they ordered all physicians to choose one of the four systems, despite the physicians' request to wait until more detailed information - and the possibility to access the systems - was available. In fact, the physicians were powerless when it came to the possibility of exerting real influence on choosing between systems (A. M. Høstgaard, 2009).

Access

The four systems possible to choose among, were not in operation at any hospital ward, therefore, it was not possible to test them in a "real live setting". This was critical, especially to the physicians as they at the beginning of the process were asked to specifically concentrate on functionalities important to clinical work practices, (e.g. configuration of the user interface, the number of mouse clicks and integration with other systems). Recognizing this problem, the physicians were offered to test prototypes of the different systems. None of the physicians were able to participate in *all* four tests because of clinical duties (no workload reduction), which meant that they were unable to compare the four systems. Thus, the tests did not provide them a basis for choosing between the systems. The fact that the four EHR systems could not be tested in a real live setting meant that clinical knowledge was not enough to chose between the systems. Technical knowledge became essential (A. M. Høstgaard, 2009).

Information

The members of the working group, who were involved from the start, were invited to different arrangements to prepare them for the different tasks they were asked to perform. The six physicians, who joined the working group 18 months after it was set up, did not receive any kind of introduction or update on the work conducted so far - or any other kind of preparation for the task. This fact, together with the fact that clinical workload reduction was not possible – meaning that the physicians had their full-time clinical work beside the work in the EHR-working group, made it impossible for the six new-comers to obtain the level of information necessary to exert real influence in decision-making (A. M. Høstgaard, 2009).

Knowledge

Because the four systems became almost alike with respect to functionalities related to clinical work practices, these were given up as criteria for the selection of an EHR system. This meant that clinical knowledge became inadequate as a basis for choosing between systems – technical knowledge was essential. Only one of the eight physicians had the necessary amount of technical knowledge to really participate in the - often very technical - debates in the working group. The old saying: "knowledge is power" thus proved to be very true. The reality was: the more technical knowledge – the more power. The lack of technical knowledge made the physicians incapable of exerting real influence on several important decisions made during the process – e.g. the final choice of EHR system (A. M. Høstgaard, 2009).

Synthesis of the Six Aspects in the Technology Carrier Analysis

When the results of the six aspects in the technology carrier analysis are synthesized, it shows that the absence of workload reduction was the main barrier for the physicians to achieve real involvement in the process, and that it affected all six conditions – interest, power, organization, information, access and knowledge – required to obtain the status of an actual social carriers of the EHR. Thus, the results of the evaluation of phase 1c and 2a showed that the physician's role during these phases was reduced to informing about physicians' needs to the requirement specifications and other documents because of lack of time. Hence, their role was reduced to clinical consultants, rather than real participants (A. M. Høstgaard, 2009).

Phase 2: Design Phase

2a) Identifying Needs

As mentioned above, the results of the evaluation of the needs analysis in the NDR case are described in the section above.

2b) Requirement Specifications

In the NDR case, it was decided to use a new way of conducting a tender process: The Competitive Dialogue Process (CDP) (fig.3), (Falch & Jensen, 2005). In NDR the CDP comprised: a) *the prequalification phase*: The EHR project management (the provider) prepared a tender notice inviting vendors to apply for the development of a new EHR for NDR. Among the applying vendors, the EHR project management -

based on criteria's decided on beforehand - choose four vendors for further dialogue. b) *The dialogue phase*: Based on experiences and knowledge from both existing technologies and work practices in NDR and other regions (provided through phase 2a), the EHR project management in cooperation with the working group prepared a document describing the provisional requirement specifications. This document constituted the basis for the initial dialogue between the working group and the four respective vendors – one at a time. c) *The quotation phase*: Next, the vendors were asked to present provisional solutions/quotations for the new EHR. These were based on the knowledge gained during the initial dialogue. The provisional solutions/quotations constituted the basis for further dialogue between the vendors and members of the working group. During this dialogue with one vendor at a time, the members of the working group gained further knowledge and insight into the possibilities for e.g. new functionalities. The dialogue process continued until the members of the working group had gained the amount of knowledge necessary to work out the final requirement specifications. d) *The decision phase*: Based on the final requirement specifications, the vendors forwarded their final quotation, and - based on certain criteria's – one vendor was chosen to develop the new EHR for NDR.

The greatest advantage of the CDP was that it provided each single member of the working group a deeper insight on – for most members in this group - unknown technological subjects by dialogue with the different vendors. Technological knowledge was– as was shown by the results of the technology carrier analysis (phase 1c) –a precondition for gaining influence on decision-making in the NDR case. The disadvantage was that many resources (time- and personnel wise) were required to organize the process. However, both the members of the working group, the EHR management and the executive board in the NDR case had a very positive attitude to the CDP and have recommended the EU to allow the use of the CDP in a broader context and not only for complex projects (Falch & Jensen, 2005). Having fulfilled its task, the EHR working group was dissolved at the end of this phase.

Phase 3: Development Phase

In the NDR case, the EHR project management sat up a working group at the Infectious disease ward in collaboration with the ward-management and the staff at the ward. This working group in close collaboration with the vendor conducted the various tasks in the development phase: Initially, they designed parts of the new EHR (e.g. the user-interface) using different games and muck-ups during a series of meetings, until all persons involved could approve the results. This approach resulted in a strong sense of ownership to the different decisions and solutions taken during this phase among the actors involved. Based on the results of this process, the vendor developed a pre-prototype of the EHR, which was implemented and pre-pilot tested at the Infectious disease ward. This test went on for several months, during which the pre-prototype was redesigned several times based on feedback from the end-users. The pre-prototype was finally developed into a proto-type of the EHR aimed at being prototype tested at four different wards during the next phase (implementation and diffusion phase).

During phase 3, the evaluators from DaCHI facilitated feedback between the different actor groups. The feedback was provided in a number of different ways: by personal contacts, through a number of meetings arranged by DaCHI between the different groups of actors and through more reports to the EHR project management and the executive board. The feedback delivered from end-users to management during this phase resulted in management deciding that the system was not yet sufficiently technically mature to be implemented on a wider basis. Thus, the feedback was of great importance for the forthcoming process, as it made management change the originally planned directions and implement a number of technical adjustments before proceeding to the next phase, phase 4 (A. M. Høstgaard, 2010).

Phase 4: Implementation and Diffusion Phase

In the NDR case, the EHR management in collaboration with the management and the staff at four different wards set up working groups at the respective wards to conduct the testing of the prototype developed during phase 3. The prototype was implemented at the four wards, thus it was tested in four different clinical contexts and adjusted according to the feedback provided from the four working groups to either the evaluators or directly to the EHR management.

During this phase, the evaluators from DaCHI provided feedback to the project management on a number of occasions, where either the system or some organizational aspects did not perform as presumed. A few examples are given in the following: a) At the Gynaecological ward, we found that the EHR project management had failed to include the Midwifes when setting up the working group at ward level. The most important work document for the midwifes was the so-called "Partogram" which is a graphical record of key data recorded during labour. Because of the midwifes not being part of the working group from the start, this record was initially not part of the EHR, which meant that the EHR did not provide any clinical benefits for this professional group. Because of the feedback to the project management at an early time in this phase, the Midwifes were included in the working group, and the EHR was expanded to include the Partogram. b) At the Emergency ward we encountered complains of a too long upstart time of the new EHR system in the different emergency rooms, resulting in the system not being used. It turned out that a certain procedure beforehand handled by the night duty staff, here re-starting all the computers during night shifts, had been closed down by mistake, when reorganizing work procedures.

This meant that when the staff entered the emergency room with patients in the morning, they had to wait for the computers to start up in order to enter the EHR. This was very time consuming and as a consequence, they did not use the system. When this was reported to the project management, the former work procedure was reintroduced, and the problem was solved c) A pocket size EHR system guide was available for all staff. However, only a few found them useful. At one of the wards, staff members had encountered a number of errors in the guide and therefore, they had lost fait in using it to solve problems. The feedback on this resulted in the guide being checked and reintroduced.

On these occasions, and all others encountered, we provided feedback between all relevant actors, thereby preventing a number of problems to occur later on in the process. During this phase we - the evaluators - had regularly meetings with the EHR project management, on which occasions we provided feedback on our observations. Our final recommendation based on observations and interviews with the end-users, was to await full implantation/diffusion until certain functionalities were better able to meet the end-users needs. NDR did adjust these functionalities and did wait another year before implementing the system to all hospital wards in the region, thereby presumably preventing a number of problems later on in the process (A. M. Høstgaard, Bertelsen, & Nøhr, 2010a).

Phase 5: Summative Evaluation and Reporting Phase

The final outcome evaluation had not yet been conducted in the NDR case, as phase 4 is still not fully completed.

SOLUTIONS AND RECOMMENDATIONS: DISCUSSION

Strengths and Limitations of the Constructive eHealth Evaluation Method Compared to other Approaches

The Constructive eHealth evaluation method has been developed to support *end-user involvement* during the *entire eHealth lifecycle*, i.e. for the *healthcare sector* specifically. No other full lifecycle frameworks for eHealth evaluation specifically, and with a specific focus on end-user involvement, have been developed before to the knowledge of this author.

Other approaches for supporting and improving end-user participation in information technology development have been proposed. However, they have not been full lifecycle frameworks, but have rather been developed with a focus on the design phase and for other organizations than the healthcare sector. The "*MUST method*" is a method for participatory design developed by Danish researchers in the 1990s (MUST is an acronym for theories of and methods for initial analysis and design activities). This method has been developed through the authors' participation in a number of projects within a range of different organizations, e.g. film companies, R/D-lab, radio-station – except for the healthcare sector. It is intended for supporting IT professionals responsible for the design phase in IT development (Bødker K., Kensing F., & Simonsen J., 2004; Kensing F., Simonsen J., & Bødker K., 1996) in contrast to the Constructive eHealth evaluation method, which is meant for eHealth management at all levels.

Full lifecycle frameworks for eHealth evaluation have been proposed by Catwell and Sheikh, Clarke et al. and van Gemert-Pijnen. However, the focus in these formative eHealth evaluation frameworks has not been on end-user involvement specifically, but on improving eHealth systems development and/or implementation by identifying and providing feedback between all groups involved on problems as they emerge (Catwell & Sheikh, 2009; Clarke et al., 1994; van Gemert-Pijnen et al., 2011). Besides, in contrast to the Constructive eHealth evaluation method, these methods do not provide any tools to guide the planning and the execution processes during the different phases in eHealth development. Finally, they do not support evaluation as an independent activity, which takes place parallel to other project activities in contrast to the Constructive eHealth evaluation method. The importance of this aspect is emphasized by both Nykänen et al. (Nykänen et al., 2011) and by this author. As mentioned earlier in this chapter, experiences from DaCHI's empirical work have clearly demonstrated the need to keep the responsibility for the evaluation separated from the responsibility for other project activities, as conflicts of interest may occur.

Also Kaufman et al. have suggested a full lifecycle evaluation framework for eHealth. Kaufman operates with a five stages system development model. The framework is a further development of an evaluation framework developed by Stead et al. in 1994(Stead, 1994). The objective is to present an evaluation framework that provides a heuristic for matching the stage of system design and the level of evaluation (Kaufman, Roberts, Merrill, Lai, & Bakken, 2006). The framework provides suggestions for data collection methods used in each of five stages (system specification, component development, integration of components into system, integration of system into a clinical setting and routine use of a system) based on the evaluation objective in each phase, and it claims to have a usercentered approach to design. However, its main objective is different from the objective of The Constructive eHealth evaluation method, as it is not to support end-user involvement during all phases in the full eHealth lifecycle. It is to provide coherence and structure to research in health informatics through rigorous evaluation in each stage in the lifecycle (Kaufman, Roberts, Merrill, Lai, & Bakken, 2006).

Constructive eHealth Evaluation

The Constructive eHealth evaluation method also offers a solution to a major problem in traditional (positivistic) evaluation besides offering a full lifecycle eHealth evaluation frameworks which supports end-user involvement during the entire eHealth lifecycle, tools to guide the process and support to evaluation as an independent activity separated from other project activities. This is the fact that evaluation in traditional evaluation is seen as scientific testing, which presuppose a number of preconditions (e.g. a fixed set of goals, stable outcomes, no intervening variables). However, these preconditions are rarely fulfilled in eHealth projects, which on the contrary are most often characterized by numerous goals, unstable outcomes and various intervening variables. According to Greenhalgh and Russell the scientific approach to eHealth evaluation might explain, why these often fail to deliver the insights expected. The authors offer an alternative approach, based on ten alternative principles for eHealth evaluation. These principle are: 1) think about your own role in the evaluation, 2) put in place a governance process, 3) provide the interpersonal and analytic space for effective dialogue, 4) take an emergent approach, 5) consider the dynamic macro level context in which the eHealth innovation is being introduced, 6) consider the different meso-level contexts 7) consider the individuals through whom the eHealth innovation will be adopted, deployed, and used, 8) consider the eHealth technologies, the expectations and constraints inscribed in them, 9) use narratives as an analytic tool and to synthesise findings, 10) consider critical events in relation to the evaluation itself. The principles are deliberately presented in an abstract and generalized way as the authors call for critique and refining by other researchers (Greenhalgh & Russell, 2010). The formative part (the first four phases) of The Constructive eHealth evaluation method is in fact build upon the same principles as Greenhalgh and Russell suggest. Besides, The Constructive eHealth evaluation method offers an actual framework for how to convert the principles into practice. Phase 5 in the Constructive eHealth evaluation method is a summative evaluation, which is often equated with scientific testing. However, in The Constructive eHealth evaluation method, the goals or outcomes are not fixed from the project start. On the contrary, they are adapted during the development process in response to experiences and feedback from the end-users and relevant actor groups in recognition of the fact that the preconditions for traditional summative evaluation can rarely be met when it comes to eHealth projects.

In line with Greenhalgh and Russell's considerations mentioned above, Cresswell, Bates and Sheikh also suggest ten important considerations for eHealth implementations to succeed. However, a fulcrum for their considerations is the importance of having focus on end-users during the entire development process. Thus, according to these authors the involvement of clinicians (end-users) in decision-making is essential in order to ensure co-ownership and commitment. The authors also stress the importance of ensuring that eHealth systems provide clinical benefits for the end-users. This is best achieved by including end-users also in high-level strategic groups and through formative evaluation methods. Thus, the authors strongly advocate a lifecycle perspective on eHealth development. According to the authors: " Real-time, longitudinal data collection strategies providing formative feedback are desirable as emerging results can be incorporated in on-going implementation activity, but this is costly and time-consuming. However, it is essential to capture user feedback about problems that are identified and respond to it in a timely manner. In our experience, investments in evaluation activities are always worth it " (Cresswell, Bates, & Sheikh, 2013)p.13. This view on eHealth evaluation is fully in line with the principles in the Constructive eHealth evaluation method. Also, the key recommendations stressing that focus must be on involving end-users is in parallel with the focus in the Constructive eHealth evaluation method.

In a recent publication, also van Gemert-Pijnen et al. points to the lack of engaging the end-users in eHealth development as a major cause of many eHealth technologies not being successful. According to the authors, this explains e.g. the incidence of usability problems, which will eventually lead to that users will simply stop using the technology, because it does not correspond with the clinical work practice (van Gemert-Pijnen et al., 2011). Thus, with a focus on end-user involvement during the full eHealth lifecycle, the Constructive eHealth evaluation method fills a knowledge gap in the current knowledge on how to best ensure successful eHealth development and implementation.

Strengths and Limitations of the Constructive eHealth Evaluation Method Used in the NDR Case

The research- and evaluation-studies, through which the Constructive eHealth evaluation method was developed, were qualitative studies using triangulation of different data collecting methods to validate the data. In qualitative studies there is a risk that the researcher has a predetermined opinion on the subject in question. There is also the risk that the researcher is "seduced" by the position taken by one group. This could be a risk in phase 1 (The research- and planning phase) and 2 (The design phase) especially, because this author had a close relation to the members of the working group for a longer period. To account for this, all activities throughout the process were thoroughly described (transparency). The fact that this author has participated throughout the planning process in all meetings and have had access to most documents – electronic as well as paper-based – has made it possible to validate interview data on e.g., time pressure and the amount of documents related to the process.

According to the framework for the Constructive eHealth evaluation method, the technology carrier analysis is to be carried through as a part of phase 1. That is, *before* identifying needs for the new eHealth technology (phase 2a). However, in the NDR case, the technology-carrier analysis was carried through during phase 2a, which means that it was carried through while the actors were identifying needs. The reason for this is the fact that phase 1 and 2 were part of a Ph.d. study with a focus on the interactions between the different actor groups involved during the process of identifying needs. However, the experience gained from this study together with experiences from former studies (A. M. Høstgaard, Bertelsen, & Nøhr, 2010b; Nøhr, Høstgaard, Botin, & Kjær-Andersen, 2004; Nøhr & Høstgaard, 2011)provided a solid basis for recommending the analysis to take place in phase 1: A number of the conflicts and problems seen in phase 2a (the identifying needs phase) in the NDR case could undoubtedly have been prevented, if informations on the conditions for the end-users to exert real influence on decision-making had been present. With this information management would have had a possibility to provide support to the end-users and to facilitate real end-user involvement. Thus, it is recommended that the technology carrier analysis be carried through in the first phase to provide information on the technology-carrier status of the end-users, as this is a good marker for their possibility for *real* involvement in decision-making in the forthcoming phases.

The Constructive eHealth evaluation method was further developed and tested through a research study in a major Danish healthcare organization. However, research show that the interactions found between the different actor groups in the NDR case are not a specific Danish phenomena, as they can be found in eHealth development in general (Berg M. & Winthereik B.R., 2004). Thus, the method will also provide eHealth management in a broader context a frame for achieving valuable information and learning during eHealth development, hence the opportunity to change direction during the process, if needed.

The Constructive eHealth evaluation method provides an evaluation method as an independent activity, which takes place in parallel to the overall project activities. This means in practice that the evaluator/evaluators cannot be identical to the project manager/project management, as conflicts of interests can occur. Examples are given in the section on " The Implementation and diffusion phase" when the method was used in NDR. More of the examples presented were directly associated to the tasks of the project management. They would possibly not have been openly presented, if the evaluation activity had been an intrinsic part of the overall project activities – rather than being a parallel and independent activity. Hence, no learning to avoid the same events to occur in the future would have taken place. Of course, a close collaboration between project management and the evaluation team is a necessity. Hence, it is important that the feedback from evaluators on events identified during the different phases in eHealth development is not considered a critique by project management, but a possibility for constructive learning. Previously in this chapter, the understanding of this is mentioned as one of the preconditions for obtaining benefits from using the method.

The most important limitation for using the Constructive eHealth evaluation method is that summative evaluation methods are traditionally preferred because of both time- and economic causes. However, as the benefits of using formative evaluation methods – also in the healthcare sector –are recognized in a wider context, this limitation is hopefully diminished. Another limitation is that upper management, as well as management at all other levels in healthcare organizations, must recognize end-user participation as a crucial success factor in eHealth development, hence for achieving the key objectives in healthcare. This implies that management at different levels must accept that their right to manage is reduced because using the method implies that end-users have a real say in decision-making.

CONCLUSION

Real end-user participation is essential for the successful outcome of eHealth development - and thus for fulfilling the key objectives for healthcare. The Constructive eHealth evaluation method presented in this chapter is a new method aiming at supporting *real* end-user participation – and thus for improving the adoption of eHealth in healthcare environments – by providing an analytical framework for achieving real end-user participation during all phases in the technological lifecycle in eHealth development. The framework offers specific methods for achieving this in each single phase in the technological lifecycle and, not least of all, on how to apply these in practice. Also, the method offers an eHealth evaluation method as an independent activity.

The Constructive eHealth evaluation method has proven effective for providing learning and feedback between end-users and management in a major region in Denmark. It has provided management at more levels on-going information and feedback from end-users allowing them to change directions during the eHealth development process, thereby supporting a successful the adoption of eHealth in the healthcare sector. However, studies show that the findings from the Danish region do not differ significantly from findings in more other countries. Therefore, the method presented in this chapter can hopefully be useful in a broader context as a frame for achieving valuable information and learning during eHealth development and thereby for supporting successful eHealth development while building on one of the most well-known success factors: the involvement of end-users in the eHealth development process.

REFERENCES

Arnstein, S. R. (2007). A ladder of citizen participation. *Journal of the American Institute of Planners, 35*(4), 216–224. doi:10.1080/01944366908977225

Ash, J., Stavre, Z., & Kuperman, G. J. (2003). A consensus statement on considerations for a successful CPOE implementation. *Journal of the American Medical Informatics Association, 10*(3), 229–234. doi:10.1197/jamia.M1204 PMID:12626376

Avison, D. E., & Fitzgerald, G. (1995). Effective technical and human implementation of computer-based system (ETHICS). In Information system development: Methodologies, techniques and tools (pp. 353-364). Berkshire, UK: The McGraw-Hill Companies.

Berg, M. (2001). Implementing information systems in health care organizations: Myths and challenges. *International Journal of Medical Informatics, 64*(2-3), 143–156. doi:10.1016/S1386-5056(01)00200-3 PMID:11734382

Berg, M., & Winthereik, B. R. (2004). Waiting for godot, episodes from the history of patient records. In M. Berg (Ed.), *Health information management: Integrating information technology in health care work* (pp. 11–44). London: Routledge.

Bijker, W. E. (2009). How is technology made?—That is the question! *Cambridge Journal of Economics, 34*(1), 63–76. doi:10.1093/cje/bep068

Black A.D., Car J., Pagliary C., Anadan C., Cresswell K., Bokun T., et al. (2011). The impact of eHealth on the quality and safety of health care: A systematic overview. *Public Library of Science (PLOS) in Medicine, 8*(1).

Bødker, K., Kensing, F., & Simonsen, J. (2004). *Participatory IT design. designing for business and workplace realities*. MIT Press.

Brandt, E. (2006). Designing exploratory design games: A framework for participation in participatory design? *Proceedings Participatory Design Conference.*

Brender, J. (2006). Handbook of evaluation methods for health informatics. Burlington, MA: Academic Press; doi:10.1145/1147261.1147271

Catwell, L., & Sheikh, A. (2009). Evaluating eHealth interventions: The need for continuous systemic evaluation. *PLoS Medicine, 6*(8), 1–6. doi:10.1371/journal.pmed.1000126 PMID:19688038

Clarke, K., O'Moore, R., Smeets, R., Talmon, J., Brender, J., & McNair, P. et al. (1994). A methodology for evaluation of knowledge-based systems in medicine. *Artificial Intelligence in Medicine*, *6*(2), 107–121. doi:10.1016/0933-3657(94)90040-X PMID:8049752

Cresswell, K., Bates, D. W., & Sheikh, A. (2013). Ten key considerations for the successful implementation and adoption of largescale health information technology. *Journal of the American Medical Informatics Association*, *20*(e1), 9–13. doi:10.1136/amiajnl-2013-001684 PMID:23599226

Edmondson, A. C. (2003). Framing for learning: Lessons in successfull technology implementation. *California Management Review*, *45*(2), 34–51. doi:10.2307/41166164

Edquist, C., & Edquist, O. (1979). Social carriers of techniques for development. *Journal of Peace Research*, *16*(4), 313–331. doi:10.1177/002234337901600403

Falch, A. M., & Jensen, F. (2005). *Erfaringer med udbudsformen "konkurrencepræget dialog" (the competitive dialogue process).* Unpublished manuscript.

Høstgaard, A. M. (2009). *Fryder forandring? casestudie af EPJ udbudsprocessen i region nord - belyst gennem en procesevaluering med fokus på lægerne som sociale bærere af den elektroniske patientjournal, EPJ* [change is the spice of life? process analysis case study of a region in Denmark]. (PhD Thesis). Aalborg Universitet.

Høstgaard, A. M. (2010). *Evaluering af præpilottest af "klinisk proces" på infektionsmedicinsk afd. aalborg sygehus syd* [evaluation of the pre-pilottest of "clinical process" at the department of infectious diseases]. Unpublished manuscript.

Høstgaard, A. M. (2012). End-user participation in health IT development: The EUPHIT method. In S. A. Zakariya Belkhamza (Ed.), *Measuring organizational information systems success: New technologies and practices* (pp. 318–340). Hershey, USA: IGI Global. doi:10.4018/978-1-4666-0170-3.ch016

Høstgaard, A. M., Bertelsen, P., & Nøhr, C. (2010a). Evaluering af pilottest af klinisk proces "vieweren" [evaluation of the 'Clinical process' electronic health record (EHR) – evaluation report]. Aalborg University.

Høstgaard, A. M., Bertelsen, P., & Nøhr, C. (2010b). How are clinicians involved in EHR planning?: A process analysis case study of a region in denmark. In C. Safran, S. Reti, & H.F. Marin (Eds.), *MEDINFO 2010: Proceedings of the 13th world congress on medical informatics* (pp. 121-125) IOS Press.

Høstgaard, A. M., Bertelsen, P., & Nøhr, C. (2011). Methods to identify, study and understand end-user involvement in HIT-development. *BioMedCentral: Medical Information and Decision Making, 11*(57).

Høstgaard, A. M., Bertelsen, P., Petersen, L. S., & Nøhr, C. (2013). *Constructive technology assessment for HIT development: Learning, feedback and user involvement.* Unpublished manuscript.

Høstgaard, A. M., & Nøhr, C. (2004a). Dealing with organizational change when implementing EHR systems. In *Medinfo 2004: Proceedings of the 11th World Congress on Medical Informatics.*

Høstgaard, A. M., & Nøhr, C. (2004b). *Metodehaandbog i forandringsparathed i forbindelse med udvikling og implementering af nye it-systemer indenfor sundhedsvæsnet [handbook in methods for change readiness in development and implementation of new IT-systems in healthcare].* Aalborg: Virtual Centre for Health Informatics.

Johnson, C. W. (2006). Why did that happen? exploring the proliferation of barely usable software in healthcare systems. *Quality & Safety in Health Care, 15*(supplement 1), i76–i81. doi:10.1136/qshc.2005.016105 PMID:17142614

Kaipio, J. (2011). *Usability in healthcare: Overcoming the mismatch between information systems and clinical work.* Aalto University, School of Science, Department of Computer Science and Engineering.

Kanstrup, A. M., & Bertelsen, P. (2011). *User innovation management.* Aalborg: Aalborg University Press.

Kanstrup, A. M., & Bertelsen, P. (2006). Participatory IT-support. *Participatory Design Conference*, pp. 87-94.

Kaplan, B., & Harris-Salamone, K. (2009). Health IT success and failure: Recommendations from literature and an AMIA workshop. *Journal of the American Medical Informatics Association, 16*(3), 291–299. doi:10.1197/jamia.M2997 PMID:19261935

Kaufman, D., Roberts, W. D., Merrill, J., Lai, T. Y., & Bakken, S. (2006). Applying an evaluation framework for health information system design, development, and implementation. *Nursing Research, 55*(2Suppl), S37–S42. doi:10.1097/00006199-200603001-00007 PMID:16601633

Kaye, R., Kokia, E., Shalev, V., Idar, D., & Chinitz, D. (2010). Barriers and success factors in health information technology: A practitioner's perspective. *Journal of Management & Marketing in Healthcare, 3*(2), 163–175. doi:10.1179/17533031 0X12736577732764

Kensing, F., & Blomberg, J. (1998). Participatory design; issues and concerns. *Computer Supported Cooperative Work*, *7*(3-4), 167–185. doi:10.1023/A:1008689307411

Kensing, F., Simonsen, J., & Bødker, K. (1996). MUST - a method for participatory design. *The Fourth Biennial Conference on Participatory Design.*

Kørnøv, L. (2007). Public participation. In L. Kørnøv, M. Thrane, A. Remmen, & H. Lund (Eds.), *Tools for sustainable development* (pp. 721–738). Aalborg, Denmark: Aalborg Universitetsforlag.

Kuanda, J. (2003). Culture and technological transformation in the south. Danmark: Samfundslitteratur Press.

Kushniruk, A., & Turner, P. (2011). Who's users? participation and empowerment in socio-technical approaches to health IT development. *International Perspectives in Health Informatics*, 280-285.

Lorentzen, A. (1994). Teknologi og udvikling i den nordjyske maskinindustri [technology and development in engineering in the northern part of Denmark]. Aalborg: Aalborg Universitetsforlag.

Mitchell, R., Agle, B., & Wood, D. (1997). Towards a therory of stakeholder identification and salience: Defining the principles of who and what really counts. *Academy of Management Review*, *22*(4), 853–886.

Muhr, T. (2004). ATLAS the knowledge workbench. V5.0 user's guide and reference. Berlin: ATLAS.ti.Scientific Software Development GmbH.

Müller, J. (1991). Hvad er teknologi? (what is technology?). In M. Rostgaard, A. Remmen, & J. Christensen (Eds.), *Samfundet i teknologien* (pp. 27–47). Aalborg: Aalborg Universitetsforlag.

Müller, J. (1990). Teknologivurdering og trovaerdighed [technology assessment and credibility]. In Cronberg T., & Friis D. (Eds.), Metoder i teknologivurdering. erfaring og fornyelse (pp. 267-279). Kobenhavn: Blytmanns forlag.

Müller, J., Kjaer-Rasmussen, J., & Nohr, C. (1989). *Proactive technology assessment as a tool in HIS development.* North Holland.

Müller, J., Kjaer-Rasmussen, J., & Nøhr, C. (1988). *Perspektiver for EDB-teknologi i sygehusvaesenet* [perspectives for IT-technology in the hospital sector]. Aalborg: Institut for Samfundsudvikling og Planlaegning, Aalborg Universitetscenter.

Mumford, E. (1983). *Designing human systems for new technology - the ETHICS method.* Manchester, UK: Manchester Business Schol.

Mumford, E., & Weir, M. (1979). *Computer systems in work design: The ETHICS method.* London: Associated Business Press.

Nielsen, J. (2005). *Ten usabiligy heuristics.* Retrieved December, 2012, from http://zonecours.hec.ca/documents/H2010-1-2357287.portionOK.pdf

Nøhr, C., & Bernstein, K. (1992). Implementation and diffusion of medical informatics; the case of electronic prescription communication. between practitioners and pharmacies. Primary Health Care Specialist Group of the British Computer Society.

Nøhr, C., Høstgaard, A. M., Botin, L., & Kjær-Andersen, S. (2004). *Evaluering af GEPKA-projektet, delrapport 2, klinisk afprovning* [evaluation of the GEPKA-project, report 2, clinical testing]. Unpublished manuscript.

Nøhr, C., & Høstgaard, A. M. (2011). *Evaluering af ABT-projektet: Genanvendelse af administrative patientdata til måling af den sundhedsfaglige kvalitet [evaluation of the ABT-project: Recycling of administrative patient data to measure health professional quality].* Denmark: Virtuel Centre for Health Informatics.

Nordjyllands Amt (The County of North Jutland). (2000). *IT-handlingsplan for sundhedsomraadet i nordjyllands amt 2002-2004* [IT-plan for the healthcare area in the county of north jutland 2002-2004]. Academic Press.

Nykänen, P., Brender, J., Talmon, J. D. K., de Keizer, N., Rigby, M., Beuscart-Zephir, M.-C., & Ammenwerth, E. (2011). Guideline for good evaluation practice in health informatics (GEP-HI). *International Journal of Medical Informatics, 80*(12), 815–927. doi:10.1016/j.ijmedinf.2011.08.004 PMID:21920809

Pagliari, C. (2007). Design and evaluation in eHealth: Challenges and implications for an interdisciplinary field. *Journal of Medical Internet Research, 9*(15). PMID:17537718

Pape-Haugaard, L., Haugaard, K., Carøe, P., & Høstgaard, A. (2013). *Exploring barriers for health visitors' adaption of the danish children's database through an empirical study.* LiU Electronic Press.

Pare, G., Sicotte, C., & Jacques, H. (2006). The effects of creating psychological ownership on physicians' acceptance of clinical information systems. *Journal of the American Medical Informatics Association, 13*(2), 197–205.

Protti, D. (2002). What can the american electronic health record (EHR) pioneers tell us about what it takes to be successful? *Health Management Forum, 15*(2), 33–35. doi:10.1016/S0840-4704(10)60578-9 PMID:12078354

Robertson, A. et al. (2010). *Implementation and adaption of nationwide electronic health records in secondary care in England: Qualitative analysis of interim results from a prospective national evaluation.* Academic Press.

Schot, J., & Rip, A. (1997). The past and future of constructive technology assessment. *Technological Forecasting and Social Change, 54*, 251–268.

Seemann, J. (2013). Interorganizational innovation in systemic networks. *The Innovation Journal: The Public Sector Innovation Journal, 18*(3), 1-1-18.

Sheikh, A., Cornford, T., & Barber, N. (2011). Implementation and adoption of nationwide electronic health record in secondary care in England: Final qualitative results from prospective national evaluation in "eraly adopter"hospitals. *British Medical Journal, 343*(d6054).

Simonsen, J., & Hertzum, J. (2006). A regional PD strategy for EPR systems: Evidence-based IT development. *Ninth Biennial Conference on Participatory Design, 2,* 125-128.

Simonsen, J., & Hertzum, J. (2008). Participative design and the challenges of large-scale systems: Estending the itereative PD approach. *Proceedings Participatory Design Conference.*

Stead, W. W. (1994). Designing medical informatics research and library: Resource projects to increase what is learned. *Journal of the American Medical Association, 1*(1), 27–33.

The European Union. (2012). *Redesigning health in Europe in 2020.* Belgium: The European Union.

Van der Meijden, M. J., Tange, H., Troost, J., & Hasman, A. (2001). Development and implementation of an EPR: How to encourage the user. *International Journal of Medical Informatics, 64*(2-3), 173–185. doi:10.1016/S1386-5056(01)00208-8 PMID:11734384

Van der Meijden, M. J., Tange, H., Troost, J., & Hasman, A. (2003). Determinants of success of inpatient clinical information systems: A literature review. *Journal of the American Medical Informatics Association, 10*(3), 235–243. doi:10.1197/jamia.M1094 PMID:12626373

van Gemert-Pijnen, J. E. W. C., Nijland, N., van Limburg, M., Ossebaard, H. C., Kelders, S. M., Eysenbach, G., & Seydel, E. R. (2011). A holistic framework to improve the uptake and impact of eHealth technologies. *Journal of Medical Internet Research, 13*(4), e111–e111. doi:10.2196/jmir.1672 PMID:22155738

Wears, R. L., & Berg, M. (2005). Computer technology and clinical work. still waiting for godot. *Journal of the American Medical Association*, *293*(10), 1261–1263. doi:10.1001/jama.293.10.1261 PMID:15755949

Yusof, M. M., Papazafeiropoulou, A., Paul, R. J., & Stergioulas, L. K. (2008). Investigating evaluation frameworks for health information systems. *International Journal of Medical Informatics*, *77*(6), 377–385. doi:10.1016/j.ijmedinf.2007.08.004 PMID:17904898

ADDITIONAL READING

Ash, J., Anderson, N. R., & Tarzy-Hornoch, P. (2008). People and organizational issues in research systems implementation. *Journal of the American Medical Informatics Association*, *15*(3), 283–289. doi:10.1197/jamia.M2582 PMID:18308986

Barki, H., & Hartwick, J. (1994). Measuring user participation, user involvement, and user attitude. *Management Information Systems Quarterly*, *18*(1), 59–82. doi:10.2307/249610

Berg, M., & Aarts, J., & Van der Lei. (2003). ICT in health care: Sociotechnical approaches. *Methods of Information in Medicine*, *42*(4), 297–301. PMID:14534625

Bødker, K., Kensing, F., & Simonsen, J. (2004). *Participatory IT design. designing for business and workplace realities*. MIT Press.

Bødker, K., & Pedersen, J. S. (1991). Workplace cultures: Looking at artifacts, symbols, and practices. In J. Greenbaum & M. Kyng (Eds.), *Design at work: Cooperative design of computer systems* (pp. 121–136). Chichester, UK: Lawrence Erlbaum associates.

Bødker S. (1994). Creating conditions for participation: Conflicts and resources in systems design. *Computer Professionals for Social Responsibility,* 13-20.

Coombs, C. R., Doherty, N. F., & Loan-Clarke, J. (2002). *The role of user ownership and positive user attitudes in the successful adoption of information systems within NHS community trusts. Advanced topics in end user computing*. PA, USA: IGI Publishing Hershey.

Dewan, N. A., & Lorenzi, N. (2000). Evaluating readiness and user acceptance. *M.B. Comput*, *4*, 50–52.

Granlien, M. F. (2009). Effect map; - a participatory tool for specifying formative effects to support mutual adaptation. *32st Information Systems Research Seminar in Scandinavia, 32,* 1-22.

Kensing, F., & Blomberg, J. (1998). Participatory design; issues and concerns. *Computer Supported Cooperative Work, 7*(3-4), 167–185. doi:10.1023/A:1008689307411

Kyng, M. (1995). Making representation work. *Communications of the ACM, 38*(9), 46–55. doi:10.1145/223248.223261

Lorenzi, N., Riley, R. T., Blyth, A. J. C., Southon, G., & Dixon, B. J. (1997). Antecedents of the people and organizational aspects of medical informatics: Review of the literature. *Journal of the American Medical Association*, 4. PMID:9067874

Olesen, F., & Markussen, R. (2003). *Reconfigured medication: Writing medicine in a sociotechnical practice (No. 11).* The Johns Hopkins University Press and the Society for Literature and Science.

Petersen, L. S., Bjørnes, C. D., & Bertelsen, P. (2010). Communication challenges in system development: Involvement of system developers in small-scale IT-projects. In C. Nøhr & J. Aarts (Eds.), *Information technology in health care: Socio-technical approaches 2010 - from safe systems to patient safety* (pp. 72–78). IOS Press.

KEY TERMS AND DEFINITIONS

eHealth: The infrastructure through which clinical and administrative information is passed in the healthcare sector EHR: In Denmark it is defined as a platform with different modules supplied by different vendors.

End-User Involvement: In this chapter the concept is used synonymous with "End-user participation."

End-User Participation: In this chapter the concept is used in the sense of enabling end-users to exert real influence in decision-making throughout the technological development process, i.e. the full eHealth lifecycle.

Social Carriers of Technology: A group of actors, or a social entity who choose the new technology and carry it forward towards the next stage during the process.

Workload Reduction: Colleagues taking over part/all of the clinical duties of the clinician involved – it does not include extra payment.

Chapter 4
Expanding Role of Telephone Systems in Healthcare:
Developments and Opportunities

Jing Shi
North Dakota State University, USA

Ergin Erdem
North Dakota State University, USA

Heping Liu
North Dakota State University, USA

ABSTRACT

The telephone systems in healthcare settings serve as a viable tool for improving the quality of service provided to patients, decreasing the cost, and improving the patient satisfaction. It can play a pivotal role for transformation of the healthcare delivery for embracing personalized and patient centered care. This chapter presents a systematic review of new developments of healthcare telephone system operations in various areas such as tele-health. Current research on topics such as tele-diagnosis, tele-nursing, tele-consultation is outlined. Specific issues associated with the emerging applications such as underreferral, legal issues, patient acceptance, on-call physician are discussed. Meanwhile, the architecture and underlying technologies for healthcare telephone systems are introduced, and the performance metrics for measuring the system operations are provided. In addition, challenges and opportunities related with improving the healthcare telephone systems are identified, and the potential opportunities of optimizing these systems are pointed out.

DOI: 10.4018/978-1-4666-9870-3.ch004

1. INTRODUCTION

Telephone systems are an indispensible part of healthcare units. Coile (1999) indicated that the conventional call centers in various healthcare settings could enhance their means for 275 million health consumers to receive better health service. The telephone systems guide the patients to receive the care, education, or related information. As such, the systems can be often considered as the entry gate for patients and other users of healthcare systems, and they present an immense opportunity to improve healthcare delivery, such as the efficient communication services for health care delivery especially in the laboratory medicine (Coiera, 2006), and supporting the functions of information technology for providing better care service (Schweiger et al., 2007).

The telephone systems in healthcare units usually involve the interaction and information exchange between the patients or their important ones and the customer service agents, nurses, or providers, with the help of telecommunication technologies. The systems can provide a variety of services such as scheduling an appointment, heath consultation, medication refills and renewals, enrollment, and co-pay. Stier (1999) indicated that the telephone systems provide substantial benefits for stakeholders in healthcare systems. Individuals who are looking for medical information to address their future health related problems or who are joining new healthcare insurance plans and would like to acquaint themselves with providers might reap substantial benefits by using those systems. In addition, hospital associates for arranging the transfer of patients within and between healthcare centers may also obtain timely and accurate information using the telephone systems. With the help of the telephone systems, the quality and efficiency of healthcare delivery systems can be significantly enhanced.

From the perspective of improving service quality and operation efficiency, this chapter reviews the new developments on telephone systems for healthcare delivery and identifies the challenges that the systems face and the potential opportunities for improvement and optimization. The organization of this chapter is as follows. In the second section, the architecture and functions of telephone systems for healthcare delivery are briefly introduced. In the third section, the indices for measuring the system performance are summarized. In the fourth section, the research progress and the expanding role of telephone systems for healthcare delivery are presented. In the fifth section, the challenges in optimizing the healthcare telephone systems are specified and analyzed. In the sixth section, the potential opportunities to improve service quality and operations efficiency are demonstrated. Finally, conclusive remarks are provided.

2. TELEPHONE SYSTEMS OPERATIONS AND TELE-HEALTH

Figure 1 illustrates the operations and activities of a typical healthcare telephone system. The schematic chart shows how a telephone system guides patients to communicate with clerks, nurses, physicians, or health counselors to obtain services. The data and education information flow is between the patients and the various units in the system. To cite an instance, a patient might provide his/her preferences on appointment date/time, and based on the data fetched from the database, a clerk/scheduler can provide the patient an appointment date/time that considers the patient preferences and the availability of clinic resources. On the other hand, the healthcare telephone systems might also be considered as a medium for dispensing information/education to the patients. For example, based on the triage algorithms implemented in the system, a nurse can decide whether the patient should be referred to another hospital. The services that can be obtained by the patients range from simple operations such as scheduling an appointment and medication refills, to complicated operations such as tele-nursing. In the telephone systems, more components such as tele-nursing, tele-counseling, tele-triage, computer telephony and computerized expert systems have been added (Mohan et al., 2004). In general, these components are also within the domain of tele-health. While the telemedicine and tele-health terms are used interchangeably in some cases (American Telemedicine Association, 2009), many believe that tele-health extends beyond the concept of telemedicine to encompass the non clinical applications which include, but are not limited to, home tele-health, remote patient monitoring, and the patient outreach programs (Darkins & Cary, 2000). New telehealth applications that aim to improve clinical outcomes associated with chronic disease management (Cassimatis & Kavanagh, 2012), and serious mental health problems (Pratt et al., 2014) are being developed. Also, recent advances in the electronics especially in sensor technology, miniaturization, and proliferation of the smart phones foster implementation of the tele-health approaches and contribute to the accessibility of the tele-health solutions (Boulos et al., 2011).

Hill and Powell (2009) indicated that medical errors cause the death of about 98,000 people per year, and the telephone systems can help significantly reduce the medical errors. The accessibility to adequate healthcare is an urgent issue for many countries. With tele-health, the geographic isolation, the scarcity of physicians and hospitals, and the difficulties of travel to medical facilities can be effectively addressed, and the patients do not need to physically visit clinics or hospitals but are able to receive proper care (Stamm & Pearce, 1995). Furthermore, tele-health can allow information to be readily communicated and shared among healthcare providers, and help curb healthcare costs over the long term. Tele-health applications

Figure 1. Typical Operations of a Healthcare Telephone System

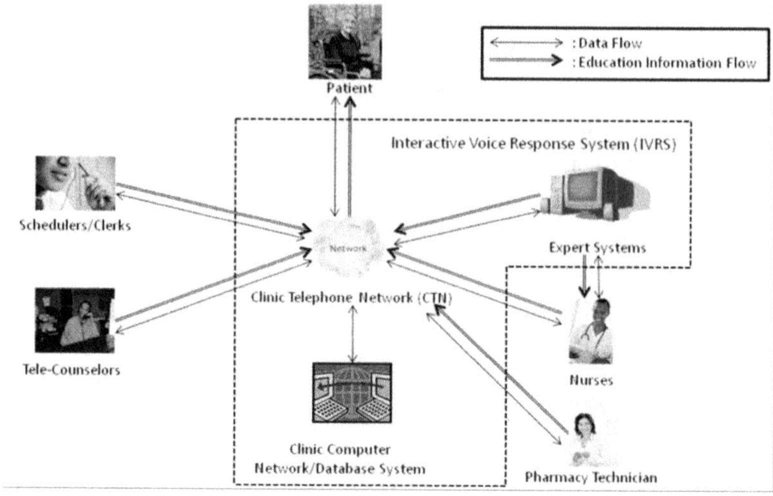

cover a wide variety of application areas for diagnostics and treatment. One application area is audiology which includes audiometry, video-otoscopy, oto-acoustic emissions, and auditory brainstem response. The intervention strategies such as hearing aid verification, counseling, and Internet-based treatment for tinnitus can also be incorporated in tele-health applications (Swanepoel & Hall III, 2010). In addition, the advent of smart phone technology paves new ways for developing new tele-health applications. In that regard, Gregoski et al. (2012) proposed a tele-health application that features photoplethysmographic acquisition and heart rate measurement. It was shown that smart phones might offer some advantages and ease of use because of the lack of electrode patches or wireless sensor telemetric straps. The tele-health applications might also be used for offering care for diseases in advanced stages. Kidd et al. (2010) discussed the applications of tele-health for providing palliative care in oncology such as out-of-hours telephone support, advice services for palliative care patients, carers and health professionals, videoconferencing for interactive case discussions, consultations and assessments, and training and education of palliative care and other health-care staff. Anderson et al. (1996) discussed how the telephone and video conferencing can be used for clinic monitoring and technician recertification for the optic neuritis research. It was shown that tele-health can be an effective cost cutting tool, and also help to attain a high visit completion rate among the patients attending the clinical trials.

Tele-health projects have been reported in many countries and districts. Suleiman (2001) demonstrated that Malaysia's tele-health initiative under the Multimedia Super Corridor project can help realize the country's health vision and goals, and meet future health challenges. Mohan and Yaacob (2004) showed that the integration of information, telecommunication, and human—machine interface technologies can assist in healthcare delivery, promote the heath status of the people. Adewale (2004) developed an Internet-based telemedicine environment for Nigeria. It supports consultations among remotely placed patients, rural health workers and specialists in the urban cities and provides a secure access to remote patient records. Barlow et al. (2006) explored the interaction among project complexity, organizational context, and project management approach during the planning and implementation phase. It was pointed out that although the organizational context would deter the researchers from drawing some general conclusions, individuals in the organizations play a vital role in the overall success of the tele-health projects. Hsu et al. (2010) illustrated the tele-health pilot project in Taiwan which uses healthcare information technology to address high healthcare costs and the shortage of healthcare providers. The project includes the home-care, community-care, and residential care models and can assist the elders in the pursuit of better healthcare and quality of life. National telehealth applications are especially important in low-income countries for improving the access of the population to the healthcare resources where there are inequitable distribution of expertise, equipment and knowledge. Setting specific goals and developing corresponding solution might help proper implementation and facilitate the access to the corresponding resources and help dissemination of the medical knowledge to the clinicians. However, significant barriers exist and the involvement of the key personnel in this endeavor is a key requirement for successful implementation as demonstrated in Zambia (Chanda & Shaw, 2010).

The adoption of tele-health will change the structures of traditional telephone systems. Hamill and Lorri (1998) showed how the clinical call centers can provide a reliable and safe homecare service for the elderly patients, and emphasized the importance of standards to ensure the efficacy of homecare related services. Koch (2006) indicated that although stand alone applications such as blood sugar monitoring, tele-cardiography have been finding wide attention, a holistic approach that assesses the effect of tele-health on the current model of healthcare delivery systems has not been taken yet. It was noted that further research is needed to address the impacts and benefits of potential solutions and overcome a number of restrictions. The restrictions include the lack of standards to combine incompatible information systems, the lack of an evaluation framework considering legal, ethical, organizational, clinical, usability and technical aspects, and the lack of proper guidelines for practical implementation of home tele-health solutions.

The continuous adoption of information technology in telephone systems has been playing a crucial role for operation improvement. As a result, tele-health has proliferated, which reflects the convergence of scientific, technological, economic and social factors (Grigsby & Sanders, 1998). Ball and Lillis (2001) demonstrated that the consumers' interest in and demand for online administrative processes, information rich Internet health portals, and access to physician web pages and e-mail has introduced a new dimension to maintain wellness and treat diseases. It was shown that these activities are redefining the relationship of physicians and patients, improving clinical decision-making, increasing efficiency, and strengthening communication between physicians and patients. Nowadays, the comprehensive telehealth applications are being integrated into the Internet health portals through personal health record for developing patient-centric healthcare model, enhancing access to care, and ensuring the responsiveness of such technologies to the preferences and circumstances of patients. Such an approach is recently implemented in the Veteran Affairs healthcare system (Hogan et al., 2011)

Prince and Herrin (2007) documented the development of a patient-centric call process using real-time, rules-based task assignment and tracking software, which enhances healthcare communications, efficiency and patient safety, guides personalized and timely response to the needs of individual patients, and allows data mining for outcome analysis. Lenz and Reichert (2007) elaborated the potential and essential limitations of IT support for healthcare processes. A broad socio-technical perspective based on scientific literature and personal experience was adopted to illustrate that the huge potential of IT to improve healthcare quality has not been fully explored by the current solutions. Tsiknakis and Kouroubali (2009) presented an application of the "Fit between Individuals, Task and Technology" framework to analyze the socio-organizational-technical factors that influence IT adoption in the healthcare domain. Lee et al. (2009) investigated the efficacy of a ubiquitous healthcare service using Zigbee and mobile phone for elderly patients with diabetes mellitus or heart diseases. It was believed that ZigBee technology could become a key component for wireless ubiquitous healthcare systems due to its advantages of lower power consumption. Adler Milstein and Bates (2010) discussed the role of IT for revolutionizing healthcare industry. It was shown how IT can be effectively used for a paperless system and how medical information can be electronically shared among various parties. Hill and Powell (2009) showed that a national electronic healthcare network is one of the most important keys to resolving this crisis, but it is underappreciated and under-exploited, and faces several formidable barriers to implementation. Recent study suggested that electronic healthcare records play a viable role for the best clinical outcomes through the clinical decision support systems. Standardization and integration of the healthcare records to the existing information systems help develop efficient and effective approaches for improving the existing clinical decision support systems, which guide the clinicians to provide the required care based on the clinical guidelines (Romano and Stafford, 2011). Electronic healthcare records are also important input for developing genomics based medicine which is a very important milestone for developing personalized healthcare solutions (Gottesman et al., 2013).

3. PERFORMANCE METRICS FOR TELEPHONE SYSTEMS

Measuring the performance of a healthcare telephone system is a critical task. By using certain metrics, the current operations can be benchmarked against the baseline and the results directly indicate if an improvement plan is needed. A number of approaches have been developed in the literature for evaluating the performance of a telephone system. Stier (1999) identified eight factors that have a significant impact on the profitability of call centers and the quality of services. The eight factors are financial viability; shared outcome requirements, a three-year migration plan, cross discipline tasking, market alignment, system integration, process redesign, leveraging high margin services and quantified outcomes, and they have universal means in the context of healthcare settings. Jack at al. (2006) developed an embedded framework to identify the trade-offs encountered during the management of a telephone system. In order to improve the performance of a telephone system, four aspects should be taken into consideration and they are the efficient deployment and use of labor, the effective use of technology, capacity management, and demand management.

Miciak and Desmarais (2001) pointed out that managers of telephone systems can use a number of performance metrics, but the metrics for measuring customer satisfaction have been lacking. It was further stated that the metrics should be based on three different facets, namely, operational characteristics, employee/customer service representative (CSR) opinions on workplace issues, and customer opinions on service quality experience. Overall, the acquisition/retention ratio, percent of total customer relationship, calls answered with live voice, call centers with unionized representatives, and average number of call center representatives constitute the metrics related with the call center operating characteristics. On the other hand, service level (percentage of the calls answered in 20 seconds or less), average length of calls, average wrap-up time, and first call resolution are the indices associated with the individual call characteristics.

Tables 1 and 2 show the performance indices widely adopted in literature. These indices are generally applicable to any general telephone system in healthcare, but they are not necessarily exhaustive considering the variations among healthcare settings. For healthcare telephone systems, some of these indices are particularly important such as abandon rates, patient waiting time, rates of mismatches, first call resolution, and average and maximum queue length of calls from patients.

Table 1. Performance Indices of Telephone Systems

	Metric	Reference
Call Center Related	Acquisition/retention ratio (%)	(Miciak and Desmarais, 2001)
	Percentage of total customer relationship at call center	(Miciak and Desmarais, 2001)
	Calls answered with live voice (%)	(Miciak and Desmarais, 2001)
	Average number of CSRs at call center	(Miciak and Desmarais, 2001)
	Service level (Percentage of calls answered within a given time frame)	(Miciak and Desmarais, 2001), (Ertogral and Bamuqabel, 2008), (Deslauriers et al., 2007)
	The number of touch-tones necessary to reach the most common transaction in the voice response system (VRU)	(Evenson et al., 1999)
	The percentage of incoming calls that are entirely handled by VRU (%)	(Evenson et al., 1999)
	Rate of outbound calls	(Deslauriers et al., 2007)
	Rate of mismatches	(Deslauriers et al., 2007)
Call Related	Average length of call in minutes	(Miciak and Desmarais, 2001)
	Average wrap-up time in minutes	(Miciak and Desmarais, 2001), (Jack et al., 2006), (Federspiel et al., 2004)
	First call resolution (%)	(Miciak and Desmarais, 2001), (Jack et al., 2006)
Customer Related	Customer waiting time	(Jack et al., 2006), (Duder and Rosenwein, 2001)
	Issue resolution time	(Jack et al., 2006)
	Customer abandon rate	(Jack et al., 2006), (Duder and Rosenwein, 2001), (Deslauriers et al., 2007)
	Short abandonment index	(Jouni et al., 2013)
	Frequency and manner the company chooses to elicit customer response	(Evenson et al., 1999)
	Average queue length of calls	(Garnet et al., 2002)
	Maximum queue length of calls	(Artelajo et al. 2007)
	Customer satisfaction rate	(Robinson and Morley, 2006)

4. NEW DEVELOPMENTS OF HEALTHCARE TELEPHONE SYSTEMS

A number of unique new developments have been witnessed in healthcare telephone systems to expand the role of nurses/providers, improve patient-centered care, and facilitate the delivery of care. The new operation developments can be categorized

Table 2. Evaluation Criteria of Staffing and Training

Metric	Reference
Call center with unionized CSRs (%)	(Miciak and Desmarais, 2001)
Average number of CSRs per supervisor	(Miciak and Desmarais, 2001)
CSRs with college degree	(Miciak and Desmarais, 2001)
CSRs with technical degree or some college	(Miciak and Desmarais, 2001)
Ratio of CSRs trained generalist/specialist	(Miciak and Desmarais, 2001), (Evenson et al., 1999)
More than 25 days of new-hire training	(Miciak and Desmarais, 2001)
More than 6 days annual ongoing training	(Miciak and Desmarais, 2001)
CSR salary	(Miciak and Desmarais, 2001)
Supervisor salary	(Miciak and Desmarais, 2001)
Total cost of new-hire CSR	(Miciak and Desmarais, 2001)
Turnover rate (the ratio of the average number of CSR leave an organization to total number of CSR in the company	(Evenson et al., 1999)
The average number of years CSR are employed in the call center	(Evenson et al., 1999)
Not utilized time (i.e. the amount of time CSR spends at work while not answering calls, training, or doing paperwork)	(Evenson et al., 1999), Deslauriers et al. (2007)
Average talk time	(Duder and Rosenwein, 2001), (Heschong Mashone Group, 2003), (Federspiel et al., 2004), (Tham and Willem, 2004), (Tham, 2004), (Wargocki et al., 2004)
Number of calls handled by CSR per unit time	(Witt, 2004)
Customer service quality (1-5 Likert scale) (self evaluation and supervisor evaluation)	(Witt, 2004), (Mcnall and Roch, 2009)
The amount of freedom given to CSR to handle calls that concern a threat to consumer defection	(Evenson et al., 1999)

into the forms of tele-counseling, tele-nursing, tele-triage, tele-diagnosis, computer telephony, interactive voice response systems (IVRS), on-call physicians, and operations of outgoing calls. In addition, national level healthcare telephone systems (call centers) are also included.

4.1 Tele-Nursing and Counseling

In recent years there has been a trend to increase the use of telephone nursing and consultation, which effectively reduce the workload of general practitioners (GPs) as well as emergency departments. Stirewalt et al. (1982) studied whether a specialized telephone service could cut down on unscheduled visits to ambulatory care and improve satisfaction with care. The results show that the telephone service, which provides a triage system for referrals as well as a source of central contact for scheduling or for complaints, helped to improve patient satisfaction and reduce the number of unscheduled visits. Similarly, McKinstry et al. (2002) showed that the use of telephone consultations for same-day appointments was associated with time saving, and did not result in lower scores of Patient Enablement Instrument which can measure patient perceptions and be used to report the willingness to use telephone consultations in the future. The possible reason is that this short-term saving is offset by higher re-consultation and less use of opportunistic health promotion. Kamei et al. (2014) conducted a meta-analysis of the existing research and showed that tele-home monitoring based tele-nursing in Chronic Obstructive Pulmonary Disease may affect the use of the healthcare services. The structure of counseling center is an important aspect for smooth operations of the tele-health applications. Russell (2012) indicated that organizing tele-counseling centers as a professional call center might pose some challenges. For instance, ambiguities over the use of skills in a system that incorporates the deployment of computer algorithms might lead to the conflicts for monitoring performance evaluation and the use of time. Tele-counseling along with the other intervention strategies might be implemented on the mobile platforms and accessed by the users using the mobile phones for different approaches for supporting preventive medicine functions such as smoking cessation (Ghorai et al., 2014).

Dale et al. (1998) reported on the evaluation of an off-hour telephone triage in general practice. A computer-based decision support tool was used to guide nurses in the assessment of patients and outcome for calls. It was found that the nurses were able to handle just over half the calls received by giving advice alone. The service was remarkably consistent in the decisions taken by nurses. Gilmour (2001) presented approaches for developing a telephone system to manage disaster and trauma, and found that without the physical contact, it is often easier to establish a closeness on telephone since the connection occurs without the initial distraction of physical cues. The perceived anonymity of callers contributes to the service quality. Callers are more open to the discussion of related matters with counselors. Bunn et al. (2005) reviewed the effects of telephone consultation on safety, service use, and patient satisfaction by using randomized controlled trials, controlled studies, controlled before/after studies, and interrupted time series of telephone consultation or triage in a general healthcare setting. The review supports that the telephone consultation and triage reduce the number of general patients visit, and at least 50% of calls can be handled by telephone advice. Zanaboni et al. (2009) studied the effect of tele-consultation on the reduction of the use of clinic resources and on the potential savings. In addition, tele-counseling applications have been developed for reducing the health risks associated with obesity through the mobile health platforms (Castelnuovo et al., 2011). Tele-counseling is also proposed as a viable method for providing follow-up psychological support for cancer survivors in the rural areas of Canada (Fuchsia et al., 2014).

4.2 Tele-Triage

A number of studies have been conducted to address the efficacy of tele-triage decisions. Telephone triage is a systematic process where the nurse screens existing symptoms for urgency, and provides the advice on whether existing symptoms require clinical center visit (Briggs, 2007) If a visit to clinic center is required, a nurse can also provide suggestions on the timing based on the urgency status. Crouch et al. (1996) indicated the importance of tele-triage even in densely populated urban centers. Devore (1999) examined the tele-triage from a perspective of midwife, pointed out the inherent difficulties of tele-triage, and provided suggestions and guidelines for improving the quality of tele-triage. A historical perspective on the development of telephone triage is presented by Breslin and Denison (2002), in which the ethical and legal implications of telephone triage are stressed, and the importance of procedures and nursing-time efficient allocation is discussed. Bunik et al. (2007) incorporated the cost concepts into tele-triage decisions by drawing the link between costs and compliance rates. Cost savings under different scenarios were discussed. Beaulieu and Humphreys (2008) conducted an observational study to assess the patient satisfaction with a nurse managed health center. It was confirmed that tele-triage might significantly reduce the number of visits made to emergency departments. The trust of the patients on the tele-triage applications is also an important factor for ensuring the efficiency and effectiveness of the service. Williams et al. (2012) showed that the users of the tele-triage services with greater self-efficacy and satisfaction with the nurse interaction are more likely to adhere to the advices for self-care. Similarly, a survey study was conducted among the patients using the tele-triage services. About 85% of the respondents indicated that they adhere to the recommendations and do not visit to the medical center. The adherence to the suggestions might reduce associated healthcare cost if the patients follow recommendations provided by the tele-triage services (Rimner et al., 2011). Mobile health platforms also contribute to the access to the healthcare resources through tele-triage functions especially for the population living in the rural areas in the developing nations (Burney et al., 2014). Tele-triage forms the backbone of the dispatch protocols and considerably improves the efficiency and effectiveness of providing medical emergency services (Alizadeh et al., 2012). Some researchers have expanded the function of tele-triage to offer the proactive care in the home-care setting. Associated with this approach, it might form the frontline for the healthcare provider network (Arnaert & Macfarlane, 2011).

Underreferral indicates the situation that nurses or providers assess the healthcare condition of callers as less serious compared to what it is. It significantly degrades the quality of healthcare delivery and puts patients at risk. Lee et al (2003b) and Kempe et al. (2003) presented studies that estimate the underreferral rate for pediatric patients. Kempe et al. (2006) used data mining techniques to sort and analyze a large collection of data to estimate the underreferral rate after hours. The findings show that the triage decisions after 11pm are more likely considered as underreferral, and adolescents and infants run the higher risks of being underreferred. Hirsh et al. (2007) calculated the underreferral rate for the patients receiving tele-triage decisions. Besides underreferral, overreferral is another important research topic about the efficiency of tele-triage decisions. Poole et al. (1993), Kempe et al. (2000b) and Hirsh et al. (2004) all indicated that healthcare call centers usually tended to overrefer patients for urgent disposition.

4.3 Tele-Diagnosis

Telephone can be used by nurses, physicians and consultants to diagnose and manage many common conditions in order to control costs, reduce appointments and visits, and maximize efficiency for patient visits. Revicki et al. (1997) evaluated the correspondence between in-person and telephone interview-derived data on affective symptoms, health-related quality of life, disability days, and medication compliance in patients with bipolar disorder. The results showed good to excellent agreement between telephone and in-person interviews. It was believed that telephone interviews are feasible and reliable for collecting data on psychiatric and other health-related outcomes in bipolar disorder patients. Feldman-Naim et al. (1997) examined the reliability and level of agreement between the telephone and face-to-face administration of two mood-rating scales in patients with rapid cycling bipolar disorder (RCBD). The results support the use of phone-administered mood ratings as a reliable and convenient method to monitor patients with RCBD. Rohde et al. (1997) examined the comparability of data obtained by telephone and face-to-face interviews for diagnosing axis I and II disorders. The agreement between telephone and face-to-face assessment was excellent for anxiety disorders, major depressive disorder, and alcohol use disorders. The findings provided qualified justification for the use of telephone interviews to collect axis I and II data. Based on an empirical research on the assessment of vulvovaginal complaints, Allen-Davis et al. (2002) examined the agreement between telephone and office management of vulvovaginal complaints and assessed the accuracy of diagnosis of vulvovaginitis. Prospective structured telephone nurse interviews of all patients with vulvovaginal complaints were conducted. The particular study challenges the notion that the telephone is an effective tool to diagnose and treat vulvovaginal complaints. Telephone systems might also support the tele-diagnosis applications for relaying the output. Muir et al. (2012) demonstrated the setting where the diagnosis obtained based on tele-dignosis applications are relayed to the medical center via telephone. It was found that the results obtained by the tele-diagnosis and face-to face diagnosis actually agree most of the time. Moreover, the agreement rate between tele-diagnosis and the final clinical diagnosis is strikingly higher (i.e., about 98%). Thomas and Kumar (2013) indicated that the telephone networks might be useful for relaying the voice, fax and data transmissions for the tele-dermatology applications. Ganapathy and Ravindra (2011) also suggested that telephone networks might play a supporting role for the tele-health applications and strongly affect the associated costs for the healthcare operations especially in the emerging economies. Novel tele-diagnosis approaches that use the existing telephone network have been developed. To cite an instance, Sakar and Kursun (2010) use the measurement of dysphonia for diagnosing the Parkinson's disease in earlier stages. Tele-diagnosis is also expanded for providing tele-dentistry functions to improve the assessment of oral health (Marino et al., 2015). Santana et al., (2012) develop a semi-automatic approach for tele-diagnosing the vascular problems. The proposed system in the first step aim to capture the relevant data using Echo-Doppler images, and the second step features the distributed tool for the collaborative diagnosis for those particular health problems.

Kathryn et al. (2003) presented a study identifying the efficacy of diagnosing the depression in outpatients. Most of the patients expressed interest in the tele-diagnosis of depression due to the various factors such as convenience and privacy. It showed that tele-diagnosis is a feasible alternative to face-to-face interviews for diagnosing the depression among cancer patients. Remschmidt et al. (2003) investigated the reliability and validity of data gathered in telephone interviews. The results indicated good reliability and underscored the validity of the collected data. Saraux et al. (2004) evaluated the agreement between a rheumatologist visit and a telephone interview, and the agreement between the two sources of data turned out to be poor for the classification criteria but satisfactory for the diagnosis. Standardized telephone interviews can accurately identify the diagnosis made by rheumatologists based on a physical examination and medical record review, whereas the agreement is poor regarding classification criteria for rheumatoid arthritis or spondyloarthropathy. Haghighat et al. (2007) demonstrated the efficiency of the tele-diagnosis system for evaluating the breast cancer related cases. The study indicated that consultants may diagnose and manage the cases successfully over a phone by using some well established diagnostic criteria, and that most of the time the findings are parallel with the findings of the specialists evaluating patients face to face.

4.4 Computer Telephony

Computer telephony is basically an integrated system combining telephone with computers to receive, transmit and process information (Edgar, 1992). It overlaps with the telephone based healthcare and telehealth (McBride & Rimer, 1999; Balas et al., 1997). The application of computer telephony dates back the late 1960's (Allen, 1969). Biem et al. (2003) conducted an exhaustive literature review by searching MEDLINE (1966-April 2003), CINAHL (1982-April 2003) and the Cochrane Central Register of Controlled Trials to identify the evidence for the medical applications of computer telephony system. The computer telephony systems, for some applications, make health care delivery more efficient by improving scheduling, communication and health information. For instance, computer telephony has been used for tracking the diet and obtaining feedback of the patients to increase the nutrition (Delichatsios et al., 2002). It has been used for evaluating the patient satisfaction (Isenberg et al., 2001). An education program based on the voice mail was developed to help the nurses for collecting administrative data (Narayan, 2001). Studies suggest that computer telephony system can actually help to improve the immunization rates (Dini, 2000) and facilitate the medical care of chronic diseases such as chronic lung diseases (Young et al., 2001) and diabetes (Piette, 2000). However, the effectiveness of computer telephony system-based management intervention is not certain. For some computer telephony applications, the controlled trials on the effectiveness based on randomized controlled trials might not be possible (Biem et al., 2004). In most of the studies, the sample size is not large enough to infer statistical conclusions or lacking follow-up studies, and the effects of computer telephony in the long run has not been fully established (Pinto et al., 2002; Rask et al., 2000). Computer telephony might also be used with the clinical longitudinal follow up studies. In that regard, Stewart et al. (2012) indicated that automated telephone contacts or web based questionnaire might be used with collecting follow-up data. It was reported that among the cohort of patients who are elderly and chronically ill, providing input using automated telephone contacts finds acceptance and might be used for longitudinal follow up studies. In addition, van der Marck et al. (2011) conducted a study in which computer telephony might be used in conjunction of reporting the falls for the elderly patients living in community-dwelling homes. It was shown that computer telephony is a suitable way of conveying the information regarding the falls for the patients. Computer telephony can be also used for providing the necessary e-coaching services for the patients that require complex care. Such approaches are very important for continuity of care for the patients suffering from serious chronic diseases (Ritchie et al., 2012), Systems that incorporate computer telephony have been proposed for various clinical settings such as the appointment reminders in clinics (Suomi et al., 2010), and reducing impulsivity among violent forensic outpatients and probationers (Berman et al., 2012).

4.5 Interactive Voice Response Systems (IVRS)

Interactive Voice Response System (IVRS) has been gaining attention in the recent years due to the ease of implementation, cost effectiveness and various other considerations. In an IVRS, a human operator is replaced by the high-quality recorded script, and the people using IVRS can be directed to various branches based on the answers provided to the system. IVRS offers advantages as compared to the human operated telephone systems. IVRS can be utilized to reach the hard-to-reach groups such as homeless people, sex workers (Alemagno et al., 1996). There is no operator bias, and human errors are eliminated. The cost per interview is likely to be small, and the detailed information using IVRS can be collected.

IVRS differs from Computer Assisted Telephone Interview (CATI) systems, although they share some technical similarities (Nicholls, 1988). In CATI, there is no person reading the questions and entering the responses into the system. Corkrey and Parkinson (2002) identified that the health related information services of IVRS in the literature are smoking cessation, depression screening, hepatitis B screening, and providing pediatric clinic information. IVRS can be used as reminder calls and handle the outbound calls for cardiac and the diabetic patients. IVRS is associated with the higher childhood immunization rates, and appointment and treatment compliance. Corkrey and Parkinson (2002) further pointed out the physical, psychological, and technical influences of voice in IVRS. For example, the soft speaker might be interpreted as less assured, the faster speaking pace might be perceived as the more convincing as compared to the slower speaking pace, the scripts recorded at the lower voice quality might hamper the intended outcome of IVRS, and the male or female voice in the scripts may have different effects.

Lee et al. (2003a) discussed the applications of (IVRS) in healthcare. It was demonstrated that the patients who interact with an IVRS through automated messages behave in a more honest manner. Combined with expert triage systems, IVRS can help healthcare providers to expand customer contracts, increase access to healthcare resources, reduce operating expenses, and increase staff efficiency. O'Brien et al. (2003) discussed the resource utilization during the clinical trial of the Viozan™ for chronic obstructive pulmonary disease. The authors indicated that IVRS can be effectively implemented to collect the resource utilization data and thus help reduce the clinical trial costs. Stritzke et al. (2005) showed that IVRS can be used to obtain daily reports of attitudes toward alcohol and tobacco use among children 9–13 years of age. Mundt et al. (2006) compared the reliability and validity of the self reported sadness and the pessimistic thought of participants in their study. A group of 60 participants were assessed using both the computer based and clinician administered versions of the Montgomery-Asberg Depression Rating Scale (MADRS). Two results turned out to be statistically insignificant. Abu-Hasaballah et al. (2007) discussed the use of IVRS as an electronic data capture tool in the clinical and behavioral research. They described how IVRS works, the advantages and pitfalls of IVRS, and some of the lessons learned from administering a number of clinical studies using IVRS. Kim et al. (2007) investigated the use of IVRS system for clinic screening of the depression along the low income, disadvantaged, urban pregnant women. It was indicated that IVRS can be a very suitable tool for prescreening and screening for the low income pregnant urban women. Compared to visiting the clinics physically, IVRS is a less costly alternative. Horton et al. (2008) discussed the compliance rate of the patients using IVRS for creating their own electronic diaries. The electronic medical diaries are considered to be a valuable tool for assessing the quantitative and qualitative mental health parameters. However, it is revealed that the excessive use of IVRS for handling outgoing calls might decrease the usefulness of IVRS. Heyworth et al. (2014) compared the interactive voice response system, patient mailing, and the mailed registry for encouraging screening for ostreoposis. It was discovered that IVRS is effective for increasing the response rate, and it remains the viable strategy for incorporating the population screening interventions. The IVRS might also be complemented with the prize based approaches. Lindsay et al. (2014) discussed enhancing the compliance of using IVRS for the cocaine addiction treatment and showed that augmenting IVRS with the prize based contingency management might produce more positive outcomes in terms of abstinence achievement. Similarly, Graham et al. (2012) found that IVRS in conjunction with the Geisinger Monitoring Program significantly reduces the 30-day readmission by 44% for the case managed Medicare population. IVRS might also be used for improving the treatment adherence for the HIV/AIDS setting in a resource limited setting for the developing countries. It is suggested that controlling access to the telephone system by providing a personal pin number might be used as an appropriate security measure for providing healthcare services for HIV/AIDS patients (Joshi et al., 2014). Telephone systems based on IVRS can also be used for collecting information regarding the patient feedback for the post clinical visits (Berner et al., 2014). The demographics of the users might have an effect on the usability of the IVRS systems. Auger et al. (2013) indicated that older users might have difficulties with using IVRS systems. Interestingly, the authors also pointed out that the education level of the users might be associated with more unsuccessful calls and lower reported usefulness.

In order to promote the acceptability for the IVRS systems especially among the elder population, the consideration of adjusting the system according to the user needs should be given. In the survey conducted among the elder population, it was discovered that the adaptive algorithms for changing the structure of the IVRS system, rather than prompting the user to adjust his/her input, is more viable method of obtaining the input of the population and gaining acceptance (Miller et al., 2011).

4.6 On-Call Physicians

On-call physicians provide services to the emergency departments, and usually screen and stabilize urgent medical conditions which require specific medical expertise and knowledge. Pike (2003) investigated the number of on-call physicians required for healthcare call centers to facilitate the smooth flow of operations. It was concluded that usually the on-call physicians are called for the house staff on the average once per night mostly on the medication type problems, and the importance of continuing medical education was emphasized to improve the effectiveness of the on-call system. Morton et al. (2004) assessed the on-call activity by performing a time-motion study of resident on-call activity at a university medical center and an urban affiliate hospital and pointed out that 25% of the total call time is spent with evaluating patients, but direct contact with patients comprised only 7% of the call night duties. Sleep deprivations, and frequent interruptions in activity are common aspects the on-call physicians and residents face during their call nights. Rudkin et al. (2004) used a mailed anonymous survey to assess the scope of problems with on-call physicians in California. It was discovered that on-call problems were more acute at night or on weekends, and patient insurance negatively affected willingness of on-call physicians to consult for at least a quarter of patients. Mohanty et al. (2006) presented a study to identify the link between the response time of on-call physicians and various factors such as the neighborhood, the type of emergency department facility and the income of corresponding healthcare facility. It was discovered that when the income of neighborhood and the corresponding healthcare facility increase, the physician response time generally decreases. McConnell et al. (2007) surveyed Oregon hospitals about the prevalence and magnitude of stipends for taking emergency call and assessed the ways in which hospitals are limiting services. The results showed that the problems with on-call coverage are prevalent in Oregon and affect hospital financing and delivery of services. Rudkin et al. (2009) reassessed the problems with on-call physician coverage in California by repeating the anonymous survey and the results showed the on-call situation in California worsened substantially. The main reasons for declining service were identified to be related to the service time (e.g., day/night of the day, whether it is a weekend coverage), and the complexity of the injury (Cantu et al., 2012). It has been reported that recent legislative changes in the on-call requirement changes contribute to the shortage of the on-call specialists. Under the Emergency Medical Treatment and Labor Act (EMTALA), the on-call physicians will be permitted to be on call simultaneously at more than one hospital. Moreover, they have the latitude of scheduling elective surgeries or other medical procedures. Additionally, hospitals have greater discretion on developing their on-call specialist list (Moran, 2014). The shortage of the on-call physicians are also confirmed with other studies as well. According to the survey among emergency department managers, about three-fourths responded that there are problems with the on-call coverage problems and sixty percent indicated that they lost around the clock 24/7 coverage for at least one specialty in the past and one-quarter reported unreliability issues (Rao et al., 2010). The level of care provided by on-call physician is also under question. Petersen et al. (2014) indicated that on-call physicians provide adequate care in 49% of the unanticipated intensive care cases. Although the sample size is small, there are similar studies confirming the worsening of on-call physician coverage. Increasing the availability of the on-call physician and improving the associated service are an important task that should be addressed promptly and carefully.

4.7 Operations of Outgoing Calls

Besides incoming calls, healthcare telephone systems can handle outgoing calls. Korcz and Moreland (1998) presented a study which utilizes a healthcare telephone system to prescreen cancer patients visiting the oncology clinic. Two clinic social workers were in charge of contacting cancer patients by telephone for prescreening purposes. The telephone prescreening can help patients/families adapt to clinic or hospital systems. It was reported that the efficiency as well as the patient satisfaction levels significantly increased after the prescreening implementation. In a similar vein, Reardon et al. (1988) discussed the effect of preadmission prescreening to access the elder people on the elective surgery list in Mt. Sinai Hospital in New York. It showed the efficiency and success of the outreach program and reported that the patients responded well and were highly satisfied with the effort to address their needs before surgery.

One more operation change in healthcare telephone systems is that a patient response platform is built to serve within a health care facility as opposed to a call center addressing the needs of outside callers. A patient response platform is essentially a computerized tool that can streamline patient care, support workflow efficiency, and enhance clinical communication and patient safety. Prince and Herrin (2007) showed that a patient response platform facilitates a 23% decrease in administration delay and it benefits the efficiency of targeted communication calls. Although the system is intended to address the request of inpatients, it can be adopted to manage the requests of outside callers. Clinic related outgoing calls is an important part of the specialty care physician trainees. For instance, a study shows that the trainee made 33 calls, each of which last 1.7 minutes on the average (Prasad et al., 2012). This indicated that a significant amount of time is spent on making outgoing calls in the clinic settings.

4.8 National Healthcare Telephone Systems

National healthcare information centers such as poisons information centers are open for inquiries from health service and the public. One of the primary tasks of the national healthcare information centers is the telephone advisory service. Hall et al. (2006) used the interview and inquires to study the structure and process of the drug information centers and the drug information services in Costa Rica. The drug information centers were designed to improve communication and offer additional information. Andrew (2006) reported the organization and functions of the poison centers located throughout Europe. Pohjanoksa-Mantyla et al. (2008) analyzed and described the utilization of a community pharmacy operated national drug information call center in Finland. The special focus was on calls concerning prescription drugs. Toverud et al. (2009) conducted a similar study to find caller satisfaction levels for people using the nation-wide poison center located in Norway, to provide the cost justification for the national call center and to evaluate the benefits to the public.

Hill and Powell (2009) pointed out the current status of the U.S. national healthcare system and illustrated how the e-health movement can help with providing a relief to the existing healthcare crisis. It was indicated that managing the electronic medical and personal health records play a key role in the implementation of the successful e-health projects. Hsu et al. (2010) discussed about how national pilot tele-health projects can have a positive impact on the hospital readmission rate, hospital visit rate, medication non-adherence rate. In addition, nosocomial infection rate and adverse drug event incident rate are also decreased by the national tele-health project. Leydon et al. (2013) indicated that for identifying the racial information and ethnic monitoring, it is worthwhile to standardize the questions by providing the list of expected answers. This approach might be useful for increasing the overall efficiency of the system. Recently national telehealth services make extensive use of technology. A national telehealth center is founded in Taiwan to battle for the hypertension that is called “Citizen Telecare Service System (CTCS)” (Lin et al., 2014). The system integrates several important features of hardware and software infrastructure, such as biometric measurement, hypertension risk assessment and clinic appointment service, etc. The national telehealth system shows significant benefits such as reducing the percentage of participants with systolic blood pressure

(SBP) above 140 mmHg from 36.38% to 27.24%, and a drop in the prevalence of SBP above 120mmHg from 75.05% to 71.24.

5. CHALLENGES AND OPPORTUNITIES

5.1 High Patient Expectations

Customers' expectations for high quality services increase the operation scale and scope of healthcare telephone systems. The new developments of telephone systems discussed above may experience difficulties during routine work. Wahlberg et al. (2003) identified the major problem areas of tele-triage implementation, which include the insufficiency of healthcare resources, no physical interaction with patients, callers overstating or understating the health status of patients, and the language problems especially related with immigrants. Also, Snooks et al. (2008) pointed out that nurses have disagreement between the job functions and the required skill sets of tele-nurses. The nurses assuming more traditional roles generally question the job functions of tele-nurses, and believe that the tight management style and computerized decision making systems cause erosion on the loss of nursing skills. Additionally, because of the high expectations of the callers, and the very nature of the healthcare delivery processes, the language choices that are realized in lexicogrammar play an indispensable role for successful development of medical telephone support (Wan, 2012). On the other hand, telemedicine might also change the relationship between the patients and the healthcare provider (Ekeland et al., 2010). This might create additional challenges in terms of satisfying the expectations of the patients.

As pointed out, one of the inherent difficulties in tele-counseling and tele-nursing is the lack of physical presence between callers and counselors (or nurses). A possible solution is that counselors and nurses can develop necessary skills to analyze the cues by listening to the voice of callers, and the e-mail based communication schemes can be implemented to follow up nursing and counseling services to improve the quality of services. Furthermore, telephone systems can become multi-channel communication centers where several new technologies can be used to provide a wide variety of services to patients. For example, fax, phone, internet, e-mail and web chat can all be used extensively to maximize opportunities of contacting with patients. Web services offer patients a non-obtrusive and easy way to get answers to their questions and patients do not need to wait in a call queue. The Internet has enabled healthcare telephone systems to yield more control to patients for the level of service desired and it can effectively reduce the cost of operations. Healthcare telephone systems have made great strides in the area of e-mail support. If patients are able to e-mail a question and get a quick reply, patients can have a very positive experience. In addition, the e-mail-based service is not real-time and it is unnecessary to staff for peak demand periods of calls, which can lead to the significant savings. Another promising technology is instant messaging that allows patients to contact nurses or doctors without waiting in phone queues.

5.2 Consistency and Efficiency of Services

The services provided need be consistent and reliable especially for national healthcare telephone systems, and the response time of healthcare telephone switchboards need to be short. Girling (2000) showed that National Health Service (NHS) of the U.K. was criticized on the grounds that the services provided to patients were inconsistent and that there were some issues with the reliability of services. Silvestro and Silvestro (2003) argued that NHS cannot bring consistency to the overall system due to the highly decentralized nature of system. With the increased complexity and reduced flexibility, aligning the decentralized call centers with each other to provide consistent and reliable services throughout the U.K. becomes increasingly difficult and the corresponding costs are increasing. The response time of hospital switchboards is critical for the quality of services. Shokrollahi et al. (2008) studied the response time of various NHS hospital switchboards and demonstrated that a maximum threshold response time of 20 seconds is deemed to be satisfactory. It was noted that automated response systems usually cannot perform well in terms of the total response time. Instead, they delay callers talking to representatives and add the expense of callers with no significant gains. Meanwhile, in the literature, Ekeland pointed out that a significant number of studies (19 out of 80) found that some evidence on the effectiveness of telemedicine exists but additional research is required. Moreover, many studies indicate that although significant benefits of the telemedicine exist, full realization of those benefits is a complex tax due to nature of complex environment and unpredictable processes associated with the telemedicine (Ekeland et al., 2010). Additional action should be taken regarding establishing licensing requirements across the states and development of standards of care associated with the tele-health applications (Martin et al., 2013).

There are some initiatives that are being taken to decrease the variation in the quality of healthcare services provided to the patients nationwide. NHS is decentralized in terms of key service design characteristics. In order to provide a consistent yet reliable service throughout the nation, the standardization of design and implementation is important. Streamlining call center operations is an effective method to improve the overall telephone systems. Silvestro and Silvestro (2003) illustrated that some necessary steps should be taken to standardize the services provided to callers. Standardization is also a way to solve the capacity management of calls. If the operations of call centers are standardized, the calls from the centers with excessive load can be transferred to the other centers with less call demand. In addition, standardization can ensure the smooth flow of operations.

5.3 Incorporating Human Factors

Incorporating human factors into a healthcare telephone system is a natural consideration. Many operations in a telephone system such as arrivals, services and abandonment reflect human behaviors. The design of telephone systems requires an integrated view of both operational and psychological considerations. Routing decisions affect customer abandonment from queue, and impatience is a psychological process. The perception from a patient of service depends on his or her interaction with a customer service representative. Therefore, operating design must be based on a proper understanding of the patient psychology and the social interactions. The operations management with the incorporation of human factors opens up a vast agenda for optimizing the operations of healthcare telephone systems. Grosjean and De Weerdt (2005) presented an ergonomic evaluation for the effect of organizational control on operators' well-being in two call centers. Mahesh and Kasturi (2006) analyzed the important aspects of the call center agents' job and the relationships between these aspects and agent effectiveness as perceived by agents' supervisors. Their study can help managers to improve the agents' performance. Croidieu et al. (2008) sought to describe call-center working conditions and call-handlers' subjective experience of their work, and confirmed the high rate of psychosocial constraints for call-handlers. Weir and Waddington (2008) investigated the emotion work in an NHS call centre in the U.K. from the perspectives of organizational psychology and sociology. Black et al. (2009) conducted a customer satisfaction survey of verbal responses provided by a pharmaceutical company's third-party medical information (MI) call center. The completeness and understanding of the medical responses were rated high, and the callers were treated in the courteous manner. The working conditions are strongly associated with the quality level of the service provided to the patients in the clinical call center. Roing and Holmstrom (2015), based on an interview with the employees and managers, noted that stress, shiftwork, fatigue, multitasking, understaffing, and factors embedded in the system affect the malpractice claims in Swedish telenursing centers. The study indicates the importance of the overall organizational commitment for improving the level of the care for telehealth applications. Those organizational approaches and improvement programs are also important for creating conductive environment for the employees.

5.4 Operation Management Tools

The qualitative and quantitative approaches in the domains of operation management, industrial engineering, and engineering management are useful to improve the efficiency of healthcare telephone systems. Simulation and analytical modeling approaches such as queuing models have been widely adopted for call center operations, and the lean principles have been introduced to re-design the healthcare telephone systems as well. A simulation model can be used to generate the operation results under "what-if" scenarios. Comparison between the simulation results and actual operation can yield valuable information which may be used to identify the system inefficiencies. Simulation may also provide a solution to analyzing the integration of human factors and operations models. Green (2006) discussed about the queuing applications that might be used in healthcare settings especially in the call center for healthcare institutions. Anton et al. (2000) elaborated the role of simulation in the call center settings and argued that healthcare call centers might benefit from improving the operations. The concept of "lean" can be introduced to healthcare telephone systems. The primary goal of lean thinking is to eliminate wastes. Despite the fact that Lean concept is originally developed for the automotive industry where the production volume is high, it has been adopted and customized by other manufacturing companies as well as service organizations (Lander & Liker 2007). Waste of money, time, supplies, or goods will negatively influence the quality of services. The applications of lean thinking in healthcare telephone systems are demonstrating a positive impact on the timely delivery of services via telephones. Needless to say, improper lean implementation may result in poorer services (Sinaiko, 1999). The warning signs include inaccurate billing and medical records, patient complaints on the service received, and low employee morality. Kim et al. (2006) consider the cultural issue as a critical important challenge in lean health care. The individually functioning units and silos in a healthcare organization should cooperate to enhance the entire process flow, and the big improvements are obtainable through continuous small changes (Spears, 2005). Applying the operations management principles in the form of re-engineering also benefits the improvement of the existing services of the telephone response systems. In that vein, Rateb et al. (2011) documented that the effect of the re-engineering in the selected check-up centers for pre-employment purposes. Six randomly selected centers were evaluated for this purpose with the re-engineering activities focusing on three main areas, namely, structure, process and outcome. The authors indicated that significant improvements (around 65% reduction) in the cycle time, and amount of the delay per customer were realized. Similarly, discrete event simulation and process improvement can also help increase patient service performance. Rohleder et al. (2013) indicated that their improvement project in the medical call center led to significant reductions in the average answering-speed (ASA) and average abandonment rate (AAR). However, the authors cautioned that the major difficulty lies with the evaluating true impact of the improvement projects because there is no control group that can be benchmarked with for evaluating the true effect of the improvement projects. Shi et al. (2014) applied the approach of discrete event simulation to improve the performance of a mini call center at a Veterans Affairs medical center. The resource pooling scenarios were proposed, and they were verified to outperform the current operations by reducing abandonment rate and balancing the resource utilizations.

5.5 Outsourcing

The potential outsourcing of calls in a healthcare telephone system is one important aspect to increase the capacity of healthcare telephone systems. The outsourcing of operations in call centers to foreign locations has been attractive (Aron et al., 2005) although the outsourcing trend brings some concerns for customer retention and loyalty. For example, advanced telecommunications systems have enabled companies such as Microsoft, Oracle, Bank of America, American Express to outsource their customers support centers to off-shore locations such as India and Philippines. Similarly, there exists the possibility to outsource the operations of healthcare telephone systems to other locations or companies (or departments). Barr (1997) discussed the role of outsourcing as part of the vision for expansion and suggested that outsourcing some functions can improve the healthcare operations and provide additional growth opportunities. Poster (2007) discussed the reasons behind the "national identity management" in outsourcing decisions where the employees are asked to subsume different national identities as part of their work. The authors indicated that this approach might be the result of various reasons such as being a tool for easing the tension between customer-agent relationship or a deliberate attempt for controlling the customers of the call center. No matter what the actual reason is, the outlined policy might be seen as a consequence of easing the tension that might stem from cultural and language differences that would be inevitably encountered during the process of receiving the service in a transnational call center.

5.6 Performance Metrics

Developing performance metrics for tele-health are of great importance. Various researchers have employed different measures to evaluate the effectiveness of the tele-health and telephone response systems. George et al. (2008) and Hirsch et al. (2007) discussed the tele-nursing from the overreferral and underreferral rates. Both underreferral and overreferral deteriorate the quality of the healthcare delivery systems, put the callers into healthcare risks, and increase the burden on the emergency departments. They should be incorporated to assess the effectiveness of the tele-nursing. Meanwhile, some studies are directed to establishing the computer telephony from cost perspective (Franzini et al., 2001). Others investigated the effect of computer telephony on the no-show rates (Piette and Schilinger, 2007), drug treatment services (Alemi et. al., 1997), medication adherence (Friedman et al, 1997), vaccination rates (Oake et al., 2009), accuracy of tele-diagnosis practices (Oztas et. al, 2007), the response rate of the clinical study (Stewart et al., 2012) The effect of tele-consultation on the reduction of the use of clinic resources and potential savings are also studied (Zanaboni et al., 2009) as well as the duration of the time to speak a live agent in emergency departments (Shokrollahi et al., 2008).

However, since tele-health is an umbrella term for a variety of different functions, developing overall performance metrics for tele-health is extremely challenging if not technically impossible. However, it should be noted that there is a substantial need for developing more comprehensive index for assessing the quality of the healthcare services delivered by the telephone systems. For this purpose, some of the performance metrics discussed in Section 3 might be borrowed and combined with the performance measures that are described in this section to construct composite indices to reflect the efficiency and effectiveness of telephone systems from a larger perspective. To cite an instance, the caller waiting time might be combined with the under referral rate for a tele-nursing applications to assess the quality of the service. Not only it would furnish the system designers, developers and analysts a powerful tool for assessing the limitations and strengths of a telephone system, but also at the same time, it would promote the transparency and accountability in the telephone response system.

6. CONCLUSIVE REMARKS

The healthcare industry faces enormous challenges of curbing costs, improving the service quality and operation efficiency. From the perspective of improving service quality and operation efficiency, it should be noted that telephone operations might provide the way for enhancing the activities of the hospital operations and might provide the base for the cost reductions during the delivery of the healthcare services. The paper in that sense systematically reviews the research progress of healthcare telephone systems and analyzes the related challenges and opportunities.

It is noted that besides traditional operations, healthcare telephone systems are being expanded to include some advanced functions, such as tele-counseling, tele-nursing, and tele-triage. These functions might be associated with improving the service of the operations, and provide the ways for bringing cost effective solutions that might be used for streamlining the patients and corresponding activities. However, the difficulties in optimizing healthcare telephone systems are also evident as the functions and complexity of these systems keep increasing. The major challenges are the high patient expectations, the potential legal issues that might arise with the remote tele-health applications. Consistency and efficiency of the services, incorporating the human factors in the telephone systems are of great importance. The chapter addresses the challenges and identifies the opportunities to improve the telephone systems in healthcare. It is expected that in the future healthcare telephone systems can serve as a better communication tool to help patients access more resources, and to assist nurses and providers to provide quality services. The lean concepts might be further applied for improving the telephone related services. The telephone system might provide a supporting role for transforming the healthcare institutions for embracing the new concepts such as the patient centered medical home and personalized care.

The recent advances in the sensor technology, miniaturization of the electronic devices, information technology, and the mobile health platforms are immensely affecting and reshaping the role of telephone systems in the healthcare industry. The telephone systems rather than being obsolete in the face of changing paradigms, play more supportive roles, and should be considered an indispensable tool for improving the access of the patients for healthcare services, and increasing the quality of the care. However, the seamless integration of the telephone systems with the rapidly developing information technology is far from being complete and additional research is called for. The telephone systems is also benefitting from the advances in related software and hardware. Those tools are viable for enriching the communication with patients due to the nature of the service and the unique expectation and needs of patients.

REFERENCES

Abu-Hasaballah, K., James, A., & Aseltine, R. H. Jr. (2007). Lessons and pitfalls of interactive voice response in medical research. *Contemporary Clinical Trials*, *28*(5), 593–602. doi:10.1016/j.cct.2007.02.007 PMID:17400520

Adewale, O. S. (2004). An Internet-based telemedicine system in Nigeria. *International Journal of Information Management*, *24*(3), 221–234. doi:10.1016/j.ijinfomgt.2003.12.014

Adler-Milstein, J., & Bates, D. W. (2010). Paperless healthcare: Progress and challenges of an IT-enabled healthcare system. *Business Horizons*, *53*(2), 119–130. doi:10.1016/j.bushor.2009.10.004

Alemagno, S. A., Cochran, D., Feucht, T. E., Stephens, R. C., Butts, J. M., & Wolfe, S. A. (1996). Assessing substance abuse treatment needs among the homeless: A telephone-based interactive voice response system. *American Journal of Public Health, 86*(11), 1626–1628. doi:10.2105/AJPH.86.11.1626 PMID:8916533

Alemi, F., Stephens, R. C., Javalghi, R. G., Dyches, H., Butts, J., & Ghadiri, A. (1996). A randomized trial of a telecommunications network for pregnant women who use cocaine. *Medical Care, 34*(suppl 10), OS10–OS20. doi:10.1097/00005650-199610003-00002 PMID:8843933

Alizadeh, R., Panahi, F., Saghafinia, M., Alizadeh, K., Barakati, N., & Khaje-Daloee, M. (2012). Impact of Trauma Dispatch Algorithm Software on the Rate of Missions of Emergency Medical Services. *Trauma Monthly, 17*(3), 319–322. doi:10.5812/traumamon.6341 PMID:24350116

Allen, S. I. (1969). The telephone as a computer input-output terminal for medical information. *Journal of the American Medical Association, 208*(4), 673–679. doi:10.1001/jama.1969.03160040081012 PMID:5818568

Allen-Davis, J. T., Beck, A., Parker, R., Ellis, J. L., & Polley, D. (2002). Assessment of vulvovaginal complaints: Accuracy of telephone triage and in-office diagnosis. *Obstetrics and Gynecology, 99*(1), 18–22. doi:10.1016/S0029-7844(01)01670-2 PMID:11777504

American Telemedicine Association. (n.d.). *What is Telemedicine & Telehealth*. Retrieved from; http://www.americantelemed.org/files/public/abouttelemedicine/What_Is_Telemedicine.pdf

Anderson, M. M., Boly, L. D., & Deck, R. W. (1996). Remote clinic/patient monitoring for multicenter trials. *Controlled Clinical Trials, 17*(5), 407–414. doi:10.1016/S0197-2456(96)00021-9 PMID:8932973

Anton, J. (2000). The past, present and future of customer access centers. *International Journal of Service Industry Management, 11*(2), 120–130. doi:10.1108/09564230010323534

Arnaert, A., & Macfarlane, F. (2011). Telehealth Nursing in Canada: Opportunities for Nurses to Shape the Future. In Telenursing (pp. 29-45). Springer London.

Aron, R., Clemons, E. K., & Reddi, S. (2005). Just right outsourcing: Understanding and managing risk. *Journal of Management Information Systems, 22*(2), 37–55.

Artalejo, J. R., Economou, A., & Corral, A. G. (2007). Applications of Maximum Queue Length for Call Center Management. *Computers & Operations Research, 34*(4), 983–996. doi:10.1016/j.cor.2005.05.020

Auger, C., Forster, A. J., Oake, N., & Tamblyn, R. (2013). Usability of a computerised drug monitoring programme to detect adverse drug events and non-compliance in outpatient ambulatory care. *BMJ Quality & Safety*, *22*(4), 306–316. doi:10.1136/bmjqs-2012-001492 PMID:23396853

Balas, E. A., Jaffrey, F., Kuperman, G. J., Boren, S. A., Brown, G. D., Pinciroli, F., & Mitchell, J. A. (1997). Electronic communication with patients. Evaluation of distance medicine technology. *Journal of the American Medical Association*, *278*(2), 152–159. doi:10.1001/jama.1997.03550020084043 PMID:9214532

Ball, M. J., & Lillis, J. (2001). E-health: transforming the physician: patient relationship. *International Journal of Medical Informatics*, *61*(1), 1–10. doi:10.1016/S1386-5056(00)00130-1 PMID:11248599

Barlow, J., Bayer, S., & Curry, R. (2006). Implementing complex innovations in fluid multi-stakeholder environments: Experiences of 'telecare'. *Technovation*, *26*(3), 396–406. doi:10.1016/j.technovation.2005.06.010

Barr, J. L., Laufenberg, S., & Sieckman, B. L. (1997). Creating a vision for your medical call center. *Healthcare Information Management: Journal of the Healthcare Information and Management Systems Society of the American Hospital Association, 12*(2), 71-85.

Beaulieu, R., & Humphreys, J. (2008). Evaluation of a telephone advice nurse in a nursing faculty managed pediatric community clinic. *Journal of Pediatric Health Care*, *22*(3), 175–181. doi:10.1016/j.pedhc.2007.05.006 PMID:18455066

Berman, A. H., Farzanfar, R., Kristiansson, M., Carlbring, P., & Friedman, R. H. (2012). Design and development of a telephone-linked care (TLC) system to reduce impulsivity among violent forensic outpatients and probationers. *Journal of Medical Systems*, *36*(3), 1031–1042. doi:10.1007/s10916-010-9565-1 PMID:20721686

Berner, E. S., Ray, M. N., Panjamapirom, A., Maisiak, R. S., Willig, J. H., English, T. M., & Schiff, G. D. et al. (2014). Exploration of an automated approach for receiving feedback after outpatient acute care visits. *Journal of General Internal Medicine*, *29*(8), 1105–1112. doi:10.1007/s11606-014-2783-3 PMID:24610308

Biem, H. J., Klimaszewski, A., & Florence, C. (2004). Computer Telephony in Healthcare. *ElectronicHealthcare*, *3*(2), 80–86. PMID:15540408

Biem, H. J., Turnell, R. W., & D'Arcy, C. (2003). Computer telephony: Automated calls for medical care. *Canadian Medical Association*, *26*(5), 259–268. PMID:14596488

Black, P., Marsh, C., & Ashworth, L. (2009). Assessment of customer satisfaction with verbal responses provided by a pharmaceutical company's third-party medical information call center. *Drug Information Journal*, *43*(3), 263–271.

Boulos, M. N., Wheeler, S., Tavares, C., & Jones, R. (2011). How smartphones are changing the face of mobile and participatory healthcare: An overview, with example from eCAALYX. *Biomedical Engineering Online*, *10*(1), 24. PMID:21466669

Breslin, E., & Denison, J. (2002). The development of telephone triage: Historical, professional and personal perspectives. *Journal of Orthopaedic Nursing*, *6*(4), 191–197. doi:10.1016/S1361-3111(02)00070-5

Briggs, J. K. (2007). *Telephone triage practices for nurses*. Lippincott Williams & Wilkins.

Bunik, M., Glazner, J. E., Chandramouli, V., Emsermann, C. B., Hegarty, T., & Kempe, A. (2007). Pediatric Telephone Call Centers: How do they affect health care use and costs? *Pediatrics*, *119*(2), 305–313. doi:10.1542/peds.2006-1511 PMID:17272593

Bunn, F., Byrne, G., & Kendall, S. (2005). The effects of telephone consultation and triage on healthcare use and patient satisfaction: A systematic review. *The British Journal of General Practice*, *55*(521), 956–961. PMID:16378566

Burney, A., Abbas, Z., Mahmood, N., & Arifeen, Q. U. (2013). Prospects for mobile health in Pakistan and other developing countries. *Advances in Internet of Things*, *3*(022A), 27–32. doi:10.4236/ait.2013.32A004

Cantu, R. V., Bell, J. E., Padula, W. V., Nahikian, K. R., & Pober, D. M. (2012). How do emergency department physicians rate their orthopaedic on-call coverage? *Journal of Orthopaedic Trauma*, *26*(1), 54–56. doi:10.1097/BOT.0b013e31821d7a81 PMID:21904223

Cassimatis, M., & Kavanagh, D. J. (2012). Effects of type 2 diabetes behavioural telehealth interventions on glycaemic control and adherence: A systematic review. *Journal of Telemedicine and Telecare*, *18*(8), 447–450. doi:10.1258/jtt.2012.GTH105 PMID:23209266

Castelnuovo, G., Manzoni, G. M., Corti, S., Cuzziol, P., Villa, V., & Molinari, E. (2011). Clinical psychology and medicine for the treatment of obesity in out-patient settings: the TECNOB project. *Telemedicine Techniques and Applications*, 257-268.

Chanda, K. L., & Shaw, J. G. (2010). The development of telehealth as a strategy to improve health care services in Zambia. *Health Information and Libraries Journal*, *27*(2), 133–139. doi:10.1111/j.1471-1842.2010.00876.x PMID:20565554

Coiera, E. (2006). Communication systems in healthcare. *The Clinical Biochemist. Reviews / Australian Association of Clinical Biochemists*, *27*(2), 89. PMID:17077879

Coile, R. C. Jr. (1999). Call centers: Phone lines, protocols, and patient care management in the 21st century. *Russ Coile's Health Trends*, *11*(5), 1–4. PMID:10351310

Corkrey, R., & Parkinson, L. (2002). Interactive voice response: Review of studies 1989–2000. *Behavior Research Methods, Instruments, & Computers*, *34*(3), 342–353. doi:10.3758/BF03195462 PMID:12395550

Croidieu, S., Charbotel, B., Vohito, M., Renaud, L., Jaussaud, J., Bourboul, C., & Bergeret, A. et al. (2008). Call-handlers' working conditions and their subjective experience of work: A transversal study. *International Archives of Occupational and Environmental Health*, *82*(1), 67–77. doi:10.1007/s00420-008-0308-2 PMID:18320205

Crouch, R., Patel, A., & Dale, J. (1996). Paediatric calls to inner city accident and emergency department: Service demand and advice given. *Accident and Emergency Nursing*, *4*(4), 170–174. doi:10.1016/S0965-2302(96)90072-7 PMID:8981836

Dale, J., Crouch, R., & Lloyd, D. (1998). Primary care: Nurse-led telephone triage and advice out of hours. *Nursing Standard*, *12*(47), 41–45. doi:10.7748/ns1998.08.12.47.39.c2520 PMID:9752159

Darkins, A. W., & Carry, M. A. (2000). *Telemedicine and telehealth. Principles, policies, performance and pitfalls*. Springer Publishing Company.

Delichatsios, H. K., Friedman, R. H., Glanz, K., Tennstedt, S., Smigelski, C., Pinto, B. M., & Killman, M. W. et al. (2001). Randomized trial of a talking computer to improve adults eating habits. *American Journal of Health Promotion*, *15*(4), 215–224. doi:10.4278/0890-1171-15.4.215 PMID:11349340

Deslauriers, A., L'Ecuyer, P., Pichitlamken, J., Ingolfsson, A., & Avramidis, A. N. (2007). Markov chain models of a telephone call center with call blending. *Computers & Operations Research*, *34*(6), 1616–1645. doi:10.1016/j.cor.2005.06.019

DeVore, N. E. (1999). Telephone triage: A challenge for practicing midwives. *Journal of Nurse-Midwifery*, *44*(5), 471–479. doi:10.1016/S0091-2182(99)00087-7 PMID:10540521

Dini, E. F., Wilkins, R. W., & Sigafoos, J. (2000). The impact of computer-generated messages on childhood immunization coverage. *American Journal of Preventive Medicine*, *18*(2), 132–139. doi:10.1016/S0749-3797(99)00086-0 PMID:10698243

Duder, J. C., & Rosenwein, M. B. (2001). Towards "zero abandonments" in call center performance. *European Journal of Operational Research, 135*(1), 50–56. doi:10.1016/S0377-2217(00)00289-7

Ekeland, A. G., Bowes, A., & Flottorp, S. (2010). Effectiveness of telemedicine: A systematic review of reviews. *International Journal of Medical Informatics, 79*(11), 736–771. doi:10.1016/j.ijmedinf.2010.08.006 PMID:20884286

Ertogral, K., & Bamuqabel, B. (2008). Developing staff schedules for a bilingual telecommunication call center with flexible workers. *Computers & Industrial Engineering, 54*(1), 118–127. doi:10.1016/j.cie.2007.06.040

Evenson, A., Harker, P. T., & Frei, F. X. (1999). *Effective Call Center Management: Evidence from Financial Services.* Working Paper 9925B. Wharton Financial Institutions Center.

Executive, N. H. S. (1999). Quality and Performance in the NHS: Clinical Indicators. Author.

Federspiel, C. C., Fisk, W. J., Price, P. N., Liu, G., Faulkner, D., Dibartolemeo, D. L., & Lahiff, M. et al. (2004). Worker performance and ventilation in a call center: Analyses of work performance data for registered nurses. *Indoor Air, 14*(s8), 41–50. doi:10.1111/j.1600-0668.2004.00299.x PMID:15663459

Feldman-Naim, S., Myers, F. S., Clark, C. H., Turner, E. H., & Leibenluft, E. (1997). Agreement between face-to-face and telephone-administered mood ratings in patients with rapid cycling bipolar disorder. *Psychological Research, 71*, 129–132. PMID:9255857

Franzini, L., Rosenthal, J., Spears, W., Martin, H. S., Balderas, L., Brown, M., & Hanson, C. et al. (2000). Cost effectiveness of childhood immunization reminder/recall systems in urban private practices. *Pediatrics, 166*, 177–183. PMID:10888689

Friedman, R. H., Kazis, L. E., & Jette, A. (1996). A telecommunications system with monitoring and counseling patients with hypertension. Impact on medication adherence and blood pressure control. *American Journal of Hypertension, 9*(4 pt 1), 285–292. doi:10.1016/0895-7061(95)00353-3 PMID:8722429

Fuchsia Howard, A., Smillie, K., Turnbull, K., Zirul, C., Munroe, D., Ward, A., & Olson, R. et al. (2014). Access to Medical and Supportive Care for Rural and Remote Cancer Survivors in Northern British Columbia. *The Journal of Rural Health, 30*(3), 311–321. doi:10.1111/jrh.12064 PMID:24483272

Ganapathy, K., & Ravindra, A. (2011). Telenursing in an emerging economy: An overview. In Telenursing (pp. 47-59). Springer London.

Garnet, O., Mandelbaum, A., & Reiman, M. (2002). Designing a call center with impatient customers. *Manufacturing & Service Operations Management*, *4*(3), 208–227. doi:10.1287/msom.4.3.208.7753

George, I. S. T., Cullen, M., Gardiner, L., Karabatsos, G., Ng, J. Y.-K., Patterson, A., & Wilson, A. (2007). Universal telenursing triage in Australia and New Zealand. *Australian Family Physician*, *37*(6), 476–479. PMID:18523705

Ghorai, K., Akter, S., Khatun, F., & Ray, P. (2014). mHealth for Smoking Cessation Programs: A Systematic Review. *Journal of Personalized Medicine*, *4*(3), 412–423. doi:10.3390/jpm4030412 PMID:25563359

Gilmour, M. B. (2001). A model for a telephone response system to disaster and trauma. *Traumatology*, *6*(3), 120–125. doi:10.1177/153476560100700304

Girling, D. (2000). Important issues in planning and conducting multi-centre randomised trials in cancer and publishing their results. *Critical Reviews in Oncology/Hematology*, *36*(1), 13–25. doi:10.1016/S1040-8428(00)00095-0 PMID:10996520

Gottesman, O., Kuivaniemi, H., Tromp, G., Faucett, W. A., Li, R., Manolio, T. A., & …, eMERGE Network, T. (2013). The Electronic Medical Records and Genomics (eMERGE) network: Past, present, and future. *Genetics in Medicine*, *15*(10), 761–771. PMID:23743551

Graham, J., Tomcavage, J., Salek, D., Sciandra, J., Davis, D. E., & Stewart, W. F. (2012). Postdischarge monitoring using interactive voice response system reduces 30-day readmission rates in a case-managed Medicare population. *Medical Care*, *50*(1), 50–57. doi:10.1097/MLR.0b013e318229433e PMID:21822152

Green, L. (2006). Queueing analysis in healthcare. In Patient flow: Reducing delay in healthcare delivery (pp. 281-307). Springer US. doi:10.1007/978-0-387-33636-7_10

Gregoski, M. J., Mueller, M., Vertegel, A., Shaporev, A., Jackson, B. B., Frenzel, R. M., & Treiber, F. A. et al. (2012). Development and validation of a smartphone heart rate acquisition application for health promotion and wellness telehealth applications. *International Journal of Telemedicine and Applications*, *2012*, 696324. PMID:22272197

Grigsby, J., & Sanders, J. H. (1998). Telemedicine: Where it is and where it's going. *Annals of Internal Medicine*, *129*(2), 123–127. doi:10.7326/0003-4819-129-2-199807150-00012 PMID:9669971

Grosjean, V., & De Weerdt, C. R. V. (2005). Towards a psycho-ergonomics study of wellbeing and emotions: The effects of organisational control in call centers. *Le Travail Humain*, *68*(4), 355–378. doi:10.3917/th.684.0355

Haghighat, S., Yunesian, M., Akbari, M. E., Ansari, M., & Montezari, A. (2007). Telephone and face-to-face consultation in breast cancer diagnosis: A comparative study. *Patient Education and Counseling*, *67*(1-2), 39–43. doi:10.1016/j.pec.2007.01.015 PMID:17467949

Hall, V., Gomez, C., & Fernandez-Llimos, F. (2006). Situation of drug information centers and services in Costa Rica. *Pharmacy Practice*, *4*(2), 83–87. PMID:25246999

Hamill, C. T., & Lorri, H.-S. (1998). 24-hour call centers and home health care. *Home Care Provider*, *3*(6), 324–325. doi:10.1016/S1084-628X(98)90012-0 PMID:10030213

Heschong Mahone Group. (2003). *Windows and offices: A study of office workers performance and the indoor environment*. California Energy Commission. Retrieved from http://www.ecw.org/sites/default/files/HMG_Windows_Offices.pdf

Heyworth, L., Kleinman, K., Oddleifson, S., Bernstein, L., Frampton, J., Lehrer, M., & Connelly, M. (2014). Comparison of interactive voice response, patient mailing, and mailed registry to encourage screening for osteoporosis: A randomized controlled trial. *Osteoporosis International*, *25*(5), 1519–1526. doi:10.1007/s00198-014-2629-1 PMID:24566584

Hill, J. W., & Powell, P. (2009). The national healthcare crisis: Is eHealth a key solution? *Business Horizons*, *52*(3), 265–277. doi:10.1016/j.bushor.2009.01.006

Hirsh, D. A., Massey, R., Simon, J., & Simon, H. (2004). Does use of a pediatric telephone triage system lead to appropriate pediatric ED utilization? *Pediatric Research*, *55*, 120A.

Hirsh, D. A., Simon, H. K., Massey, R., Thomton, L., & Simon, J. E. (2007). The Host Hospital 24-Hour Underreferral Rate: An Automated Measure of Call-Center Safety. *Pediatrics*, *119*(6), 1139–1144. doi:10.1542/peds.2006-1986 PMID:17545381

Hogan, T. P., Wakefield, B., Nazi, K. M., Houston, T. K., & Weaver, F. M. (2011). Promoting access through complementary eHealth technologies: Recommendations for VA's Home Telehealth and personal health record programs. *Journal of General Internal Medicine*, *26*(2), 628–635. doi:10.1007/s11606-011-1765-y PMID:21989614

Horton, R. C., Minniti, A., Mireylees, S., & McEntegart, D. (2008). A randomized trial to determine the impact on compliance of a psychophysical peripheral cue based on the Elaboration Likelihood Model. *Contemporary Clinical Trials*, *29*(6), 823–828. doi:10.1016/j.cct.2008.08.005 PMID:18805509

Hsu, M. H., Chu, T. B., Yen, J. C., Chiu, W. T., Yeh, G. C., Chen, T. J., & Li, Y. C. J. (2010). Development and implementation of a national telehealth project for long-term care: A preliminary study. *Computer Methods and Programs in Biomedicine*, *97*(3), 286–292. doi:10.1016/j.cmpb.2009.12.008 PMID:20092907

Hyman, D. J., Ho, K. S., Dunn, J. K., & Simons-Morton, D. (1998). Dietary intervention for cholesterol reduction in public clinic patients. *American Journal of Preventive Medicine*, *15*(2), 139–145. doi:10.1016/S0749-3797(98)00038-5 PMID:9713670

Isenberg, S. F., Davis, C. L., Adams, C. E., Isenberg, J. S., & Isenberg, M. A. (2001). Incentivized Digital Outcomes Collection. *American Journal of Medical Quality*, *16*(6), 202–211. doi:10.1177/106286060101600604 PMID:11816851

Jack, E. P., Bedics, T. A., & McCary, C. E. (2006). Operational challenges in the call center industry: A case study and resource-based framework. *Managing Service Quality*, *16*(5), 477–500. doi:10.1108/09604520610686142

Joshi, A., Rane, M., Roy, D., Emmadi, N., Srinivasan, P., Kumarasamy, N., & Rutten, R. et al. (2014, April). Supporting treatment of people living with HIV/AIDS in resource limited settings with IVRs. In *Proceedings of the 32nd annual ACM conference on Human Factors in Computing Systems* (pp. 1595-1604). ACM. doi:10.1145/2556288.2557236

Jouini, O., Koole, G., & Roubos, A. (2013). Performance indicators for call centers with impatient customers. *IIE Transactions*, *45*(3), 341–354. doi:10.1080/0740817X.2012.712241

Kamei, T., Yamamoto, Y., Kajii, F., Nakayama, Y., & Kawakami, C. (2013). Systematic review and meta-analysis of studies involving telehome monitoring-based telenursing for patients with chronic obstructive pulmonary disease. *Japan Journal of Nursing Science*, *10*(2), 180–192. doi:10.1111/j.1742-7924.2012.00228.x PMID:24373441

Kathryn, A., Cull, A., & Sharpe, M. (2003). Diagnosing medical depression in medical outpatient: Acceptability of telephone interviews. *Journal of Psychosomatic Research*, *55*(4), 385–387. doi:10.1016/S0022-3999(02)00637-2 PMID:14507551

Kempe, A., Bunik, M., Ellis, J., Magid, D., Hegarty, T., Dickinson, L. M., & Steiner, J. F. (2006). How safe is triage by an after-hours telephone call center? *Pediatrics*, *118*(2), 457–463. doi:10.1542/peds.2005-3073 PMID:16882795

Kempe, A., Dempsey, C., Hegarty, T., Frei, N., Chandramouli, V., & Poole, S. R. (2000a). Reducing after-hours referrals by an after-hours call center with second-level physician triage. *Pediatrics*, *106*(1), 226–230. PMID:10888697

Kempe, A., Dempsey, C., Whitefield, C., Bothner, T., Mackenzie, T., & Poole, S. (2000b). Appropriateness of urgent referrals by nurses at a hospital-based pediatric call center. *Archives of Pediatrics & Adolescent Medicine*, *154*(4), 355–360. doi:10.1001/archpedi.154.4.355 PMID:10768672

Kempe, A., Luberti, A. A., Hertz, A. R., Sherman, H. B., Amin, H. B., Dempsey, C., & Hegarthy, T. W. et al. (2001). Delivery of pediatric after-hours care by call centers: A multicenter study of parental perceptions and compliance. *Pediatrics*, *108*(6), 111–117. doi:10.1542/peds.108.6.e111 PMID:11731638

Khamis, A.-H., James, A., & Aseltine, R. H. (2007). Lessons and pitfalls of interactive voice response in medical research. *Contemporary Clinical Trials*, *28*(5), 593–602. doi:10.1016/j.cct.2007.02.007 PMID:17400520

Kidd, L., Cayless, S., Johnston, B., & Wengstrom, Y. (2010). Telehealth in palliative care in the UK: A review of the evidence. *Journal of Telemedicine and Telecare*, *16*(7), 394–402. PMID:20813893

Kim, C. S., Spahlinger, D. A., Kin, J. M., & Billi, J. E. (2006). Lean health care: What can hospitals learn from a world-class automaker? *Journal of Hospital Medicine*, *1*(3), 191–199. doi:10.1002/jhm.68 PMID:17219493

Kim, H., Bracha, A., & Tipnis, A. (2007). Automated depression screening in disadvantaged pregnant women in an urban obstetric clinic. *Archives of Women's Mental Health*, *10*(4), 163–169. doi:10.1007/s00737-007-0189-5 PMID:17593320

Koch, S. (2006). Home telehealth-Current state and future trends. *International Journal of Medical Informatics*, *75*(8), 565–576. doi:10.1016/j.ijmedinf.2005.09.002 PMID:16298545

Korcz, I. P., & Moreland, S. (1998). Telephone prescreening: Enhancing a model for proactive healthcare practice. *Cancer Practice*, *6*(5), 270–275. doi:10.1046/j.1523-5394.1998.00021.x PMID:9767345

Kwan, S. K., Davis, M. M., & Greenwood, A. G. (1988). A simulation model for determining variable worker requirements in a service operation with time-dependent customer demand. *Queueing Systems*, *3*(3), 265–276. doi:10.1007/BF01161218

Lander, E., & Liker, J. K. (2007). The Toyota production system and art: Making highly customized and creative products the Toyota way. *International Journal of Production Research*, *45*(16), 3681–3698. doi:10.1080/00207540701223519

Lee, H., Friedman, M. E., Cukor, P., & Ahern, D. (2003). Interactive Voice Response System (IVRS) in Health Care Services. *Nursing Outlook*, *51*(6), 277–283. doi:10.1016/S0029-6554(03)00161-1 PMID:14688763

Lee, H. J., Lee, S. H., Ha, K.-S., Jang, H. C., Chung, H. C., Kim, H. C., & Yoo, D. H. et al. (2009). Ubiquitous healthcare service using Zigbee and mobile phone for elderly patients. *International Journal of Medical Informatics*, *78*(3), 193–198. doi:10.1016/j.ijmedinf.2008.07.005 PMID:18760959

Lee, T. J., Baraff, L. J., Guzy, J., Johnson, D., & Woo, H. (2003b). Does telephone triage delay significant medical treatment? *Archives of Pediatrics & Adolescent Medicine*, *157*(7), 635–641. doi:10.1001/archpedi.157.7.635 PMID:12860783

Lenz, R., & Manfred, R. (2006). IT support for healthcare processes– premises, challenges, perspectives. *Data & Knowledge Engineering*, *61*(1), 39–58. doi:10.1016/j.datak.2006.04.007

Leydon, G. M., Ekberg, K., Kelly, M., & Drew, P. (2013). Improving ethnic monitoring for telephone-based healthcare: A conversation analytic study. *BMJ Open*, *3*(6e002676), 1–7. doi:10.1136/bmjopen-2013-002676 PMID:23811170

Lin, C. W., Pan, C. J., Paranjape, K., Yu, C., & Feng, P. (2014). Taipei Citizen Telecare Service System for Hypertension Management in Elders. In *2014 Annual SRII Global Conference (SRII)* (pp. 157-180). IEEE.

Lindsay, J. A., Minard, C. G., Hudson, S., Green, C. E., & Schmitz, J. M. (2014). Using prize-based incentives to enhance daily interactive voice response (IVR) compliance: A feasibility study. *Journal of Substance Abuse Treatment*, *46*(1), 74–77. doi:10.1016/j.jsat.2013.08.003 PMID:24029622

Mahesh, V. S., & Kasturi, A. (2006). Improving call centre agent performance - A UK-India study based on the agents' point of view. *International Journal of Service Industry Management*, *17*(2), 136–157. doi:10.1108/09564230610656971

Mariño, R., Clarke, K., Manton, D. J., Stranieri, A., Collmann, R., Kellet, H., & Borda, A. (2015). Teleconsultation and Telediagnosis for Oral Health Assessment: An Australian Perspective. In Teledentistry (pp. 101-112). Springer International Publishing.

Martin, A. C. (2013). Legal, clinical, and ethical issues in teletherapy.*Psychoanalysis Online: Mental Health, Teletherapy, and Training*, 75.

McBride, C. M., & Rimer, B. K. (1999). Using the telephone to improve health behavior and health service delivery. *Patient Education and Counseling*, *37*(1), 3–18. doi:10.1016/S0738-3991(98)00098-6 PMID:10640115

McConnell, K. J., Johnson, L. A., Arab, N., Richards, C. F., Newgard, C. D., & Edlund, T. (2007). The on-call crisis: A statewide assessment of the costs of providing on-call specialist coverage. *Annals of Emergency Medicine*, *49*(6), 727–733. doi:10.1016/j.annemergmed.2006.10.017 PMID:17210209

McDaniel, J. G. (1995). Discrete event simulation of a wide area health care network. *Journal of the American Medical Informatics Association*, *2*(4), 220–237. doi:10.1136/jamia.1995.96010391 PMID:7583646

McKinstry, B., Walker, J., Campbell, C., Heaney, D., & Wyke, S. (2002). Telephone consultations to manage requests for same-day appointments: A randomized controlled trial in two practices. *The British Journal of General Practice*, *52*(477), 306–310. PMID:11942448

McNall, L. A., & Roch, S. G. (2009). A social exchange model of employee reactions to electronic performance monitoring. *Human Performance*, *22*(3), 204–224. doi:10.1080/08959280902970385

McNemish, J., Lyle, D., McCowan, M., Emmerson, S., McAuley, S., & Reilly, J. (2007). Post-discharge surgical site infection surveillance by automated telephony. *Journal of Hospital Telephony*, *66*(3), 232–236. doi:10.1016/j.jhin.2007.04.003 PMID:17544545

Miciak, A., & Desmarais, M. (2001). Benchmarking service quality performance at business-to-business and business-to-consumer call centers. *Journal of Business and Industrial Marketing*, *16*(5), 340–353. doi:10.1108/08858620110400205

Miller, D. I., Bruce, H., Gagnon, M., Talbot, V., & Messier, C. (2011). Improving older adults' experience with interactive voice response systems. *Telemedicine Journal and e-Health*, *17*(6), 452–455. doi:10.1089/tmj.2010.0204 PMID:21631386

Mohan, J., Razali, R., & Yaacob, R. (2003). The Malaysian telehealth flagship application: A national approach to health data protection and utilisation and consumer rights. *International Journal of Medical Informatics*, *73*(3), 217–227. doi:10.1016/j.ijmedinf.2003.11.023 PMID:15066550

Mohanty, S. A., Donna, L., Washington, S., Lambe, S., Fink, A., & Asch, S. M. (2006). Predictors of on-call specialist response times in California emergency departments. *Academic Emergency Medicine*, *13*(5), 505–512. doi:10.1111/j.1553-2712.2006.tb01000.x PMID:16609102

Moran, M. (2014). Rule change on emergency care could reduce specialty coverage. *Psychiatr News, 38*, 10-28. Retrieved from http://pn.psychiatryonline.org/cgi/content/full/38/22/10?etoc

Morrissey, J. (1999). FHS hooks up with Access Health Group. Calif. HMO will outsource its telephone medical advice services to Colo. Company. *Modern Healthcare*, *29*(4), 36. PMID:10345464

Morton, J. M., Baker, C. C., Farrell, T. M., Yohe, M. H., Kimple, R. J., Herman, D. C., & Meyer, A. et al. (2004). What do surgery residents do on their call nights? *American Journal of Surgery*, *188*(3), 225–229. doi:10.1016/j.amjsurg.2004.06.011 PMID:15450824

Muir, J., Xu, C., Paul, S., Staib, A., McNeill, I., Singh, P., & Sinnott, M. (2011). Incorporating teledermatology into emergency medicine. *Emergency Medicine Australasia*, *23*(5), 562–568. doi:10.1111/j.1742-6723.2011.01443.x PMID:21995470

Mundt, J. C., Katzelnick, D. J., Kennedy, S. H., Eisfeld, B. S., Bouffard, B. B., & Greist, J. H. (2006). Validation of an IVRS version of the MADRS. *Journal of Psychiatric Research*, *40*(3), 243–246. doi:10.1016/j.jpsychires.2005.05.002 PMID:15979643

Narayan, M. C. (2001). Oasis Voice Mailbox InServices. *Home Healthcare Nurse*, *19*(9), 542–548. doi:10.1097/00004045-200109000-00011 PMID:11982193

Nicholls, W. L. (1988). Computer-assisted telephone interviewing: A general introduction. In R. M. Groves, P. P. Biemer, L. E. Lyberg, J. T. Massey, W. L. Nicholls, & J. Waksberg (Eds.), *Telephone Survey Methodology* (pp. 377–385). New York: Wiley.

O'Brien, J. A., Ward, A. J., Jones, M. K. C., McMillan, C., & Lordan, L. (2003). Utilization of health care services by patients with chronic obstructive pulmonary disease. *Respiratory Medicine*, *97*(S1), S53–S58. doi:10.1016/S0954-6111(03)80015-X PMID:12564611

Oake, N., Jennings, A., van Walrayen, C., & Forster, A. J. (2009). Interactive Voice Response Systems for Improving Delivery of Ambulatory Care. *The American Journal of Managed Care*, *15*(6), 283–291. PMID:19514804

Oztas, M. O., Calikoglu, E., Baz, K., Birol, A., Onder, M., Calikoglu, T., & Kitapci, M. T. (2004). Reliability of Web-based teledermatology consultations. *Journal of Telemedicine and Telecare*, *10*(1), 25–28. doi:10.1258/135763304322764158 PMID:15006212

Petersen, J. A., Mackel, R., Antonsen, K., & Rasmussen, L. S. (2014). Serious adverse events in a hospital using *early warning score*–What went wrong? *Resuscitation, 85*(12), 1699–1703. doi:10.1016/j.resuscitation.2014.08.037 PMID:25238741

Piette, J. D. (2000). Perceived Access Problems among patients with diabetes in two public systems of care. *Journal of General Internal Medicine, 15*(11), 797–804. doi:10.1046/j.1525-1497.2000.91107.x PMID:11119172

Piette, J. D., & Schilinger, D. (2007). *Medical management of vulnerable and underserved patients. Principles, practices and populations. Mc* Graw Hill Companies.

Pike, J. H. (2003). Nature of After-Hours Calls at a Tertiary-Level Rehabilitation Center. *Archives of Physical Medicine and Rehabilitation, 84*(7), 1039–1042. doi:10.1016/S0003-9993(03)00028-5 PMID:12881831

Pinto, B. M., Friedman, R., Marcus, B. H., Kelley, H., Tennstedt, S., & Gillman, M. W. (2002). Effects of a computer based telephone-counseling system on physical activity. *American Journal of Preventive Medicine, 23*(2), 113–120. doi:10.1016/S0749-3797(02)00441-5 PMID:12121799

Pohjanoksa-Mantyla, M. K., Antila, J., Eerikainen, S., Enakoski, M., Hannuksela, O., Pietila, K., & Airaksinen, M. (2008). Utilization of a community pharmacy-operated national drug information call center in Finland. *Research in Social & Administrative Pharmacy, 4*(2), 144–152. doi:10.1016/j.sapharm.2007.05.001 PMID:18555967

Poole, S. R., Schmitt, B. D., Carruth, T., Peterson-Smith, A., & Slusarski, M. (1993). After-hours telephone coverage: The application of an area-wide telephone triage and advice system for pediatric practices. *Pediatrics, 92*(5), 670–679. PMID:8414853

Poster, W. R. (2007). Who's On the Line? Indian Call Center Agents Pose as Americans for US-Outsourced Firms. *Industrial Relations, 46*(2), 271–304. doi:10.1111/j.1468-232X.2007.00468.x

Prasad, M. K. S., Mahmood, S., Gregson, B. A., & Mitchell, P. (2012). Telephone logs of neurosurgery specialty trainees: A time study. *British Journal of Neurosurgery, 26*(2), 195–198. doi:10.3109/02688697.2011.633643 PMID:22149539

Pratt, S. I., Naslund, J. A., Wolfe, R. S., Santos, M., & Bartels, S. J. (2014). Automated telehealth for managing psychiatric instability in people with serious mental illness. *Journal of Mental Health*, 1-5.

Prince, S. B., & Herrin, D. M. (2007). The role of information technology in healthcare communications, efficiency, and patient safety. *The Journal of Nursing Administration, 37*(4), 184–187. doi:10.1097/01.NNA.0000266841.46684.50 PMID:17415105

Rao, M. B., Lerro, C., & Gross, C. P. (2010). The Shortage of On-call Surgical Specialist Coverage: A National Survey of Emergency Department Directors. *Academic Emergency Medicine*, *17*(12), 1374–1382. doi:10.1111/j.1553-2712.2010.00927.x PMID:21091822

Rask, K. J., LeBaron, C. W., & Starnes, D. M. (2001). The Cost of Registry-Based Immunization Based Interventions. *American Journal of Preventive Medicine*, *21*(4), 267–271. doi:10.1016/S0749-3797(01)00370-1 PMID:11701296

Rateb, S. A. H., El Nouman, A. A. R., Rateb, M. A. H., Asar, M. N., El Amin, A. M., & Mohamed, M. S. E. (2011). Re-engineering pre-employment check-up systems: A model for improving health services. *International Journal of Health Care Quality Assurance*, *24*(6), 484–497. doi:10.1108/09526861111150734 PMID:21916149

Reardon, G. T., Blumenfield, S., Weissman, A., & Rosenberg, G. (1988). Findings and implications from preadmission screening of elderly patients waiting for elective surgery. *Social Work in Health Care*, *13*(3), 51–63. doi:10.1300/J010v13n03_05 PMID:2852851

Remschmidt, H., Hirsch, O., & Mattejat, F. (2003). Reliability and validity of evaluation data collected by telephone. *Zeitschrift fur Kinder- und Jugendpsychiatrie und Psychotherapie*, *31*(1), 35–49. doi:10.1024/1422-4917.31.1.35 PMID:12616747

Revicki, D. A., Tohen, M., Gyulai, L., Thompson, C., Pike, S., Davis-Vogel, A., & Zarate, C. (1997). Telephone versus in-person clinical and health assessment interviews in patients with bipolar disorder. *Harvard Review of Psychiatry*, *5*(2), 75–81. doi:10.3109/10673229709034730 PMID:9385024

Rimner, T., Blozik, E., Begley, C., Grandchamp, C., & von Overbeck, J. (2011). Patient adherence to recommendations after teleconsultation: Survey of patients from a telemedicine centre in Switzerland. *Journal of Telemedicine and Telecare*, *17*(5), 235–239. doi:10.1258/jtt.2011.101013 PMID:21565847

Ritchie, C., Richman, J., Sobko, H., Bodner, E., Phillips, B., & Houston, T. (2012). The E-Coach transition support computer telephony implementation study: Protocol of a randomized trial. *Contemporary Clinical Trials*, *33*(6), 1172–1179. doi:10.1016/j.cct.2012.08.007 PMID:22922245

Robinson, G., & Morley, C. (2006). Call centre management: Responsibilities and performance. *International Journal of Service Industry Management*, *17*(3), 284–300. doi:10.1108/09564230610667122

Rohde, P., Lewinsohn, P. M., & Seeley, J. R. (1997). Comparability of telephone and face-to-face interviews in assessing axis I and II disorders. *The American Journal of Psychiatry*, *154*(11), 1593–1598. doi:10.1176/ajp.154.11.1593 PMID:9356570

Rohleder, T., Bailey, B., Crum, B., Faber, T., Johnson, B., Montgomery, L., & Pringnitz, R. (2013). Improving a patient appointment call center at Mayo Clinic. *International Journal of Health Care Quality Assurance*, *26*(8), 714–728. doi:10.1108/IJHCQA-11-2011-0068 PMID:24422261

Röing, M., & Holmström, I. K. (2015). Malpractice Claims in Swedish Telenursing: Lessons Learned From Interviews With Telenurses and Managers. *Nursing Research*, *64*(1), 35–43. doi:10.1097/NNR.0000000000000063 PMID:25502059

Romano, M. J., & Stafford, R. S. (2011). Electronic health records and clinical decision support systems: Impact on national ambulatory care quality. *Archives of Internal Medicine*, *171*(10), 897–903. doi:10.1001/archinternmed.2010.527 PMID:21263077

Rudkin, S. E., Langdorf, M. I., Oman, J. A., Kahn, C. A., White, H., & Anderson, C. L. (2009). The worsening of ED on-call coverage in California: 6-year trend. *The American Journal of Emergency Medicine*, *27*(7), 785–791. doi:10.1016/j.ajem.2008.06.012 PMID:19683105

Rudkin, S. E., Oman, J., Langdorf, M. I., Hill, M., Bauche, J., Kivela, P., & Johnson, L. (2004). The state of ED on-call coverage in California. *The American Journal of Emergency Medicine*, *22*(7), 578–581. doi:10.1016/j.ajem.2004.08.001 PMID:15666264

Russell, B. (2012). Professional call centres, professional workers and the paradox of the algorithm: The case of telenursing. *Work, Employment and Society*, *26*(2), 195–210. doi:10.1177/0950017011433155

Sakar, C. O., & Kursun, O. (2010). Telediagnosis of Parkinson's disease using measurements of dysphonia. *Journal of Medical Systems*, *34*(4), 591–599. doi:10.1007/s10916-009-9272-y PMID:20703913

Santana, M. A. S., Aupet, J. B., Betbeder, M. L., Lapayre, J. C., & Ibarrola, J. A. C. (2012). Adaptive collaborative environment for vascular problems telediagnosis. In *Ambient Assisted Living and Home Care* (pp. 1–8). Springer Berlin Heidelberg. doi:10.1007/978-3-642-35395-6_1

Saraux, A., Guillemin, F., Fardellone, P., Guggenbuhl, P., Behier, J. M., Cantagrel, A., & Coste, J. et al. (2004). Agreement between rheumatologist visit and lay interviewer telephone survey for screening for rheumatoid arthritis and spondyloarthropathy. *Joint, Bone, Spine*, *71*(1), 44–50. doi:10.1016/S1297-319X(03)00092-7 PMID:14769520

Schweiger, A., Sunyaev, A., Leimeister, J. M., & Krcmar, H. (2007). Information systems and healthcare XX: Toward seamless healthcare with software agents. *Communications of the Association for Information Systems*, *19*(1), 33.

Shi, J., Peng, Y., Erdem, E., & Woodbridge, P. (2014, September). Simulation analysis on patient visit efficiency of a typical VA primary care clinic with complex characteristics. *Simulation Modelling Practice and Theory*, *47*, 165–181. doi:10.1016/j.simpat.2014.06.003

Shokrollahi, K., Tadiparthi, S., & Jayagopal, S. (2008). How fast is fast enough? An audit and league table of response times of acute hospital NHS Trust switchboards in England. *Journal of the Royal Society of Medicine*, *101*(7), 364–371. doi:10.1258/jrsm.2008.080006 PMID:18591690

Silvestro, R., & Silvestro, C. (2003). New service design in NHS: An evaluation of the strategic alignment of NHS Direct. *International Journal of Operations & Production Management*, *23*(4), 401–417. doi:10.1108/01443570310467320

Sinaiko, J. E. (1999). The danger of being too lean. Warning signs that your health care organization has cut too much. *Cost & Quality: CQ*, *5*(4), 29–31. PMID:11066613

Snooks, H. A., Williams, A. M., Griffiths, L. J., Peconi, J., Rance, J., Snelgrove, S., & Cheung, W. Y. et al. (2008). Real nursing? The development of telenursing. *Journal of Advanced Nursing*, *62*(6), 631–640. doi:10.1111/j.1365-2648.2007.04546.x PMID:18302604

Spear, S. J. (2005). Fixing health care from inside. *Harvard Business Review*, *83*(9), 78–91. PMID:16171213

Stanberry, B. (2001). Legal and Ethical Issues in Telemedicine. *Computer Methods and Programs in Telemedicine*, *64*(3), 225–233. doi:10.1016/S0169-2607(00)00142-5 PMID:11226620

Stewart, J. I., Moyle, S., Criner, G. J., Wilson, C., Tanner, R., Bowler, R. P., & Regan, E. A et al.. (2012). Automated telecommunication to obtain longitudinal follow-up in a multicenter cross-sectional COPD study. *COPD: Journal of Chronic Obstructive Pulmonary Disease*, *9*(5), 466–472. doi:10.3109/15412555.2012.690010 PMID:22676387

Stier, R. D. (1999). The medical call center. *Marketing Health Services*, *19*(2), 25–28. PMID:10557751

Stirewalt, C. F., Linn, M. W., Godoy, G., Knopka, F., & Linn, B. S. (1982). Effectiveness of an ambulatory care telephone service in reducing drop-in visits and improving satisfaction with care. *Medical Care*, *20*(7), 739–748. doi:10.1097/00005650-198207000-00009 PMID:7121093

Stritzke, W. G. K., Dandy, J., Durkin, K., & Houghton, S. (2005). Use of interactive voice response (IVR) technology in health research with children. *Behavior Research Methods*, *37*(1), 119–126. doi:10.3758/BF03206405 PMID:16097351

Suleiman, A. B. (2001). The untapped potential of tele-health. *International Journal of Medical Informatics*, *61*(2-3), 103–112. doi:10.1016/S1386-5056(01)00132-0 PMID:11311664

Suomi, R., Serkkola, A., & Mikkonen, M. (2010). Automated Telephone Services in Dentist Appointment Management. *Informatics in Oral Medicine: Advanced Techniques in Clinical and Diagnostic Technologies*, 269-276.

Swanepoel, D. W., & Hall, J. W. III. (2010). A systematic review of telehealth applications in audiology. *Telemedicine Journal and e-Health*, *16*(2), 181–200. doi:10.1089/tmj.2009.0111 PMID:20187743

Tham, K. W. (2004). Effects of temperature and outdoor air supply rate on the performance of call center operators in the tropics. *Indoor Air*, *14*(s7), 119–125. doi:10.1111/j.1600-0668.2004.00280.x PMID:15330779

Tham, K. W., & Willem, H. C. (2004). *Effects of reported neurobehavioral symptoms on call center operator performance in the tropics*. In RoomVentilation Conference, Coimbra, Portugal

Thomas, J., & Kumar, P. (2013). The scope of teledermatology in India. *Indian Dermatology Online Journal*, *4*(2), 82. doi:10.4103/2229-5178.110579 PMID:23741661

Toverud, E. L., Pike, E., & Walloe, E. (2009). The national poison center in Norway: User satisfaction and health economic evaluation. *European Journal of Clinical Pharmacology*, *65*(9), 935–940. doi:10.1007/s00228-009-0693-9 PMID:19590863

Tsiknakis, M., & Kouroubali, A. (2009). Organizational factors affecting successful adoption of innovative eHealth services: A case study employing the FITT framework. *International Journal of Medical Informatics*, *78*(1), 39–52. doi:10.1016/j.ijmedinf.2008.07.001 PMID:18723389 van der Marck, M. A., Overeem, S., Klok, P., Bloem, B. R., & Munneke, M. (2011). Evaluation of the falls telephone: An automated system for enduring assessment of falls. *Journal of the American Geriatrics Society*, *59*(2), 340–344. doi:10.1111/j.1532-5415.2010.03263.x PMID:21314652

Wahlberg, A., Anna, C., Cedersund, E., & Wredling, R. (2003). Telephone nurses' experience of problems with telephone advice in Sweden. *Journal of Clinical Nursing*, *12*(1), 37–45. doi:10.1046/j.1365-2702.2003.00702.x PMID:12519248

Wan, Y. N. (2012). *Call centre communication: an analysis of interpersonal meaning*. (Master's thesis). The Hong Kong Polytechnic University.

Wargocki, P., Wyon, D. P., & Fanger, P. O. (2004). The performance and subjective responses of call-center operators with new and used supply air filters at two outdoor air supply rates. *Indoor Air*, *14*(s8Suppl. 8), 7–16. doi:10.1111/j.1600-0668.2004.00304.x PMID:15663456

Weir, H., & Waddington, K. (2008). Continuities in caring? Emotion work in a NHS Direct call centre. *Nursing Inquiry*, *15*(1), 67–77. doi:10.1111/j.1440-1800.2008.00391.x PMID:18271792

Williams, B., Warren, S., McKim, R., & Janzen, W. (2012). Caller self-care decisions following teletriage advice. *Journal of Clinical Nursing*, *21*(7-8), 1041–1050. doi:10.1111/j.1365-2702.2011.03986.x PMID:22283747

Witt, L. A., Andrews, M. C., & Carlson, D. S. (2004). When conscientiousness isn't enough: Emotional exhaustion and performance among call center customer service representatives. *Journal of Management*, *30*(1), 149–160. doi:10.1016/j.jm.2003.01.007

Young, M., Sparrow, D., Gottlieb, D., Selim, A., & Friedman, R. (2001). A telephone linked computer system for COPD care. *Chest*, *119*(5), 1565–1575. doi:10.1378/chest.119.5.1565 PMID:11348968

Zanaboni, P., Scalvini, S., Bernocchi, P., Borghi, G., Tridico, C., & Masella, C. (2009). Teleconsultation service to improve healthcare in rural areas: Acceptance, organizational impact and appropriateness. *BMC Health Services Research*, *9*(1), 238. doi:10.1186/1472-6963-9-238 PMID:20021651

KEY TERMS AND DEFINITIONS

Healthcare Telephone System: Part of the healthcare system that is intended for providing service to the callers/patients over various clinical and non-clinical matters.

IVRS: Telecommunication system that is based on Interactive Voice Response technology to interact with the callers by using the voice and the dual tone multi frequency signaling.

On-Call Physician: The physician, who according to the current practices, is supposed to provide the healthcare service in pre-specified amount of time after he/she is contacted or paged.

Tele-Diagnosis: The diagnosis of the related healthcare problems, symptoms, issues over a distance using the telecommunication technologies.

Tele-Health: Method of delivery for the health related services via various telecommunication technologies.

Telephone-Triage: It is a nursing service that is intended to provide the service of prioritizing the patient's treatments based on person's health condition over distance using the telecommunication technologies.

Underreferral: A situation where medical situation, problem, or symptom is deemed less important than it is.

Chapter 5
Evaluating and Managing Electronic Commerce and Outsourcing Projects in Hospitals

Chad Lin
Curtin University, Australia

Geoffrey Jalleh
Curtin University, Australia

Yu-An Huang
National Chi Nan University, Taiwan

ABSTRACT

Despite the huge popularity of outsourcing in electronic commerce/IT in the past two decades, many hospitals have failed to realize the expected benefits from their outsourcing projects. Not surprisingly, the management of electronic commerce/IT outsourcing contracts has become one of the top management issues for hospitals executives in recent years. Hence, the purpose of this study was to provide an overview of outsourcing in electronic commerce/IT investment evaluation and benefits realization processes and practices in Australian and Taiwanese hospitals. Inherent in this study was the opportunity to compare such practices between a developed economy (Australia) and a newly industrialized economy (Taiwan). Several key electronic commerce/IT investment evaluation and outsourcing issues and challenges faced by Australian and Taiwanese hospitals will be presented. The results will assist hospital executives to develop their own approaches and strategies to better manage the opportunities and threats that exist in undertaking electronic commerce/IT outsourcing projects in Australian and Taiwanese hospitals.

DOI: 10.4018/978-1-4666-9870-3.ch005

INTRODUCTION

Electronic commerce has revolutionized the way business is conducted. According to eMarketer (2014), worldwide electronic commerce sale is likely to increase by 20.1% to reach US$1.5 trillion in 2014. It utilizes information technology (IT) (e.g. the Web, the Internet, intranets, extranets) in support of commercial activities (Cao, Lu, Gupta, & Yang, 2015; Standing & Lin, 2007). Electronic commerce can enhance hospitals' competitive advantage via increased efficiency and reduced costs. The main characteristics of electronic commerce include: externalities and exponential growth; critical mass; customer cohesion; content and category depth; broadening and deepening hub services; and disintermediation (Zeng, Wen, & Yen, 2003). It is able to assist organizations in lowering the cost of entry and in expanding the market reach for a variety of business activities. The innovative electronic commerce as an Internet-based option provides a means of achieving the desired degree of interconnectivity without a huge investment and greater technical complexity (Chau & Jim, 2002). Its implementation allows business partners to access their internal business systems via the Internet (Lee, Lim, & Tan, 1999). Electronic commerce provides an efficient and effective channel for information exchange and sharing and enables organizations to trade on a 24x7x365 basis (Lee et al., 1999; Tsao, Lin, & Lin, 2004). It also helps organizations such as hospitals and healthcare companies to use it as a wide-coverage, high-functionality, low-cost tool for venturing into new markets in the global economy (Lin, Huang, Jalleh, Liu, & Tung, 2010; Raisinghani et al., 2005).

Hospitals and healthcare organizations must make good use of their IT/electronic commerce systems through both internal and non-internal sourcing activities in order to remain competitive. According to Gartner, worldwide IT outsourcing spending is forecast to grow by a 5.9% compound annual growth rate from 2013 to 2018 (Britz et al., 2014). IT outsourcing spending accounted for 10.6% of the total IT budget among organizations undertaking outsourcing in 2013 (Computer Economics, 2013). However, only 39% of healthcare organizations engaged in IT outsourcing activities, which was well below the average for all sectors at 60% in the same year (Computer Economics, 2013). Hence, the management of electronic commerce/IT outsourcing contracts has become one of the top management issues for hospitals executives in recent years. However, difficulty in measuring and monitoring the performance of the electronic commerce/IT outsourcing contracts is one of the major problems for hospitals. Despite the benefits of electronic commerce/IT, organizations need to evaluate to determine whether their outsourcing efforts are paying off (Cutler & Sterne, 2000). Although the effective leverage and evaluation of electronic commerce investments can result in improved organizational performance (Melville, Kraemer, & Gurbaxani, 2004), there is little doubt that the less precisely bounded environment of electronic commerce technology adds more complexity to the traditional IT measurement problem as this type of investment is physically distributed between suppliers and vendors, making the evaluation process even more difficult (Zhuang, 2005). The problem becomes more evident as electronic commerce is used to link the supply chain or to change the structure of industries, since costs and benefits have to be tracked across functional and organizational boundaries (Barua, Konana, & Whinston, 2004; Liu, Huang, & Lin, 2012). Existing business models are unequal to this task and planning for such systems has to encompass capabilities for managing and evaluating organizational capabilities to create value across the network of alliances and hence requires evolutionary approaches which can be tailored to business needs at different stages of organizational maturity (Lin, Huang, & Burn, 2007). Needless to say, many organizations find these issues challenging and evaluation methodologies are required to measure and monitor the performance of such investments (Lin, Pervan, Lin, & Tsao, 2008).

Successful benefits realization is strongly associated with organizational performance and hence, the adoption and formulation of the target IT/electronic commerce investments benefits are often regarded as the first and critical step in the benefit management (Chih, & Zwikael, 2015). The adoption of benefits realization methodologies or processes has been extremely difficult and time consuming for most organizations (Lin & Pervan, 2000). It is also a continuing problem that there is a lack of empirical research studies on benefits realization practices and processes (Hellang, Flak, & Päivärinta, 2013). The issue of realization of electronic commerce/IT benefits has generated a significant amount of debate in the IT and electronic commerce literature among the researchers, academics, and practitioners (Brynjolfsson & Hitt, 2003; Hellang et al., 2013; Lin, Pervan, & McDermid, 2002). Some researchers (e.g. (Brynjolfsson & Hitt, 2003; Byrd, Lewis, & Bryan, 2006)) take the position that the confusion over the realization of electronic commerce/IT benefits is due to, among other things, poor IT evaluation processes and poor outsourcing management practices. In particular, the practices and processes of electronic commerce/IT evaluation and outsourcing in Australian and Taiwanese hospitals remain poorly understood and relatively under-researched. Therefore, the case study approach is conducted to investigate the electronic commerce investment evaluation and outsourcing practices in Australian and Taiwanese hospitals. Hence, the main objectives of this study are: (1) to examine current practices and norms in managing and evaluating electronic commerce/IT investments and outsourcing contracts in Australian and Taiwanese hospitals; and (2) to identify key issues or challenges in managing and evaluating electronic commerce/IT investments and outsourcing contracts in Australian and Taiwanese hospitals. A key contribution of this study is the identification and examination of key electronic commerce investment evaluation and outsourcing practices issues and challenges faced by the Australian and Taiwanese hospitals. The results will assist hospital executives to develop their own approaches and strategies to better manage the opportunities and threats that exist in undertaking electronic commerce/IT outsourcing projects in Australian and Taiwanese hospitals.

BACKGROUND

The socio-technical systems theory examines the introduction of innovations (e.g. electronic commerce and IT outsourcing) into organizations from both the social and technical subsystems (Trist, Murray, & Pollack, 1963). Hence, the theory was drawn in this study to the identified issues and problems emerged from the analysis of the case study data. The theory allows organizations to understand why results are meaningful and how the integration of the social and technical systems leads to improved results (Shani & Sena, 1994). STS has particular relevance to understand hospitals where social and technical issues have been identified as some of the key evaluation and benefits realization issues and problems in the implementation of electronic commerce/IT outsourcing projects (Doherty, 2014; Heeks, 2002). The theory provides the foundation for an investigation of the organizational, social, and technological perspectives (e.g. electronic commerce/IT investment evaluation and benefits realization, electronic commerce/IT outsourcing, user participation, top management support, user information requirements determination, perceived time pressure, and strategic alignment and cultural similarity) that might affect the implementation of electronic commerce and IT outsourcing projects in hospitals.

Evaluation and Benefits Realization of Electronic Commerce/IT

Evaluation of health technologies is important for hospitals and healthcare organizations (Claxton, Paulden, Gravelle, Brouwer, & Culyer, 2011; Lin et al., 2014). It is a critical success factor for implementation of electronic commerce/IT in healthcare (Peute, Aarts, Bakker, & Jaspers, 2010). The need to justify expenditure, to identify potential benefits, and/or to judge the effectiveness of an electronic commerce/IT system is a common facet of evaluation (Chao, Lin, Lin, Shen, & Wang, 2012; Karthik & Kumar, 2013; Lin, 2002; Mitra, Sambamurthy, & Westerman., 2011). Although there is now a well-established field of research concerned with evaluation in electronic commerce/IT (Lin & Huang, 2007; Lin, Lin, Huang, & Kuo, 2006), there has been limited academic and practice based work undertaken on in the domain of healthcare setting (Brender, 1997). Traditionally, electronic commerce/IT evaluation studies in the healthcare setting focuses mainly on technical or clinical correctness (Brender, 1997; Coiera, 2003). Evaluation of electronic commerce/

IT are usually carried out in main systems development life cycle (SDLC) phases (Brender, 1997; Norton, Coulson-Thomas, Coulson-Thomas, & Ashurst, 2013). However, more recent electronic commerce/IT evaluation studies in healthcare have begun to also examine the aspects of human/organizational and business processes which involve various stakeholders such as system developers, IT professionals, patients, medical professionals, and system users (Walston, Bennett, & Al-Harbi, 2014; Yusof, Papazafeiropoulou, Paul, & Stergioulas, 2008a). The evaluation and benefits realization mechanisms can expedite the organizational learning process and help make electronic commerce/IT work to the benefit of all customers and external partners, whether viewed from a narrow buyer/seller perspective or a broader supply chain perspective (Huang, Phau, & Lin, 2010; McGaughey, 2002). A good evaluation of electronic commerce/IT can help healthcare organizations and hospitals to, for example, improve quality of their systems, achieve greater clinical efficiency, reduce operating costs, improve the quality of care and effectiveness of the health information systems, and investigate electronic commerce/IT failures and learn from previous mistakes (Friedman & Wyatt, 1997; Kuhn, Giuse, & Talmon, 2003). However, the adoption of IT investment evaluation methodologies by healthcare organizations and hospitals alone could not produce electronic commerce/IT benefits and they must be used by hospitals in conjunction with other organizations factors in order to realize expected benefits (Lin et al., 2014).

Many organizations fail to realize expect benefits from their electronic commerce/IT systems (Coombs, 2015). The adoption of suitable evaluation methods can assist organizations in achieving their objectives (Ozkan, Baykal, & Sincan, 2012; Sadoughi & Aminpour, 2011). Nevertheless, evaluation is often not carried out effectively by healthcare organizations and hospitals (Yusof et al., 2008a). As a result, hospitals are under increasing pressure to find a way to evaluate the contribution of their electronic commerce/IT to business performance, as well as to find reliable ways to ensure that the business benefits from electronic commerce/IT are actually realized (Yusof, Kuljis, Papazafeiropoulou, & Stergioulas, 2008b). Only a very tiny portion of electronic commerce/IT projects can be considered totally successful (Doherty, 2014). Therefore, the selection of a formal electronic commerce/IT evaluation methodology or process which a hospital can implement is crucial in improving its performance (Ammenwerth et al., 2004; Doherty, 2014). In addition, obtaining users' acceptance and their information requirements of the new and/or outsourced electronic commerce/IT evaluation can be instrumental in enhancing business performance (Liu,, Chen, Chen, & Sheu, 2011; Yusoft et al., 2008a).

A review of the relevant literature reveals that many organizations had no measures of success and most did not carry out post-implementation reviews for their electronic commerce/IT investments (e.g., McKay and Marshall, 2004). In addition, research has delivered contradictory findings on the effect of the electronic commerce expenditures on organizational productivity (Thatcher & Pingry, 2004). Therefore, it is not surprising to see that the measurement of the business value of IT investment in electronic commerce has been the subject of considerable debate by many academics and practitioners (Sugumaran & Arogyaswamy, 2004). Although some IT productivity studies have produced inconclusive and negative results, or the interpretation of results may depend on many factors (e.g. mismeasurement of outputs and inputs, the difficulty of establishing the overall value of IT, the choice of inappropriate methods of evaluation, and lags in learning and adjustments) (e.g., Stratopoulos & Dehning, 2000), a number of researchers have indicated that electronic commerce/IT spending is directly related to organizational performance (e.g. Brynjolfsson & Hitt, 2003) with effective leverage and evaluation of such investments resulting in improved organizational performance (Melville et al., 2004). According to Lee & Runge (2001), organizations that evaluate their IT adoption and investments are better able to exploit the Internet's potential for their organization, and thus create short-term competitive advantages.

The major benefits organizations can gain from electronic commerce investments are inherently qualitative and cannot be easily assessed beforehand and calculated in monetary terms (Giaglis, Paul, & Doukidis, 1999). The problem becomes more evident as IT is used to link the supply chain or to change the structure of industries, and costs and benefits have to be tracked across functional and organizational boundaries (Lin, Huang, & Stockdale, 2011; McKay & Marshall, 2004). The less precisely bounded environment of electronic commerce technology adds more complexity to the measurement problem as this type of investment is physically distributed between suppliers and customers (Standing, Standing, & Lin, 2008; Torkzadeh & Dhillon, 2002). Thus, failure to plan for and, evaluate the benefits from an electronic commerce investment and consideration of other aspects of human/organizational and business processes which involve main stakeholders can have detrimental consequences on organizational performance (Doherty, 2014).

Despite the fact that evaluation of electronic commerce/IT investment is crucial for the success of organizations, it is still insufficient in terms of ensuring that the expected benefits are eventually realized and delivered to the organizations (Ward & Griffiths, 1996). Assessing the effective delivery of useful benefits from these services to the business is very difficult (Remenyi & Whittaker, 1996). Benefits realization comprises of a range of management activities designed to ensure that an organization realized the benefits it plans to achieve from an electronic commerce/IT investment (Love, Irani, Standing, Lin, & Burn, 2005). Benefits may be considered as the effect of the changes, i.e. management of changes - the difference between the current and proposed way that work is done (Ward & Griffiths, 1996). It has been found that there is a clear indication of the benefits that flow from being able to compare the impacts of a specific electronic commerce/IT investment against a set of underlying objectives with the possibility of introducing corrective action (e.g. post-implementation review) if necessary (Tallon, Kraemer, & Gurbaxani, 2000). Benefits need to be actively and regularly reviewed throughout the full system life-cycle via an on-going benefits realization program or process (Doherty, 2014).

Outsourcing of Electronic Commerce/IT

Government regulations and intensive competition can have a significant effect on the decision of hospitals to outsourcing their some of their electronic commerce/IT systems (Ferdosi et al., 2013). Other motivation and benefits contributing to the growth of the outsourcing in the healthcare industry include cost saving, improved customer satisfaction, focus of core competencies, reduction in staff turnover, access to requisite skills, improved services and efficiency, increased flexibility, and economies of scale (Danvers & Nikolov, 2010; Hsiao, Pai, & Chiu, 2009; Johnson, Murphy, McNeese, Reddy, & Purao, 2013; Menachemi, Burke, & Diana, 2007; Sujata, Reddy, & Jayalakshmi, 2013). However, despite the promised savings and benefits from the electronic commerce/IT outsourcing contracts, there have been risks and disadvantages for healthcare organizations to undertake outsourcing. These include costs increase for the patients, employee resistance, poor strategic similarity between outsourcing hospitals and external outsourcing contractors, inability to manage outsourcing contracts, dependency on external outsourcing contractors, inexperienced employees by external contractors, hidden costs, and government regulations (Hsiao et al., 2009; Karimi, Agharahimi, & Yaghoubi, 2012; Lawrence & Firth, 2013; Ondo & Smith, 2006).

Electronic commerce/IT can play an important part in providing quality services to clients and patients in hospitals and other healthcare organizations (Johnson et al., 2013). Many believe that extensive IT outsourcing by both healthcare and non-healthcare organizations can bring in benefits such as cost reduction, improved quality of patient care, improved patients' privacy, access to required technical expertise and knowledge, reduction of risks, reduced medical errors, improved decision-making process, enhanced competitive advantage, increased user satisfaction, and rapid introduction of new products and services (Aggelidis & Chatzoglou, 2012; Alaghehband, Rivard, Wu, & Goyette, 2011; Gorla & Somers, 2014; Moon, Choe, Chung, Jung, & Swar, 2014; Mudambi & Tallman, 2010; Samantra, Datta, & Mahapatra, 2014; Sujata et al., 2013; Yu, 2010). However, complexity and scope of electronic commerce/IT outsourcing are often the major constraints and difficulties in evaluation and benefits realization processes (Doherty, Ashurst, & Peppard, 2012; Lin & Pervan, 2001; Tallon et al., 2000). One reason for this is that most healthcare organizations fail to properly monitor and evaluate their electronic commerce/IT outsourcing contracts or projects (Low & Chen, 2012). Indeed, most organizations do not have formal process to evaluate their electronic commerce/IT outsourcing decision and, instead, relied on limited cost analysis associated with the outsourcing decision (McIvor, 2000). Organizations that make extensive use of electronic commerce/IT evaluation methodologies or measures have higher perceived payoffs (Tallon et al., 2000). Misra (2004) found that outsourcing organizations need to choose the evaluation methodologies which: (1) can be aligned with mutual strategic alignment, expectations, and business objectives; (2) are within the external outsourcing contractors' control; (3) can be easily measured by both the outsourcing organizations and external outsourcing contractors; (4) can be measured by objective criteria rather than subjective criteria; and (5) lead to the desired behavior by both outsourcing organizations and external outsourcing contractors.

User Participation and Top Management Support

One of the major factors contributing to the failures of IT/electronic commerce is the lack of user participation. By failing to involve them during the initial system development stages, the users might feel frustrated and disillusioned when they perceive new technologies or outsourced systems as the threatening creations of outsiders. This usually results in resistance and conflicts between the analysts and the users (Abelein & Paech, 2014; Bano & Zowghi, 2015; Durugbo, 2012). Lack of user participation often results in distrust between the users and the senior executives, resulting in reduced job satisfaction and less than adequate systems (Lin & Lin, 2011). On the other hand, there are a number of advantages that can come from users being involved in the process such as increased system efficiency, enhanced system quality, greater user knowledge about the system, and gaining user acceptance (Abelein & Paech, 2014; Durugbo, 2012; de Waal & Batenburg, 2014).

Top management support has been described as the degree to which senior executives understands the importance of the IT/electronic commerce function and the extent to which it is involved in IT/electronic commerce projects (Ragu-Nathana, Apigian, Ragu-Nathana, & Tu, 2004). It can influence an organization's electronic commerce/IT capability as well as the implementation of IT strategies (Yeh, Lee, & Pai, 2014). It has been identified as one of the most important contributing factors for IT system success (e.g., Norton et al., 2013; Young & Jordan, 2008). Several studies believe that top management support is crucial and will most certainly enhance the probability of IT system success (e.g., Ragu-Nathana et al., 2004). For example, the presence of strong top management support facilitates organization establishing vertical IT instead of processing information through the existing hierarchical channels and, thus such efforts will increase the system capacity of the organization (Ramezan, 2011). Past research also suggests that successful introduction of new or outsourced IT/electronic commerce systems is less likely without top management support. Support from top management is required to overcome the communication and coordination barriers between interdepartmental collaboration (Lee & Kim, 2007). Another benefit of top management support is to deal with user resistance to, for example, the implementation of new or outsourced IT/electronic commerce systems which are likely to bring in new innovation.

Strategic Alignment and Cultural Similarity

The alignment between various business and IT functions is crucial for the successful implementation of any electronic commerce/IT system (Rahim, Kurnia, Samson, & Singh, 2014). The lack of strategic alignment between business and IT can have a great impact on the value of all IT outsourcing effort (Aversano, Grasso, & Tortorella, 2013; Lin, 2002). Parker (1996) has suggested that IT strategy should both derive from and shape business strategy in a dynamic environment. Strategic fit recognizes that both business and IT domains (i.e. "Business" and "Information Technology") should be managed and positioned in terms of their respective IT and business focuses. Functional integration focuses on the connection between strategy and execution and deals with the link: (1) between business strategy and IT strategy; and (2) between business operations and IT execution. The capabilities embedded in IT can open up additional possibilities for generating and delivering value to the organizations. Drawing upon the findings of the previous studies reviewed, Yayla & Hu (2012) have also found that organizations with higher levels of alignment of their strategies and control mechanisms perform better than those with lower levels of alignment. Such mutual alignment between outsourcing hospitals and external contractors can also assist in utilizing and integrating their various IT resources effectively to support their business strategies and to realize the maximum benefits of their outsourcing contracts (Huang, Lin, Liu, & Tung, 2013; Kuo, Lin, Hsu, & Huang, 2006; Li, 2012). Organizations with a high IT strategic alignment have been found to exhibit better performance (Chan, Huff, Barclay, & Copeland, 1997).

The impact of culture similarity or divergence on organizational performance is an important research area for researchers (Hahn & Bunyaratavej, 2010; Ralston, Holt, Terpstra, & Kai-Cheng, 2008; Peute et al., 2010). According to Hofstede (1997), the cultural divergence or distance between two entities with different cultures can be explained in terms of factors such as individualism/collectivism, masculinity/femininity, power distance, and uncertainty avoidance. Organizations from different cultures understand, and judge the nature of the world in systematically different ways (Han & Lee, 2012). Similarly, cultural differences between two organizations or countries can be significant as people (e.g. IT professionals and users) from different cultures understand and judge the nature of the world in systematically different ways (Licht, 2004). In the context of outsourcing, this can increase the costs of transaction, risks, and uncertainty since it is likely that external outsourcing contractors might not fully understand outsourcing hospitals' business culture or its needs (Han & Lee, 2012).

Perceived Time Pressure

Some recent attention has been placed on the adverse effects of coping with perceived time pressure in IT literature as completion by deadline is one of the most frequently used measurements of project success (Thomas, Fugate, & Koukova, 2011; Syrek, Apostel, & Antoni, 2013). Perceived time pressure happens as the perception of a limited time to complete a given task is created and this can result in negative effects for the entire IT project team (Thomas et al., 2011). When the time required to complete a given task exceeds the available time, an information overload occurs (Schick, Gordon, & Haka, 1990). High level of perceived time pressure can lead to stress, errors, passivity and avoidance as well as result in a negative effect on business decision making process and performance (Kocher & Sutter, 2006; Rissler, 1994). It is an important driving force for work progress (Zika-Viktorsson, Sundstrom, & Engwall, 2006).

A review of the relevant literature revealed that there is a variety of different coping mechanisms have been posited for organizational executives dealing with time pressure. For example, the use of filtering mechanisms has been advocated by Schultze & Vandenbosch (1998) who studied users of LotusNotes in an organization. Paul & Nazareth (2010) demonstrated that the use of appropriate decision aids such as schema that synthesized prior decisions can alleviate the problem of overload. Therefore, it is likely that an increase in the perceived time pressure can have a positive impact on the level of electronic commerce/IT outsourcing by hospitals. However, it is also likely that if outsourcing does not help hospital IT professionals to cope with perceived time pressure it would have a negative effect on the building of better relationship, communication, and trust with their external outsourcing contractors.

Information Requirements Determination (IRD)

Organizations which solicit feedback about users' business requirements and processes are likely to better understand their task needs (Babar, Wong, & Abedin, 2014; Shuraida & Barki, 2013). The information requirements determination (IRD) process is a critical phase within the SDLC. IRD has generated a lot of interest and debate among researchers and practitioners as a potential means for improving the success rates of ISD projects (Hsu, Lin, Zheng, & Hung, 2012; Liu et al., 2011; Wu & Shen, 2006). The IRD process which Browne &

Ramesh (2002, p. 625) defined as "a set of activities used by a systems analyst when assessing the functionality required in a proposed system", has become increasingly important in obtaining the correct and complete set of user requirements. However, with today's rapid changes of technology and customer driven environments and needs, IRD have become increasingly difficult for systems analysts to elicit and predict (Gorschek, Svahnberg, Borg, Loconsole, & Sandahl, 2007). There are two types of requirement uncertainty –requirements diversity and requirements instability (Liu et al., 2011). This IRD uncertainty can result in interpersonal conflict among stakeholders since system users desire changes to reflect environmental changes whereas IT professionals desperately need to lock-in requirements so that the project or contract can be delivered within budget and on time (Liu et al., 2011). This in turn can lead to poor project or contract performance. Hence, the successful IRD process during the ISD project is a critical factor for project or contract success.

A review of the relevant literature revealed that the IRD phase of an ISD project is a problematic process and in many cases, budget blowouts and missed deadlines occur (Lin & Lin, 2011; Urquhart, 2001). Too often, initial design and programming is followed by a reassessment of needs, redesign and then more programming. However, many ISD project failures have little to do with technical or programming issues. The source of many of these problems lies with one or a combination of the following factors: incomplete and/or inaccurate requirement specifications, lack of users' involvement, lack of flexibility of computer-based information systems, poor communication, worldviews of the systems analysts, lack of common knowledge, and lack of harmonious relationships between users and systems analysts. Incomplete and/or inaccurate requirements specifications can often lead an organization to address the wrong problem or identify the incorrect information needs and this may ultimately lead to electronic commerce/IT project failures (Khalil & Elkordy, 2005). In this case, high levels of common knowledge and harmonious relationship between systems analysts and users can assist in obtaining complete user IRD which in turn can result in better project/contract performance (Hsu et al., 2012).

After all, the main reason why it was difficult to obtain accurate and complete user IRD is due to the constraints on humans as information processors and problem solvers (Land, 1987). Finally, according to Browne & Ramesh (2002), the following challenges should be recognized by both systems analysts and users when they are dealing with each other: (a) there can never be a complete, correct set of user information requirements; (b) requirements are not stable over time, but are in a constant process of evolution; (c) the facilitation skills of systems analysts are crucial to the effective management of the IRD process; and (d) systems analysts work in a highly political contexts.

METHODS

The purpose of this study was to provide an overview of outsourcing in electronic commerce/IT investment evaluation and benefits realization processes and practices in Australian and Taiwanese hospitals. Inherent in this study was the opportunity to compare such practices between a developed economy (Australia) and a newly industrialized economy (Taiwan). Hospitals in Australia and Taiwan were chosen for this study because electronic commerce investment and outsourcing have been extremely popular within the hospital industry in both countries. However, electronic commerce/IT investment evaluation and benefits realization processes and practices in outsourcing Australian and Taiwanese hospitals remain poorly understood. To the best of our knowledge, we have not found any comprehensive studies reported in the literature focusing on electronic commerce investment evaluation and outsourcing in both Australian and Taiwanese hospitals. Therefore, better understanding of the electronic commerce investment evaluation and outsourcing practices is warranted. Case studies were conducted with IT professionals and users from 10 Australian hospitals and 10 Taiwanese hospitals.

All of the hospitals interviewed had been using at least an electronic commerce system for more than five years. In recent years, both Australian and Taiwanese hospitals have come to realize that they can only compete with competitors through the efficient use of their IT resources such as electronic commerce systems and health information systems. Hospitals executives in both countries are becoming increasingly aware of challenges and opportunities in order to be more efficient and effective in delivering healthcare services to their patients. To remain competitive, hospitals must enhance and maintain their IT/electronic commerce systems through both internal and non-internal sourcing activities (Hsiao et al., 2009).

Driven by concerns about low electronic commerce uptake and escalating procurement costs within the industry, several electronic commerce initiatives have been launched by Australian Federal and State governments during the last decade to develop better ways of, among other things, ordering and procuring medical supplies electronically within the Australian hospitals and healthcare industry (e.g. Project Electronic Commerce and Communication (PECC) and the Pharmaceutical Extranet Gateway (PEG) in 1998 (More & McGrath, 2002), the Monash Pharmacy Project under the Victorian Government's e-Commerce Exhibition Projects Program (ECEPP) in 2003 (GS1 Australia, 2005), and GS1Locatenet GLN Directory for Healthcare in 2010 (NEHTA, 2010)). These initiatives have attempted to assist in the integration of electronic commerce/supply chain functionality with other Australian hospital and healthcare IT systems. However, despite substantial amount of resources being spent by the Australian Federal and State governments, these initiatives have achieved only limited success so far.

Due to the financial difficulties within the national health care system in Taiwan, the costs and revenue of these hospitals and healthcare providers have been closely monitored by Bureau of National Health Insurance (BNHI) (Lee & Jones, 2004). BNHI's fixed-budget policy has resulted in reimbursement prices that made many hospitals unsustainable. That is, the payments to hospitals, have been decreasing markedly each year while, at the same time, their costs have been increasing rapidly. The reimbursement prices by the BNHI are among the lowest in the world (Shapiro, 2009). Under the twin pressures of BNHI reimbursement price constraints and the intense competition among hospitals, the total number of hospitals in Taiwan has decreased by more than 30% (from 835 to 530) between 1986 and 2007 (Shapiro, 2009; THRF, 2011).

These twenty cases were deliberately chosen in order to focus efforts on theoretically useful cases (following the theoretical, non-random sampling strategy by Eisenhardt (1989)). The data collection at these twenty cases continued until a point of theoretical saturation, which is when the value of an additional interview was considered to be negligible (Eisenhardt, 1989). The case study method enabled the researcher to examine how both Australian and Taiwanese hospitals evaluated their IT/electronic commerce investments and to what extent their electronic commerce benefits were realized. The questions asked during the interviews included the practices and processes of electronic commerce evaluation and benefits realization and their impact on electronic commerce benefits and user satisfaction in Taiwanese hospitals, as well as other electronic commerce adoption and IT outsourcing issues. Multiple data sources were used and included hospital documents and annual reports. Extensive notes were taken during the interviews and they were later were coded and analyzed. This serves as a method of triangulation of research data and ensures that the questions and answers are properly understood by repeating or rephrasing the questions and through paraphrasing the responses back to the interview participants (Silverman, 2001).

Qualitative content analysis by Miles & Huberman (1994) was then used to analyze the data from the case study. The analysis of the case study results was conducted in a cyclical manner and the results were checked by other experts in the field. The external experts were asked to trace the logical flow of the research study, research questions, case findings and analysis and identification of constructs and thereby identifying any gaps in the chain of evidence (Yin, 2002). The findings from these information gathering approaches were analyzed iteratively by the researchers on an individual level, differences reconciled and then a judgment made on each of the major themes. Questions relating to a particular research theme, for example, level of B2B e-commerce, were examined as a cluster. Divergent views within the same company were assessed in terms of the relative strength of the perspective according to the numbers of responses falling in particular categories. This was done as a form of in-case analysis and to develop general explanations and interpretations (Eisenhardt, 1989). These steps enhance the construct validity, reliability and overall quality of the research (Yin, 2002). Furthermore, multiple sources of information and data were sought for each case study. Where some participants' accounts did not reflect other participants' accounts or the researchers own observation and understanding, alternative explanations were sought from the participants themselves. The extensive notes were then re-examined and deeper interpretation of observation was produced.

FINDINGS

Drawing on the socio-technical systems theory, the study attempts to identify and examine the following organizational issues: electronic commerce/IT investment evaluation and benefits realization, electronic commerce/IT outsourcing, user participation, top management support, user information requirements determination, perceived time pressure, and strategic alignment and cultural similarity. As mentioned earlier, qualitative content analysis was used as a powerful tool to analyze the data collected for this study. Hospitals participated in this study had outsourced at least part of their electronic commerce and IT functions. The findings revealed that while a great proportion of the Australian and Taiwanese hospitals (70% vs 80%) had used a formal or semi-formal IT investment evaluation methodology or process to evaluate their outsourced electronic commerce investments, the same cannot be said about their electronic commerce benefits realization practices. About 60% of Australian hospitals had used a formal or semi-formal IT benefits realization methodology or process on their electronic commerce investments and only 40% of Taiwanese hospitals had adopted the above-mentioned methodology or process. Of those who had adopted the methodologies or processes, most of them indicated that they were in most cases neither effective in ensuring successful electronic commerce systems nor they were widely used in these hospitals.

Cost reduction and efficiency improvement were the two main reasons for both Australian and Taiwanese hospitals to outsource their electronic commerce functions. There were also differences for Australian and Taiwanese hospitals to undertake outsourcing. For Australian hospitals, outsourcing gave rise to greater business focus and increased justification of costs against often measurable business unit outcomes as well as to decrease the power of the union. For Taiwanese hospitals, outsourcing was often used as one way to overcome lack of resources and to downsize their labor force. A number of issues and problems emerged from the analysis of the text data and some of the key issues surrounding the electronic commerce/IT outsourcing contracts and projects are presented below in some detail.

Lack of Strong User Participation and Top Management Support

Both user participation and top management support are important for electronic commerce/IT outsourcing projects in healthcare (Rise, Solbjør, & Steinsbekk, 2014; Wolf et al., 2014). A review of the relevant revealed that there is a positive association between user participation, top management support, and system success (Abelein & Paech, 2013; Petter, DeLone, & McLean, 2013; Spears & Barki, 2010; Young & Jordan, 2008). In other words, the effectiveness of a system depends heavily on the participation of all relevant users and stakeholders and their willingness to use it (Doherty, 2014). There are a number of advantages that can come from users being involved in the process such as increased system efficiency, enhanced system quality, greater user knowledge about the system, and gaining user acceptance (Abelein & Paech, 2014; Durugbo, 2012; de Waal & Batenburg, 2014). However, much of the outsourcing and adoption of the new IT systems by the hospitals interviewed were generally forced upon the employees or users by the senior management. Many employees and users within the hospitals interviewed said they were not extensively consulted beforehand and were not involved in the outsourcing, designing and adoption of these systems. Those hospitals which kept the users and customers in the dark would tend to result in user resistance or have low usage for their new IT systems. Moreover, many benefits expected from the outsourcing and adoption of these systems were mainly tailored for the senior managers. Furthermore, there was a positive relationship between hospitals which had adopted IT investment evaluation and benefits realization methodologies and those which had extensively consulted with system users before the outsourcing or adoption of implementing their IT systems.

Similarly, there are a number of advantages that can come from top management support such as minimization of the communication and coordination barriers between interdepartmental collaboration, minimization of user resistance, and increased product/service quality. According to hospitals interview respondents, it had appeared that there was a lack of strong top management support and commitment for most of the new and outsourced the electronic commerce/IT projects in most hospitals. Those electronic commerce/IT projects which had received strong top management support and commitment tended to provide more training for users. More training had resulted in greater skill with the systems or projects by the users. This in turn had led to more user involvement and familiarity with the electronic commerce/IT systems and projects. Those users which were deeply involved with the projects tended to perceive fewer system barriers and more benefits than those with less involvement. Again, there was a positive relationship between hospitals which had adopted IT investment evaluation and benefits realization methodologies and those projects which had received strong top management support and commitment. One IT manager stated: *"......the methodology has allowed us to produce the evidence and key performance measures to show our top management that these projects will have long-term strategic benefits to the hospital......"* After all, the use of these methodologies had allowed hospital executives to determine if a particular project had significant long-term benefit(s) to the organization.

Inability to Cope with Perceived Time Pressure

Perceived time pressure is an important factor to consider when negotiating an electronic commerce/IT outsourcing contract (Saorín-Iborra, Redondo-Cano, Revuelto-Taboada, & Vogler, 2015). Too much perceived time pressure can lead to stress, errors, passivity and avoidance as well as result in a negative effect on business decision making process and performance (Kocher & Sutter, 2006; Rissler, 1994). The results of the study indicated that high level of perceived time pressure particularly from the participants in Taiwanese hospitals had led to high level of psychological stress and employee turnover in the workplace. In many instances, they responded by trying to minimize risks as well as to work faster and this had appeared to have a negative effect on the relationships and trust with their external outsourcing contractors. One IT manager in a Taiwanese hospital revealed that: *"......we simply do not have enough manpower and time to complete the many projects we have at the moment......this is a real problem for us and our external outsourcing contractors."* Many participants complained that no proper training and procedures were put in place by hospital executives to assist them in coping with perceived time pressure. For example, the ambiguity in task distribution by outsourcing hospitals did not help in reducing the level of perceived time pressure among IT project team involved in electronic commerce outsourcing and this in turn had a negative effect on the building of better relationship, communication, and trust with their external outsourcing contractors. This problem appeared to be more prevalent among participating Taiwanese hospitals.

Cultural Divergence between Outsourcing Hospitals and Contractors

The issue of culture similarity can have a significant impact on the relationship between governance and opportunism in outsourcing relationships (Handley & Angst, 2015). Australian and Taiwanese hospitals participated in this study outsourced their electronic commerce systems to external outsourcing contractors in the hope to realize the benefits such as cost savings, higher service quality, and improved business efficiency. However, not all hospitals were able to realize these expected benefits due to cultural divergence or distance between the hospitals and the external outsourcing contractors (Han & Lee, 2012). According to Hofstede (1997), the cultural divergence or distance between two entities with different cultures can be explained in terms of factors such as individualism/collectivism, power distance, and uncertainty avoidance. For example, based on the individualism-collectivism index proposed by Hofstede (1997), Australia is an individualistic country whereas Taiwan represents a collectivistic country. Most western and individualistic cultures tend to perceive themselves as distinct from each other whereas many Asian countries are characterized by high collectivism. Asian countries with high collectivism usually focus more on community, society, or nation and are concerned with cohesion within the social group.

Taiwanese society is characterized by high collectivism, high uncertainty avoidance, and high power distance. This was particularly the issue for the Taiwanese hospitals where the entire Taiwanese IT outsourcing market was dominated by Western outsourcing companies. Organizations from different cultures understand, and judge the nature of the world in systematically different ways (Han & Lee, 2012). Some of the problems encountered by both of the Taiwanese hospitals and their external outsourcing contractors related to the different shared values and methods of achieving and managing projects and goals. Although for Taiwanese hospitals to enter into electronic commerce outsourcing contracts with foreign contractors were likely to gain global synergies, this had also created a high degree of uncertainty for these outsourcing hospitals since the foreign outsourcing contractors may not fully understand their business culture and values. It was not surprising to find that there was often a cultural clash between the Taiwanese public hospitals in particular and their foreign external outsourcing contractors on their expectation of the outsourcing contracts. This was especially true for the Taiwanese public hospitals which expected better and efficient services in line with government regulations and directives. For example, an IT manager of a Taiwanese public hospital said: *"As a public hospital, the reason for outsourcing was often more to do with providing better services in line with government directives rather than simply cost saving and generating revenue......but our outsourcing contractor appears to be only interested in making money out of us from the outsourced ......system......we also seem to have different cultures in managing things and achieving the stated goals..."* In addition, the selection of right external outsourcing contractors was an important part of IT investment evaluation process for the Taiwanese hospitals to undertake. It came down to whether an outsourcing relationship worked best when the cultural distance between hospitals and outsourcing contractors was small. Those hospitals which did not undertake proper IT investment evaluation process at the pre-project stage on their outsourcing projects to determine the cultural distance between themselves and their external outsourcing contractors tended to have more cultural related issues after the contracts were signed. On the other hand, this was a lesser problem for the Australian hospitals where the Australian IT outsourcing market was dominated by domestic or foreign contractors owned by companies located in western countries. This smaller overall cultural distance was an important factor for Australian hospitals having less cultural related problems with their external outsourcing contractors.

Lack of Mutual Strategic Alignment and Expectations

Hospitals need to ensure the alignment of their business strategies and expectations in order to respond to the competitive environment affecting the quality, efficiency and costs of health service delivery as well as cope with technological advancements (Mettler, Fitterer, Rohner, & Winter, 2014). Organizations with higher levels of alignment of their strategies and control mechanisms perform better than those with lower levels of alignment (Yayla & Hu, 2012). Similarly, such mutual alignment between outsourcing hospitals and external contractors can also assist in utilizing and integrating their various IT resources effectively to support their business strategies and to realize the maximum benefits of their outsourcing contracts (Li, 2012; Lin & Lin, 2011). However, most participating hospitals admitted that it was not easy to achieve such alignment. This was due to the fact that from the pre-project justification stage an external outsourcing contractor had to be evaluated and then selected based on not only outsourcing hospital's organizational and service requirements but also areas of similarity in terms of its strategic alignment, visions, and expectation between both parties. One IT manager commented: *"......a lot of time and resources had been spent...... to make sure that our (outsourcing hospital and contractor's) strategies and control mechanism are properly aligned......"* In other words, sufficient time and resources for a proper IT investment evaluation methodology or process had to be allocated at the pre-project justification stage. Outsourcing hospitals also needed to communicate and agree to the strategic alignment, visions, and expectations with their external outsourcing contractors before the signing of the contracts. The lack of mutually agreed strategic alignment, visions, and expectation between the outsourcing hospitals and their contractors can often lead to unfulfilled goals and requirements for both parties. This can affect the quality and user satisfaction of the outsourced electronic commerce systems developed by the contractors. For Australian hospitals lack of funding was often the most mentioned reason for not achieving such alignment while for Taiwanese hospitals the number one reason was lack of expertise and time in conducting a properly IT investment evaluation at the pre-project justification stage to ensure that a contractor with similar strategic alignment was selected.

Inaccurate Information Requirements Determination (IRD) Process

Organizations matching their information requirement determination process with their electronic commerce/IT capabilities perform better (Dutot,, Bergeron, & Raymond, 2014). Indeed, getting accurate and complete user IRD is one of the most critical aspects for a successful ISD process and most of the errors from the ISD can be traced back to the IRD stage (Hsu et al., 2012; Lin & Lin, 2011). This is critical given that the main purpose of users engaging in the ISD process is to contribute their know-how and experience to determine actual requirements of the new systems and/or outsourcing contracts so that both users and developer requirements can be incorporated into the new system design (He & King, 2008). If key users and stakeholders are involved and updated during the outsourcing process, they may view the outsourced systems as their own systems (Nakatsu & Iacovou, 2009). This can assist hospitals in, for example, communicating, sharing, and clarifying organizational and business objectives as well as in resolving issues arising from outsourcing contracts and projects. However, it appeared that few responding hospitals had paid sufficient attention to the potentially problematic user IRD process. For example, one IT procurement manager stated: *"......It was difficult to obtain complete requirements from users......they were changing all the time...... We couldn't do much about it."* In many cases, this had led to mismatch between user requirements and business outcomes from the electronic commerce outsourcing contracts since most of hospital know-how and experience integration process does not go through the established or documented procedures. One of the major reasons for this was that outsourcing hospitals often failed to allocate sufficient resources to properly manage and monitor the IRD process for their electronic commerce outsourcing contracts. Several other reasons were identified by the participants and the researchers: (1) outsourcing hospitals and external outsourcing contractors had conflicting agendas; (2) lack of effective communication between the top management of outsourcing hospitals and the users; (3) user requirements were not stable over time and kept changing; and (4) lack of experience of system analysts and developers to obtain accurate and complete user information requirements. In addition, many outsourcing hospitals and external outsourcing contractors simply did not allocate sufficient resources to set up a proper governance mechanism as well as to obtain sufficient competencies to manage and assess their IRD processes. To make the matter worse, many participating hospitals failed to involve users and stakeholders during the electronic commerce outsourcing contract process as well as to provide most current information to users in order to counter uncertainties (e.g. job loss and resistance to change) arising from the electronic commerce outsourcing contracts.

It is not surprising that many potential problems were not properly identified before the commencement of the electronic commerce outsourcing contracts and the development of new electronic commerce systems. These had resulted in schedule delays, budget blowout, system flaws, and inappropriate design functions in later stages of the projects and contracts. Extra time and costs were often needed to undertake the remedial work to fix the system flaws and defects and in many cases, resulting in poor system and contract performance. However, there were differences for Australian and Taiwanese hospitals in engaging users and stakeholders during the electronic commerce outsourcing process. Australian hospitals executives tended to spend more time and allocate resources than their Taiwanese counterparts in involving and obtaining users requirements. For Australian hospitals, outsourcing gave rise to increased justification costs against measurable business unit outcomes. For Taiwanese hospitals, decision to outsource was often undertaken by the senior executives without consulting with the key users and stakeholders and was often used as one way to overcome lack of resources and to downsize their labor force.

DISCUSSIONS AND CONCLUSION

The primary focus of this research was to identify key issues in managing and evaluating electronic commerce/IT investments and outsourcing contracts in order to assist hospital executives in Australian and Taiwanese hospitals in developing a better understanding of their electronic commerce/IT outsourcing projects. This, in turn, will also help them to formulate their own approaches and strategies to better manage the opportunities and threats that exist in undertaking electronic commerce/IT outsourcing projects. While there are other issues that might influence the management and evaluation of electronic commerce/IT investments and outsourcing projects, only key issues identified in the study have been explored and examined.

The findings support the view that having a greater business focus was often one of the major reasons for Australian hospitals to outsource their electronic commerce systems while for Taiwanese hospitals electronic commerce outsourcing was often adopted to overcome lack of resources as well as to downsize their labor force. The findings also revealed that while a large proportion of the Australian and Taiwanese hospitals (70% vs 80%) had used a formal or semi-formal IT investment evaluation methodology or process to evaluate their electronic commerce investments, the same cannot be said about their electronic commerce benefits realization practices. About 60% of Australian hospitals had used a formal or semi-formal IT benefits realization methodology or process on their electronic commerce investments and only 40% of Taiwanese hospitals had adopted the above-mentioned methodology or process. The other key issues identified in this study are: (1) lack of strong user participation and top management support; (2) inability to cope with perceived time pressure; (3) cultural divergence between outsourcing hospitals and contractors; (4) lack of mutual strategic alignment and expectations; and (5) inaccurate information requirements determination process. Results showed that much of the outsourcing and adoption of the new IT systems by the hospitals interviewed were generally forced upon the employees or users by the senior management. Many employees and users within the hospitals interviewed said they were not extensively consulted beforehand and were not involved in the outsourcing, designing and adoption of these systems. According to hospitals interview respondents, it had appeared that there was a lack of strong top management support and commitment for most of the new and outsourced the electronic commerce/IT projects in most hospitals. Those electronic commerce/IT projects which had received strong top management support and commitment tended to provide more training for users. The results of the study also indicated that high level of perceived time pressure particularly from the participants in Taiwanese hospitals had led to high level of psychological stress and employee turnover in the workplace. In many instances, they responded by trying to minimize risks as well as to work faster and this had appeared to have a negative effect on the relationships and trust with their external outsourcing contractors. This problem appeared to be more prevalent among participating Taiwanese hospitals than their Australian counterparts.

In order to minimize for example the perceived time pressure among IT professionals and users, hospitals can: (1) provide them with appropriate training in explicit communication among system users; (2) reduce the ambiguity in their task distribution; and (3) provide timely assistance in crisis and critical situations. Although it is unlikely for both the outsourcing hospitals and their external contractors to have exactly the same strategic goals, visions, and expectations, they nevertheless should be communicated and understood by both parties during the contract negotiation process. These should also be linked to the terms and conditions contained within the service level agreements and where possible, apply best practices across all stages of electronic commerce outsourcing processes. They need to be continuously monitored and evaluated after the contract is signed. Moreover, outsourcing hospitals should take initiatives in further strengthening the communication process with their external contractors and put in place a mechanism in monitoring and evaluating their objectives in outsourcing their electronic commerce systems in the first place. After all, the performance and outcomes of the outsourcing contracts may suffer and deteriorate quickly if the strategic alignment, visions, and expectation become off-balance between the two parties.

In addition, cultural divergence was particularly the issue for the Taiwanese hospitals where the entire Taiwanese IT outsourcing market was dominated by Western outsourcing companies. Some of the problems encountered by both of the

Taiwanese hospitals and their external outsourcing contractors related to the different shared values and methods of achieving and managing projects and goals. Although for Taiwanese hospitals to enter into electronic commerce outsourcing contracts with foreign contractors were likely to gain global synergies, this had also created a high degree of uncertainty for these outsourcing hospitals since the foreign outsourcing contractors may not fully understand their business culture and values. On the other hand, this was a lesser problem for the Australian hospitals where the Australian IT outsourcing market was dominated by domestic or foreign contractors owned by companies located in western countries. Moreover, most participating hospitals admitted that it was not easy to achieve alignment of their strategies and control mechanism with external contractors in terms of their outsourcing contracts. The lack of mutually agreed strategic alignment, visions, and expectation between the outsourcing hospitals and their contractors can often lead to unfulfilled goals and requirements for both parties. This can affect the quality and user satisfaction of the outsourced electronic commerce systems developed by the contractors. For Australian hospitals lack of funding was often the most mentioned reason for not achieving such alignment while for Taiwanese hospitals the number one reason was lack of expertise and time in conducting a properly IT investment evaluation at the pre-project justification stage to ensure that a contractor with similar strategic alignment was selected. Getting accurate and complete user IRD is one of the most critical aspects for a successful ISD process and most of the errors from the ISD can be traced back to the IRD stage. However, it appeared that few outsourcing hospitals had paid sufficient attention to the potentially problematic user IRD process. In addition, there were differences for Australian and Taiwanese hospitals in engaging users and stakeholders during the electronic commerce outsourcing process. Australian hospitals executives tended to spend more time and allocate resources than their Taiwanese counterparts in involving and obtaining users requirements. For Australian hospitals, outsourcing gave rise to increased justification costs against measurable business unit outcomes. For Taiwanese hospitals, decision to outsource was often undertaken by the senior executives without consulting with the key users and stakeholders and was often used as one way to overcome lack of resources and to downsize their labor force.

Arguably, these findings have the potential to assist hospitals and other healthcare organizations in enhancing the understanding of their IT evaluation and benefits realization practices and processes. Paying close attention to their IT evaluation and benefits realization practices and processes is likely to enable hospitals and other healthcare organizations to reap benefits from their electronic commerce investments. These salient issues should be a top priority for hospital managers, researchers, and practitioners to pay close attention to. Indeed, it is imperative for the senior executives of the hospitals to carefully examine these key issues in order to obtain expected electronic commerce benefits from their outsourcing contracts. However, this does not mean that other behavioral, attitudinal and organizational issues should be neglected. For example, understanding the reactions of their users toward the newly acquired electronic commerce systems and their subsequent behavior can assist hospital executives in devising the appropriate intervention strategies, policies, and programs to maximize their use and their effects on the hospitals. These deliberate steps must be identified to achieve desirable outcomes and increase the pace of electronic commerce dissemination within the hospitals. For instance, relevant project champions should be identified to assist in minimizing the uncertainty of others in adopting new electronic commerce investments.

The study's contribution is not only to identify and examine key electronic commerce investment evaluation and outsourcing issues, but also to highlight the challenges by which hospitals can overcome in order to better manage the electronic commerce/IT outsourcing projects. As suspected, there are striking similarities between the Australian and Taiwanese hospitals. For example, a large proportion of the Australian and Taiwanese hospitals had used an IT investment evaluation methodology or process to measure and manage their outsourced projects. Finally, electronic commerce/IT also allows hospitals to target or communicate with their stakeholders such as customers (e.g., patients), external contractors (e.g., IT outsourcing contractors), or users (E.g., IT professionals) at a much lower cost (Huang, Phau, Lin, Chung, & Lin, 2008). Therefore, hospital executives need to make more informed decisions on how to invest in various types of electronic commerce/IT initiatives and systems in order to increase their efficiency and growth through building relationship with their customers and online users. Hospitals should spend more time, effort, and resources to develop effective long-term electronic commerce/IT marketing strategies in order to enhance stakeholder loyalty and improve efficiency. Similar to those strategies and programs employed in health promotion and advertising, through the participation of the online communities (e.g., Facebook, LinkedIn, MySpace, Twitter), intensive public awareness campaigns (e.g., posters) or other promotional events, the level of awareness and positive image of the electronic commerce/IT investments and services offered by the hospitals can be enhanced for both the existing and potential stakeholders (Donovan, Jalleh, Clarkson, & Giles-Corti, 1999; Donovan, Boulter, Borland, Jalleh, & Carter, 2003; Economo et al., 2010; Heydon, Kennington, Jalleh, & Lin, 2012; Jalleh et al., 2010; Jalleh, Donovan, Lin, & Slevin, 2008; Johnson et al., 2013). For existing stakeholders, these activities may facilitate them to form a sense of identity from being a valuable affiliate or member of the hospital, resulting in enhanced loyalty towards the hospital. Online word-of-mouth recommendations, for example, by these stakeholders can help to boost hospitals' financial and operational performance (Carter, Donovan, & Jalleh, 2011; Stringam & Gerdes Jr., 2010).

FUTURE RESEARCH DIRECTIONS AND STUDY LIMITATIONS

A lot of resources have been invested in implementing new and updated electronic commerce/IT systems across Australian and Taiwanese hospitals. Despite this, electronic commerce/IT systems within the hospital industry are generally not mature enough and they tend to struggle with the ability to utilize these resources into improved quality and efficiency for patients and other stakeholders. Due to the limited electronic commerce/IT sophistication between hospitals and other healthcare organizations, distributors, suppliers, and business partners in the past, they are lagging behind the bigger players in other industries in using electronic commerce applications to create competitive business networks. Nevertheless, electronic commerce systems and applications are creating a more level playing field for all industry players. It is expected that future electronic commerce systems and applications will bring about faster and more efficient business to hospitals by providing their users and patients more convenience and variety. Other areas that can benefits from electronic commerce systems and applications are legal counsels and external suppliers. It can also be applied in managing relationships with external organizations such as electronic intermediaries and other members of product and service value chain.

Finally, additional research is required to identify other issues which might influence the management and evaluation of electronic commerce/IT investment projects. Also, the study findings are based on 20 hospitals in Australia and Taiwan only. It would be interesting to conduct the research in other countries and with different healthcare systems and applications. This research relied on the information provided at a particular point in time. Further research could take a longitudinal approach as the hospitals' electronic commerce or IT investment evaluation and benefits realization practices and processes are likely to change over time. Alternatively, the study could be replicated in a few years' time to examine how electronic commerce/IT investment evaluation and benefits realization practices and processes in Australian and Taiwanese hospitals have changed and are being managed and evaluated in light of new or emerging electronic commerce technologies.

REFERENCES

Abelein, U., & Paech, B. (2013). Understanding the Influence of User Participation & Involvement on System Success–a Systematic Mapping Study. *Empirical Software Engineering*, 1–54.

Abelein, U., & Paech, B. (2014). State of Practice of User-Developer Communication in Large-Scale IT Projects. In *Requirements Engineering: Foundation for Software Quality* (pp. 95–111). Springer International Publishing. doi:10.1007/978-3-319-05843-6_8

Aggelidis, V. P., & Chatzoglou, P. D. (2012). Hospital information systems: Measuring end user computing satisfaction (EUCS). *Journal of Biomedical Informatics, 45*(3), 566–579. doi:10.1016/j.jbi.2012.02.009 PMID:22426283

Alaghehband, F. K., Rivard, S., Wu, S., & Goyette, S. (2011). An Assessment of the Use of Transaction Cost Theory in Information Technology Outsourcing. *The Journal of Strategic Information Systems, 20*(2), 125–138. doi:10.1016/j.jsis.2011.04.003

Ammenwerth, E., Brender, J., Nykanen, P., Prokosch, H. U., Rigby, M., & Talmon, J. (2004). HIS-EVAL workshop participants. Visions & strategies to improve evaluation of health information systems: Reflections & lessons based on the HIS-EVAL workshop in Innsbruck. *International Journal of Medical Informatics, 73*(6), 479–491. doi:10.1016/j.ijmedinf.2004.04.004 PMID:15171977

Aversano, L., Grasso, C., & Tortorella, M. (2013). A Literature Review of Business/IT Alignment Strategies. *Lecture Notes in Business Information Processing, 141*, 471–488. doi:10.1007/978-3-642-40654-6_28

Babar, A., Wong, B., & Abedin, B. (2014). Investigating the role of business analysts competencies into strategic business requirements gathering. *The 18th Pacific Asia Conference on Information Systems (PACIS 2014).*

Bano, M., & Zowghi, D. (2015). A systematic review on the relationship between user involvement and system success. *Information and Software Technology, 58*, 148–169. doi:10.1016/j.infsof.2014.06.011

Barua, A., Konana, P., & Whinston, A. B. (2004). An Empirical Investigation of Net-Enabled Business Value. *Management Information Systems Quarterly, 28*(4), 585–620.

Brender, J. (1997). *Methodology for Assessment of Medical IT-Based Systems.* IOS Press.

Britz, B., Petri, G., Tramacere, G., Roy, A., Ng, F., & Blackmore, D. et al. (2014). Forecast Analysis: IT Outsourcing, Worldwide, 1Q14 Update. *Gartner Report, G00261935*, 14.

Browne, G. J., & Ramesh, V. (2002). Improving Information Requirements Determination: A Cognitive Perspective. *Information & Management, 39*(8), 625–645. doi:10.1016/S0378-7206(02)00014-9

Brynjolfsson, E., & Hitt, L. M. (2003). Computing Productivity: Firm-Level Evidence. *The Review of Economics and Statistics*, *85*(4), 793–808. doi:10.1162/003465303772815736

Byrd, T. A., Lewis, B. R., & Bryan, R. W. (2006). The Leveraging Influence of Strategic Alignment on IT Investment: An Empirical Examination. *Information & Management*, *43*(3), 308–321. doi:10.1016/j.im.2005.07.002

Cao, Y., Lu, Y., Gupta, S., & Yang, S. (2015). The effects of differences between e–commerce and m–commerce on the consumers' usage transfer from online to mobile channel. *International Journal of Mobile Communications*, *13*(1), 51–70. doi:10.1504/IJMC.2015.065890

Carter, O., Donovan, R. J., & Jalleh, G. (2011). Using Viral e-mails to Distribute Tobacco Control Advertisements to Young Adults: An Experimental Investigation. *Journal of Health Communication*, *16*(7), 698–707. doi:10.1080/10810730.2011.551998 PMID:21432712

Chan, Y. E., Huff, S. L., Barclay, D. W., & Copeland, D. G. (1997). Business strategy orientation. *Information Systems Research*, *8*(2), 125–150. doi:10.1287/isre.8.2.125

Chao, C. J., Lin, C., Lin, K., Shen, C. L., & Wang, C. H. (2012). Using the Analytic Hierarchy Process Methodology to Assess the Drivers Affecting the Implementation of Interactive Digital Television as a Commerce Platform. *International Journal of Wireless Networks and Broadband Technologies*, *2*(3), 42–51. doi:10.4018/ijwnbt.2012070104

Chau, P. Y. K., & Jim, C. C. F. (2002). Adoption of Electronic Data Interchange in Small & Medium Sized Enterprises. *Journal of Global Information Management*, *10*(4), 61–85. doi:10.4018/jgim.2002100104

Chih, Y. Y., & Zwikael, O. (2015). Project benefit management: A conceptual framework of target benefit formulation. *International Journal of Project Management*, *33*(2), 352–362. doi:10.1016/j.ijproman.2014.06.002

Claxton, K., Paulden, M., Gravelle, H., Brouwer, W., & Culyer, A. J. (2011). Discounting & Decision Making in the Economic Evaluation of Health-Care Technologies. *Health Economics*, *20*(1), 2–15. doi:10.1002/hec.1612 PMID:21154521

Coiera, E. (2003). *Guide to Health Informatics*. Hodder Arnold. doi:10.1201/b13618

Coombs, C. R. (2015). When planned IS/IT project benefits are not realized: A study of inhibitors and facilitators to benefits realization. *International Journal of Project Management*, *33*(2), 363–379. doi:10.1016/j.ijproman.2014.06.012

Cutler, M., & Sterne, J. (2000). *E-Metrics: Business Metrics for the New Economy*. NetGenesis. Retrieved from http://www.netgen.com/emetrics/

Danvers, K., & Nikolov, P. (2010). Does Outsourcing Affect Hospital Profitability? *Journal of Health Care Finance*, *37*(1), 13–29. PMID:20973370

de Waal, B. M., & Batenburg, R. (2014). The process & structure of user participation: A BPM system implementation case study. *Business Process Management Journal*, *20*(1), 107–128. doi:10.1108/BPMJ-05-2012-0045

Doherty, N. F. (2014). The Role of Socio-technical Principles in Leveraging Meaningful Benefits from IT Investments. *Applied Ergonomics*, *45*(2), 181–187. doi:10.1016/j.apergo.2012.11.012 PMID:23305923

Doherty, N. F., Ashurst, C., & Peppard, J. (2012). Factors Affecting the Successful Realisation of Benefits from Systems Development Projects: Findings from Three Case Studies. *Journal of Information Technology*, *27*(1), 1–16. doi:10.1057/jit.2011.8

Donovan, R. J., Boulter, J., Borland, B., Jalleh, G., & Carter, O. (2003). Continuous Tracking of the Australian National Tobacco Campaign: Advertising Effects on Recall, Recognition, Cognitions, & Behaviour. *Tobacco Control*, *12*(90002Suppl II), ii30–ii39. doi:10.1136/tc.12.suppl_2.ii30 PMID:12878771

Donovan, R. J., Jalleh, G., Clarkson, J., & Giles-Corti, B. (1999). Evidence for effectiveness of sponsorship as a health promotion tool. *Australian Journal of Primary Health*, *5*(3), 82–92.

Durugbo, C. (2012). Modelling User Participation in Organisations as Networks. *Expert Systems with Applications*, *39*(10), 9230–9245. doi:10.1016/j.eswa.2012.02.082

Dutot, V., Bergeron, F., & Raymond, L. (2014). Information management for the internationalization of SMEs: An exploratory study based on a strategic alignment perspective. *International Journal of Information Management*, *34*(5), 672–681. doi:10.1016/j.ijinfomgt.2014.06.006

Economics, C. (2013). *IT Outsourcing Statistics: 2013/2014*. Irvine, CA: Computer Economics Inc.

Economo, K., Stewart, S., Sullivan, D., Jalleh, G., Carter, O., & Lin, C. (2010). The Importance of Public Education Campaigns in Raising Awareness & Support for Smoke-free Car Legislation in Western Australia. *Australian and New Zealand Journal of Public Health*, *34*(1), 92–93. doi:10.1111/j.1753-6405.2010.00483.x PMID:20920115

Eisenhardt, K. M. (1989). Building Theories From Case Study Research. *Academy of Management Review*, *14*(4), 532–550.

eMarketer. (2014). *Global B2C Ecommerce Sales to Hit $1.5 Trillion This Year Driven by Growth in Emerging Markets: Asia-Pacific leapfrogs North America to become world's largest regional ecommerce market*. eMaketer Inc.

Ferdosi, M., Farahabadi, E., Mofid, M., Rejalian, F., Haghighat, M., & Naghdi, P. (2013). Evaluation of Outsourcing in Nursing Services: A Case Study of Kashani Hospital, Isfahan in 2011. *Materia Socio-Medica*, *25*(1), 37–39. PMID:23678338

Friedman, C. P., & Wyatt, J. C. (1997). *Evaluation Methods in Medical Informatics*. New York: Springer-Verlag. doi:10.1007/978-1-4757-2685-5

GS1 Australia. (2005). *Hospital Pharmaceutical eCommerce Looks Healthy*. Media Press Release. GS1 Australia.

Giaglis, G. M., Paul, R. J., & Doukidis, G. I. (1999). Dynamic Modelling to Assess the Business Value of Electronic Commerce. *International Journal of Electronic Commerce*, *3*(3), 35–51. doi:10.1080/10864415.1999.11518340

Gorla, N., & Somers, T. M. (2014). The Impact of IT Outsourcing on Information Systems Success. *Information & Management*, *51*(3), 320–335. doi:10.1016/j.im.2013.12.002

Gorschek, T., Svahnberg, M., Borg, A., Loconsole, A., & Sandahl, K. (2007). A controlled empirical evaluation of a requirements abstraction model. *Information and Software Technology*, *49*(7), 790–805. doi:10.1016/j.infsof.2006.09.003

Hahn, E. D., & Bunyaratavej, K. (2010). Services cultural alignment in offshoring: The impact of cultural dimensions on offshoring location choices. *Journal of Operations Management*, *28*(3), 186–193. doi:10.1016/j.jom.2009.10.005

Han, J., & Lee, S. T. (2012). Impact of Vendor Selection on Firms' IT Outsourcing: The Korea Experience. *Journal of Global Information Management*, *20*(2), 25–43. doi:10.4018/jgim.2012040102

Handley, S. M., & Angst, C. M. (2015). The Impact Of Culture On The Relationship Between Governance And Opportunism In Outsourcing Relationships. *Strategic Management Journal*, *36*(9), 1412–1434. doi:10.1002/smj.2300

He, J., & King, W. R. (2008). The role of user participation in information systems development: Implications from a meta-analysis. *Journal of Management Information Systems*, *25*(1), 301–331. doi:10.2753/MIS0742-1222250111

Heeks, R. (1999). *Reinventing government in the information age: international practice in IT-enabled public sector reform*. London: Routledge. doi:10.4324/9780203204962

Hellang, Ø., Flak, L. S., & Päivärinta, T. (2013). Diverging Approaches to Benefits Realization from Public ICT Investments: A Study of Benefits Realization Methods in Norway. *Transforming Government: People. Process & Policy*, *7*(1), 93–108.

Heydon, N., Kennington, K. S., Jalleh, G., & Lin, C. (2012). Western Australian Smokers' Strongly Support Regulations on the Use of Chemicals and Additives in Cigarettes. *Tobacco Control*, *21*(3), 381–382. doi:10.1136/tobaccocontrol-2011-050302 PMID:22170334

Hofstede, G. H. (1997). *Cultures & organizations: Software of the mind*. New York, NY: McGraw-Hill.

Hsiao, C., Pai, J., & Chiu, H. (2009). The Study on the Outsourcing of Taiwan's Hospitals: A Questionnaire Survey Research. *BMC Health Services Research*, *9*(1), 78. doi:10.1186/1472-6963-9-78 PMID:19435526

Hsu, J. S., Lin, T., Zheng, G., & Hung, Y. (2012). Users as knowledge co-producers in the information system development project. *International Journal of Project Management*, *30*(1), 27–36. doi:10.1016/j.ijproman.2011.05.008

Huang, Y., Lin, C., Liu, Y., & Tung, M. (2013). The Effects of IT Resource Alignment and Organizational Dynamism on Alliance Performance in Hemodialysis Centers, *International Technology. Management Review*, *3*(2), 105–115.

Huang, Y., Phau, I., & Lin, C. (2010). Consumer Animosity, Economic Hardship, & Normative Influence: How Do They Affect Consumer's Purchase Intention? *European Journal of Marketing*, *44*(7/8), 909–937. doi:10.1108/03090561011047463

Huang, Y., Phau, I., Lin, C., Chung, H., & Lin, K. (2008). Allocentrism & Consumer Ethnocentrism: Social Identity on Purchase Intention, *Social Behavior & Personality. International Journal (Toronto, Ont.)*, *36*(8), 1097–1110.

Jalleh, G., Donovan, R. J., Lin, C., & Slevin, T. (2008). Changing Perceptions of Solaria & Cancer Risk: The Role of the Media. *The Medical Journal of Australia*, *188*(12), 735–735. PMID:18558905

Jalleh, G., Donovan, R. J., Lin, C., Slevin, T., Clayforth, C., Pratt, S., & Ledger, M. (2010). Beliefs about Bowel Cancer among the Target Group for the National Bowel Cancer Screening Program in Australia. *Australian and New Zealand Journal of Public Health*, *34*(2), 187–192. doi:10.1111/j.1753-6405.2010.00505.x PMID:23331364

Johnson, N., Murphy, A., McNeese, N., Reddy, M., & Purao, S. (2013). A Survey of Rural Hospitals' Perspectives on Health Information Technology Outsourcing. In *AMIA Annual Symposium Proceedings*. American Medical Informatics Association.

Johnson, R., Jalleh, G., Pratt, I. S., Donovan, R. J., Lin, C., Saunders, C., & Slevin, T. (2013). Online advertising by three commercial breast imaging services: Message takeout and effectiveness. *The Breast*, *22*(5), 780–786. doi:10.1016/j.breast.2013.01.013 PMID:23422256

Karimi, S., Agharahimi, Z., & Yaghoubi, M. (2012). Impacts of Outsourcing in Educational Hospitals in Iran: A Study on Isfahan University of Medical Sciences-2010. *Journal of Education & Health Promotion*, *1*(1), 25. doi:10.4103/2277-9531.99959 PMID:23555128

Karthik, V., & Kumar, S. (2013). Investigating 'Degree of Adoption' Effects on e–procurement Benefits. *International Journal of Procurement Management*, *6*(2), 211–234. doi:10.1504/IJPM.2013.052470

Khalil, O. E. M., & Elkordy, M. M. (2005). EIS Information: Use & Quality Determination. *Information Resources Management Journal*, *18*(2), 68–93. doi:10.4018/irmj.2005040104

Kocher, M. G., & Sutter, M. (2006). Time is Money: Time Pressure, Incentives, & the Quality of Decision Making. *Journal of Economic Behavior & Organization*, *61*(3), 375–392. doi:10.1016/j.jebo.2004.11.013

Kuhn, K. A., Giuse, D. A., & Talmon, J. L. (2003). The Heidelberg Conference: Setting an Agenda for the IMIA Working Group on Health Information Systems. *International Journal of Medical Informatics*, *69*(2–3), 77–82. doi:10.1016/S1386-5056(02)00097-7 PMID:12810112

Kuo, W., Lin, C., Hsu, G., & Huang, Y. (2006). An Empirical Study of Resource Contribution in SMEs Alliance. *Journal of Global Business Management*, *2*(2), 103–111.

Land, F. (1987). Adapting to Changing User Requirements. In R. D. Galliers (Ed.), *Information Analysis: Selected Readings*. Sydney: Addison - Wesley.

Lawrence, C., & Firth, D. (2013). Improving Healthcare Administration: Real Time Locations Systems or Outsourcing? *Information Systems Education Journal*, *11*(5), 49.

Lee, J., & Runge, J. (2001). Adoption of Information Technology in Small Business: Testing Drivers of Adoption for Entrepreneurs. *Journal of Computer Information Systems*, *42*(1), 44–57.

Lee, K. S., Lim, G. H., & Tan, S. J. (1999). Dealing with Resource Disadvantage: Generic Strategies for SMEs. *Small Business Economics, 12*(4), 299–311. doi:10.1023/A:1008085310245

Lee, M., & Jones, A. M. (2004). How Did Dentists Respond to the Introduction of Global Budgets in Taiwan? An Evaluation Using Individual Panel Data. *International Journal of Health Care Finance and Economics, 4*(4), 307–326. doi:10.1023/B:IHFE.0000043760.57999.36 PMID:15467407

Lee, S., & Kim, K.-J. (2007). Factors affecting the implementation success of Internet-based information systems. *Computers in Human Behavior, 23*(4), 1853–1880. doi:10.1016/j.chb.2005.12.001

Li, J. J. (2012). The alignment between organizational control mechanisms & outsourcing strategies: A commentary essay. *Journal of Business Research, 65*(9), 1384–1386. doi:10.1016/j.jbusres.2011.09.020

Licht, A. N. (2004). Legal plug-Ins: Cultural distance, cross-listing, & corporate governance reform. *Berkeley Journal of International Law, 22*, 195–239.

Lin, C. (2002). *An Investigation of the Process of IS/IT Investment Evaluation & Benefits Realisation in Large Australian Organisations*. (PhD Thesis). Curtin University of Technology, Perth, Western Australia. Retrieved from http://adt.curtin.edu.au/theses/available/adt-WCU20030826.094151/

Lin, C., & Huang, Y. (2007). An Integrated Framework for Managing eCRM Evaluation Process. *International Journal of Electronic Business, 5*(4), 340–359. doi:10.1504/IJEB.2007.014782

Lin, C., Huang, Y., & Burn, J. (2007). Realising B2B e-Commerce Benefits: The Link with IT Maturity, Evaluation Practices, & B2B e-Commerce Adoption Readiness. *European Journal of Information Systems, 16*(6), 806–819. doi:10.1057/palgrave.ejis.3000724

Lin, C., Huang, Y., Jalleh, G., Liu, Y., & Tung, M. (2010). An Exploratory Study of Factors Affecting Adoption & Implementation of B2B E-Commerce in Australian Health Care Organizations. *International Journal of Electronic Commerce Studies, 1*(2), 77–96.

Lin, C., Huang, Y., & Stockdale, R. (2011). Developing a B2B Website Effectiveness Model for SMEs. *Internet Research, 21*(3), 304–325. doi:10.1108/10662241111139327

Lin, C., Lin, H. K., Huang, Y., Jalleh, G., Liu, Y. C., Huang, Y-H., … Chao, C. (2014). Towards a B2B E-Commerce Evaluation Management Model to Assess Organizational Drivers in Hospitals. *International Technology Management Review*, *4*(3), 115-132.

Lin, C., & Lin, K. (2011). A Study of Information Requirement Determination Process of an Executive Information System. In Enterprise Information Systems: Concepts, Methodologies, Tools & Applications. IGI Publishing.

Lin, C., Lin, K., Huang, Y., & Kuo, W. (2006). Evaluation of Electronic Customer Relationship Management: The Critical Success Factors. *The Business Review, Cambridge*, *6*(2), 206–212.

Lin, C., & Pervan, G. (2000) Realising the Benefits of IS/IT Investments in Australian Organisations. *Proceedings of the Eleventh Australasian Conference on Information Systems (ACIS 2000)*.

Lin, C., & Pervan, G. (2001) IS/IT Investment Evaluation & Benefits Realisation Issues in a Government Organisation. *Proceedings of the Twelfth Australasian Conference on Information Systems (ACIS 2001)*.

Lin, C., Pervan, G., Lin, K., & Tsao, H. (2008). An Investigation into Business-to-Business Electronic Commerce Organizations. *Journal of Research & Practice in Information Technology*, *40*(1), 3–18.

Lin, C., Pervan, G., & McDermid, D. (2002). Research on IS/IT Investment Evaluation & Benefits Realization in Australia. In W. Van Grembergen (Ed.), *Information Systems Evaluation Management* (pp. 244–254). Hershey, PA: IRM Press. doi:10.4018/978-1-931777-18-6.ch015

Liu, J. Y., Chen, H., Chen, C., & Sheu, T. S. (2011). Relationships among Interpersonal Conflict, Requirements Uncertainty, & Software Project Performance. *International Journal of Project Management*, *29*(5), 547–556. doi:10.1016/j.ijproman.2010.04.007

Liu, Y., Huang, Y., & Lin, C. (2012). Organizational Factors' Effects on The Success of E-Learning System & Organizational Benefits - An Empirical Study in Taiwan. *International Review of Research in Open and Distance Learning*, *13*(4), 130–151.

Love, P. E. D., Irani, Z., Standing, C., Lin, C., & Burn, J. (2005). The Enigma of Evaluation: Benefits, Costs & Risks of IT in Small-Medium Sized Enterprises. *Information & Management*, *42*(7), 947–964. doi:10.1016/j.im.2004.10.004

Low, C., & Chen, Y. H. (2012). Criteria for the Evaluation of a Cloud-based Hospital Information System Outsourcing Provider. *Journal of Medical Systems*, *36*(6), 3543–3553. doi:10.1007/s10916-012-9829-z PMID:22366976

McGaughey, R. E. (2002). Benchmarking Business-to-business Electronic Commerce, *Benchmarking. International Journal (Toronto, Ont.)*, *9*(5), 471–484.

McIvor, R. (2000). A practical framework for understanding the outsourcing process. *Supply Chain Management: An International Journal*, *5*(1), 22–36. doi:10.1108/13598540010312945

McKay, J., & Marshall, P. (2004). Strategic Management of eBusiness, John Wiley & Sons Australia, Ltd, Queensland.

Melville, N., Kraemer, K., & Gurbaxani, V. (2004). Review: Information Technology & Organizational Performance: An integrative Model of IT Business Value. *Management Information Systems Quarterly*, *28*(2), 283–322.

Menachemi, N., Burke, D., & Diana, M. (2007). Characteristics of Hospitals that Outsource Information. System Functions. *Journal of Healthcare Information Management*, *19*(1), 63–69. PMID:15682678

Mettler, T., Fitterer, R., Rohner, P., & Winter, R. (2014). Does a hospital's IT architecture fit with its strategy? An approach to measure the alignment of health information technology. *Health Systems*, *3*(1), 29–42.

Miles, M. B., & Huberman, A. M. (1994). *Qualitative Data Analysis: An Expanded Sourcebook*. California: Sage Publications.

Misra, R. B. (2004). Global IT Outsourcing: Metrics for Success of All Parties. *Journal of Information Technology Cases & Applications*, *6*(3), 21–34. doi:10.1080/15228053.2004.10856047

Mitra, S., Sambamurthy, V., & Westerman, G. (2011). Measuring IT Performance & Communicating Value. *MIS Quarterly Executive*, *10*(1), 47–59.

Moon, J., Choe, Y. C., Chung, M., Jung, G. H., & Swar, B. (2014). IT outsourcing success in the public sector lessons from e-government practices in Korea. *Information Development*, *0266666914528930*, 1–19.

More, E., & McGrath, M. (2002). An Australian Case in e-Health Communication & Change. *Journal of Management Development*, *21*(7/8), 612–632.

Mudambi, S. M., & Tallman, S. (2010). Make, buy or ally? Theoretical perspectives on knowledge process outsourcing through alliances. *Journal of Management Studies*, *47*(8), 1434–1456. doi:10.1111/j.1467-6486.2010.00944.x

Nakatsu, R. T., & Iacovou, C. L. (2009). A Comparative Study of Important Risk Factors Involved in Offshore & Domestic Outsourcing of Software Development Projects: A Two-Panel Delphi Study. *Information & Management*, *46*(1), 57–68. doi:10.1016/j.im.2008.11.005

NEHTA. (2010). *Australia Launches Leading Edge e-Health Supply Chain Location Directory – NEHTA*. National E-Health Transition Authority, Media Press Release. Retrieved from http://www.nehta.gov.au/

Norton, A. L., Coulson-Thomas, Y. M., Coulson-Thomas, C. J., & Ashurst, C. (2013). Ensuring Benefits Realisation from ERP II: The CSF Phasing Model. *Journal of Enterprise Information Management*, *26*(3), 218–234. doi:10.1108/17410391311325207

Ondo, K., & Smith, M. (2006). Outside IT the Case for Full IT Outsourcing: Study Findings Indicate Many Hospitals Are Turning to Full IT Outsourcing to Achieve IT Excellence. What's the Best Approach for Your Organization? *Healthcare Financial Management*, (February): 1–3.

Ozkan, S., Baykal, N., & Sincan, M. (2012). *Process-Based Evaluation of Hospital Information Systems: Application of an Information System Success Model (PRISE) in the Healthcare Domain. In Health Information Systems: Concepts, Methodologies, Tools, and Applications* (pp. 339–355). Hershey, PA: IGI Global.

Parker, M. M. (1996). *Strategic Transformation & Information Technology*. Upper Saddle River, NJ: Prentice-Hall.

Paul, S., & Nazareth, D. L. (2010). Input information complexity, perceived time pressure, & information processing in GSS-based work groups: An experimental investigation using a decision schema to alleviate information overload conditions. *Decision Support Systems*, *49*(1), 31–40. doi:10.1016/j.dss.2009.12.007

Petter, S., DeLone, W., & McLean, E. R. (2013). Information Systems Success: The Quest for the Independent Variables. *Journal of Management Information Systems*, *29*(4), 7–62. doi:10.2753/MIS0742-1222290401

Peute, L. W., Aarts, J., Bakker, P. J., & Jaspers, M. W. (2010). Anatomy of a failure: A sociotechnical evaluation of a laboratory physician order entry system implementation. *International Journal of Medical Informatics*, *79*(4), e58–e70. doi:10.1016/j.ijmedinf.2009.06.008 PMID:19640778

Ragu-Nathana, B. S., Apigian, C. H., Ragu-Nathana, T. S., & Tu, Q. (2004). A path analytic study of the effect of top management support for information systems performance. *Omega*, *32*(6), 459–471. doi:10.1016/j.omega.2004.03.001

Rahim, M. M., Kurnia, S., Samson, D., & Singh, P. (2014). Developing an IT Maturity Model for Sustainable Supply Chain Management Implementation. *The 18th Pacific Asia Conference on Information Systems (PACIS 2014).*

Raisinghani, M. S., Melemez, T., Zhou, L., Paslowski, C., Kikvidze, I., Taha, S., & Simons, K. (2005). E-Business Models in B2B: Process Based Categorization & Analysis of B2B Models. *International Journal of E-Business Research*, *1*(1), 16–36. doi:10.4018/jebr.2005010102

Ralston, D. A., Holt, D. H., Terpstra, R. H., & Kai-Cheng, Y. (2008). The impact of national culture & economic ideology on managerial work values: A study of the United States, Russia, Japan, & China. *Journal of International Business Studies*, *39*(1), 8–26. doi:10.1057/palgrave.jibs.8400330

Ramezan, M. (2011). Intellectual capital & organizational organic structure in knowledge society:How are these concepts related? *International Journal of Information Management*, *31*(1), 88–95. doi:10.1016/j.ijinfomgt.2010.10.004

Remenyi, D., & Whittaker, L. (1996). The Evaluation of Business Process Reengineering Projects. In L. Willcocks (Ed.), *Investing in information systems: evaluation & management* (pp. 143–167). Chapman & Hall.

Rise, M. B., Solbjør, M., & Steinsbekk, A. (2014). Experiences from the implementation of a comprehensive development plan for user involvement in a mental health hospital: A qualitative case study. *The International Journal of Social Psychiatry*, *60*(4), 387–395. doi:10.1177/0020764013491739 PMID:23812411

Rissler, A. (1994). Extended periods of challenging demands in high tech work. Consequences for efficiency, quality of life & health. In G. E. Bradley & H. W. Hendrick (Eds.), *Human factors in organizational design & management* (vol. 4, pp. 727–732). Amsterdam: Elsevier.

Sadoughi, F., & Aminpour, F. (2011). A Review on the Evaluation Methods of Health Information Systems. *Indian Journal of Medical Education*, *10*(5), 1077–1086.

Samantra, C., Datta, S., & Mahapatra, S. S. (2014). Risk Assessment in IT Outsourcing using Fuzzy Decision-making Approach: An Indian Perspective. *Expert Systems with Applications*, *41*(8), 4010–4022. doi:10.1016/j.eswa.2013.12.024

Saorín-Iborra, M. C., Redondo-Cano, A., Revuelto-Taboada, L., & Vogler, É. (2015). Negotiating behavior in service outsourcing. An exploratory case study analysis. *Service Business*, 1–31. doi:10.1007/s11628-014-0259-5

Schick, A. G., Gordon, L. A., & Haka, S. (1990). Information overload: A temporal approach. *Accounting, Organizations and Society*, *15*(3), 199–220. doi:10.1016/0361-3682(90)90005-F

Schultze, U., & Vandenbosch, B. (1998). Information overload in a groupware environment: Now you see it, now you don't. *Journal of Organizational Computing and Electronic Commerce*, *8*(2), 127–148. doi:10.1207/s15327744joce0802_3

Shani, A. B., & Sena, J. A. (1994). Information technology & the integration of change: Sociotechnical system approach. *The Journal of Applied Behavioral Science*, *30*(2), 247–261. doi:10.1177/0021886394302007

Shapiro, D. (2009). Examining Taiwan's hospitals. *Topics*, *39*(3).

Shuraida, S., & Barki, H. (2013). The Influence of Analyst Communication in IS Projects. *Journal of the Association for Information Systems*, *14*(9), 482–520.

Silverman, D. (2001). *Interpreting qualitative data* (2nd ed.). London: Sage.

Spears, J. L., & Barki, H. (2010). User Participation in Information Systems Security Risk Management. *Management Information Systems Quarterly*, *34*(3), 503–528.

Standing, C., & Lin, C. (2007). Organizational Evaluation of the Benefits, Constraints & Satisfaction with Business-To-Business Electronic Commerce. *International Journal of Electronic Commerce*, *11*(3), 107–153. doi:10.2753/JEC1086-4415110304

Standing, S., Standing, C., & Lin, C. (2008). A Framework for Managing Knowledge in Strategic Alliances in the Biotechnology Sector. *Systems Research and Behavioral Science*, *25*(6), 783–796. doi:10.1002/sres.861

Stratopoulos, T., & Dehning, B. (2000). Does Successful Investments in Information Technology Solve the Productivity Paradox? *Information & Management*, *38*(2), 103–117. doi:10.1016/S0378-7206(00)00058-6

Stringham, B. B., & Gerdes, J. Jr. (2010). An Analysis of Word-of-Mouse Ratings & Guest Comments of Online Hotel Distribution Sites. *Journal of Hospitality Marketing & Management*, *19*(7), 773–796. doi:10.1080/19368623.2010.508009

Sugumaran, V., & Arogyaswamy, B. (2004). Measuring IT Performance: "Contingency" Variables & Value Modes. *Journal of Computer Information Systems*, *44*(2), 79–86.

Sujata, T. L., Reddy, B. K., & Jayalakshmi, C. (2013). Hospitals Outsourcing Complete Departments: A Study. *International Journal of Research in Commerce & Management*, *4*(9), 1–4.

Syrek, C. J., Apostel, E., & Antoni, C. H. (2013). Stress in Highly Demanding IT Jobs: Transformational Leadership Moderates the Impact of Time Pressure on Exhaustion & Work–life Balance. *Journal of Occupational Health Psychology*, *18*(3), 252–261. doi:10.1037/a0033085 PMID:23834443

Tallon, P. P., Kraemer, K. L., & Gurbaxani, V. (2000). Executives' Perceptions of the Business Value of Information Technology: A Process-Oriented Approach. *Journal of Management Information Systems*, *16*(4), 145–173. doi:10.1080/07421222.2000.11518269

Thatcher, M. D., & Pingry, D. E. (2004). Understanding the Business Value of Information Technology Investments: Theoretical Evidence from Alternative Market & Cost Structure. *Journal of Management Information Systems*, *21*(2), 61–85.

Thomas, R. W., Fugate, B. S., & Koukova, N. T. (2011). Coping with Time Pressure & Knowledge Sharing in Buyer-Supplier Relationships. *Journal of Supply Chain Management*, *47*(3), 22–42. doi:10.1111/j.1745-493X.2011.03229.x

THRF. (2011). *Hospital Finance: The Financial Supervision for the Health Institutions in Taiwan*. Taipei, Taiwan: Taiwan Healthcare Reform Foundation.

Torkzadeh, G., & Dhillon, G. (2002). Measuring Factors that Influence the Success of Internet Commerce. *Information Systems Research*, *13*(2), 187–204. doi:10.1287/isre.13.2.187.87

Trist, E. H., Murray, B. J., & Pollack, A. (1963). *Organizational Choice*. London: Tavistock.

Tsao, H., Lin, K., & Lin, C. (2004). An Investigation of Critical Success Factors in the Adoption of B2BEC by Taiwanese Companies. *The Journal of American Academy of Business, Cambridge*, *5*(1/2), 198–202.

Urquhart, C. (2001). Analysts & Clients in Organizational Context: A Conversational Perspective. *The Journal of Strategic Information Systems*, *10*(3), 243–262. doi:10.1016/S0963-8687(01)00046-4

Walston, S. L., Bennett, C. J., & Al-Harbi, A. (2014). Understanding the Factors Affecting Employees' Perceived Benefits of Healthcare Information Technology. *International Journal of Healthcare Management*, *7*(1), 35–44. doi:10.1179/2047971913Y.0000000051

Ward, J., & Griffiths, P. (1996). *Strategic Planning For Information Systems*. Chichester, UK: John Wiley & Sons Ltd.

Wolf, M. S., Seligman, H., Davis, T. C., Fleming, D. A., Curtis, L. M., & Pandit, A. U. et al. (2014). Clinic-Based Versus Outsourced Implementation of a Diabetes Health Literacy Intervention. *Journal of General Internal Medicine*, *29*(1), 59–67. doi:10.1007/s11606-013-2582-2 PMID:24002623

Wu, I., & Shen, Y. (2006). A Model for Exploring the Impact of Purchasing Strategies on User Requirements determination of e-SRM. *Information & Management*, *43*(4), 411–422. doi:10.1016/j.im.2004.11.004

Yayla, A. A., & Hu, Q. (2012). The impact of IT-business strategic alignment on firm performance in a developing country setting: Exploring moderating roles of environmental uncertainty & strategic orientation. *European Journal of Information Systems*, *21*(4), 373–387. doi:10.1057/ejis.2011.52

Yeh, C. H., Lee, G. G., & Pai, J. C. (2014). Using a technology-organization-environment framework to investigate the factors influencing e-business information technology capabilities. *Information Development*.

Yin, R. K. (2002). *Case Study Research, Design & Methods* (3rd ed.). Newbury Park, CA: Sage Publications.

Young, R., & Jordan, E. (2008). Top management support: Mantra or necessity. *International Journal of Project Management*, *26*(7), 713–725. doi:10.1016/j.ijproman.2008.06.001

Yu, P. (2010). A multi-method approach to evaluate health information systems. *World Congress on Medical Informatics* (pp. 1231-1235). Amsterdam: IOS Press.

Yusof, M. M., Kuljis, J., Papazafeiropoulou, A., & Stergioulas, L. K. (2008b). An Evaluation Framework for Health Information Systems: Human, Organization & Technology-fit Factors (HOT-fit). *International Journal of Medical Informatics*, *77*(6), 386–398. doi:10.1016/j.ijmedinf.2007.08.011 PMID:17964851

Yusof, M. M., Papazafeiropoulou, A., Paul, R. J., & Stergioulas, L. K. (2008a). Investigating Evaluation Frameworks for Health Information Systems. *International Journal of Medical Informatics*, *77*(6), 377–385. doi:10.1016/j.ijmedinf.2007.08.004 PMID:17904898

Zeng, Y. E., Wen, H. J., & Yen, D. C. (2003). Customer Relationship Management (CRM) in Business-to-business (B2B) E-commerce. *Information Management & Computer Security*, *11*(1), 39–44. doi:10.1108/09685220310463722

Zhuang, Y. (2005). Does Electronic Business Create Value For Firms? An Organizational Innovation Perspective. *Journal of Electronic Commerce Research*, *6*(2), 146–159.

Zika-Viktorsson, A., Sundstrom, P., & Engwall, M. (2006). Project overload: An exploratory study of work & management in multi-project settings. *International Journal of Project Management*, *24*(5), 385–394. doi:10.1016/j.ijproman.2006.02.010

ADDITIONAL READING

Carver, C. S. (1996). Emergent integration in contemporary personality psychology. *Journal of Research in Personality*, *30*(3), 319–334. doi:10.1006/jrpe.1996.0022

Farbey, B. F., Land, F., & Targett, D. (1999). The Moving Staircase: Problems of Appraisal & Evaluation in a Turbulent Environment. *Information Technology & People*, *12*(3), 238–252. doi:10.1108/09593849910278196

Galliers, R. D., & Sutherland, A. R. (1991). Information Systems Management & Strategy Formulation: The 'Stages of Growth' Model Revisited. *Journal of Information Systems*, *1*(1), 89–114. doi:10.1111/j.1365-2575.1991.tb00030.x

Haley, D. (2004). A Case for Outsourcing Medical Device Reprocessing. *AORN Journal*, *79*(4), 806–808. doi:10.1016/S0001-2092(06)60821-1 PMID:15115351

Hirschheim, R., Earl, M., Feeny, D., & Lockett, M. (1988). An Exploration Into the Management of the Information Function: Key issues & an Evolutionary Model, *Proceedings of Information Technology Management for Productivity & Strategic Advantage*, IFIP TC-8 Open Conference, Singapore, March.

Huang, Y., Phau, I., & Lin, C. (2010). Effects of Animosity & Allocentrism on Consumer Ethnocentrism: Social Identity on Consumer Willingness to Purchase, *Asia Pacific. Management Review*, *15*(3), 359–376.

Jalleh, G., Donovan, R. J., Slevin, T., & Lin, C. (2009). Efficacy of Breast Cancer Appeals for Promoting Physical Activity. *Journal of Cancer Education*, *24*(1), 33–35. doi:10.1080/08858190802664313 PMID:19259863

Kaplan, B., & Shaw, N. (2002). People, organizational & social issues: evaluation as an Exemplar, in: R. Haux, C. Kulikowski (Eds.), Yearbook of Medical Infomatics, 91–102.

Lin, C., Huang, Y., & Jalleh, G. (2008). Improving Alliance Satisfaction: The Resource Alignment of IT Competency in Small Healthcare Centers, *International Technology. Management Review*, *1*(2), 25–42.

Lin, C., & Pervan, G. (2003). The Practice of IS/IT Benefits Management in Large Australian Organizations. *Information & Management*, *41*(1), 13–24. doi:10.1016/S0378-7206(03)00002-8

Lin, C., Pervan, G., & McDermid, D. (2005). IS/IT Investment Evaluation & Benefits Realization Issues in Australia. *Journal of Research & Practices in Information Technology*, *37*(3), 235–251.

Liu, X., Hotchkiss, D. R., & Bose, S. (2008). The Effectiveness of Contracting out Primary Health Care Services in Developing Countries: A Review of the Evidence. *Health Policy and Planning*, *23*(1), 1–13. doi:10.1093/heapol/czm042 PMID:17999986

Liu, Y., & Lin, C. (2008). How Are Public Sector Organizations Assessing their IT Investments & Benefits - An Understanding of Issues For Benchmarking. *International Journal of Advanced Information Technologies*, *2*(2), 86–100.

Lorence, D. P., & Spink, A. (2004). Healthcare Information Systems Outsourcing. *International Journal of Information Management*, *24*(2), 131–145. doi:10.1016/j.ijinfomgt.2003.12.011

Marshall, P., & McKay, J. (2002). Evaluating the Benefits of Electronic Commerce in Small & Medium Enterprises. *The Australian Journal of Information Systems*, *9*(2).

Meyers, S. (2004). ED Outsourcing: Is It Good for Patient Care? *Trustee*, *57*, 12–14. PMID:15119060

Moschuris, S. J., & Kondylis, M. N. (2006). Outsourcing in Public Hospitals: A Greek Perspective. *Journal of Health Organization and Management*, *20*(1), 4–14. doi:10.1108/14777260610656534 PMID:16703840

Pennington, R., & Tuttle, B. (2007). The Effects of Information Overload on Software Project Risk Assessment. *Decision Sciences*, *38*(3), 489–526. doi:10.1111/j.1540-5915.2007.00167.x

Ranganathan, C., & Balaji, S. (2007). Critical capabilities for offshore outsourcing of IS. *MIS Quarterly Executive*, *6*(3), 147–164.

Roberts, V. (2001). Managing Strategic Outsourcing in the Healthcare Industry. *Journal of Healthcare Management*, *46*(4), 239–249. PMID:11482242

Standing, C., Guilfoyle, A., Lin, C., & Love, P. E. D. (2006). The Attribution of Success & Failure in IT Projects. *Industrial Management & Data Systems, 106*(8), 1148–1165. doi:10.1108/02635570610710809

Ward, J., Taylor, P., & Bond, P. (1996). Evaluation & Realization of IS/IT Benefits: An Empirical Study of Current Practice. *European Journal of Information Systems, 4*(4), 214–225. doi:10.1057/ejis.1996.3

Willcocks, L., & Lester, S. (1997). Assessing IT Productivity: Any Way Out of the Labyrinth? In L. Willcocks, D. F. Feeny, & G. Islei (Eds.), *Managing IT as a Strategic Resource, Ch4* (pp. 64–93). London: The McGraw-Hill Company.

KEY TERMS AND DEFINITIONS

Electronic Commerce: It refers to the utilization of information and communication technologies (e.g. the Web, the Internet, intranets, extranets) in support of all business activities. It is a business model that is conducted over the Internet in which clients are able to participate in all phases of a purchase decision. Electronic commerce can be between two businesses transmitting funds, goods, services or between a business and a customer.

IRD: The information requirements determination. It is a set of activities used by a systems analyst when assessing the functionality required in a proposed system.

Information Technology (IT): Any computer-based tool that users use to work with information and support the information needs of an organization.

Information Technology Outsourcing: The practice of transferring IT systems, assets, staff, and management responsibility for delivery of services from internal IT functions to external contractors.

IT Investment Evaluation Methodologies: Approaches that are used to evaluate and monitor organizations' IT investments.

Methodology: An organized, documented set of guidelines and procedures for one or more phases of the systems development life cycle, such as analysis or design.

Top Management Support: It is the degree to which senior executives understand the importance of the IT/electronic commerce function and the extent to which it is involved in IT/electronic commerce projects.

Chapter 6
Waseda University's E-School:
10 Years of E-Education in Japan

Shoji Nishimura
Waseda University, Japan

Douglass J. Scott
Waseda University, Japan

ABSTRACT

In 2003, the School of Human Sciences, Waseda University (Japan), established the e-School, Japan's first complete undergraduate program enabling students to earn their bachelor degrees solely through e-learning. Supported by the availability of high-speed Internet connections, it has become possible to economically transmit high-quality videotaped lectures across Japan and throughout the world. Waseda's e-School has many features that contribute to its success, among these are that lecture contents are transmitted with an image quality that allows students to easily read what is written on the blackboard. In addition, online classes are relatively small—21 students on average—and new classes are created to respond to students' needs and interests. This chapter outlines the e-School's first 10 years of operation: Its history, curriculum, administration, and management learning system. Data are also presented for student engagement with the e-School system for the first ten years of operation (2003-2012).

DOI: 10.4018/978-1-4666-9870-3.ch006

INTRODUCTION

Waseda University, one of Japan's oldest private universities, started to issue "*Waseda kougiroku*" ("Waseda lecture transcripts") for off-campus students in 1886, only four years after the University was founded. *Waseda kougiroku* continued to be issued until 1957 and was ultimately distributed to a total of 2.7 million students. Such students include many distinguished researchers and scholars in Japan, such as Soukichi Tsuda, the famous historian specializing in Japanese and Chinese intellectual histories. *Waseda kougiroku*, along with the "itinerant lectures" given in various regions in Japan, deserves special mention in the history of lifelong education in Japan (Waseda Daigaku 1972).

Since 1949, Waseda University was engaged in providing continuing education through its School of Political Science and Economics II (closed in 1973), the School of Law II (closed in 1973), the School of Letters, Arts and Sciences II, the School of Commerce II (closed in 1973), and the School of Science and Engineering II (closed in 1968), all of which taught evening courses, as well as the School of Social Sciences (established in 1966) which offered classes both in the daytime and evenings. However, these courses were offered on-campus and the University had no correspondence courses as a university under the post-war system. The advent of widely-available Internet connections was to greatly change the University's educational delivery options (Waseda Daigaku 2007).

Aoki and Bray (2006) explained that the Japanese Ministry of Education recognized correspondence and distance learning schools starting in 1950. This recognition granted accredited schools the authority to issue degrees to graduating students. The authors note that while distance-learning programs could receive accreditation, the Ministry of Education maintained separate systems for these new programs and traditional campus-based institutions (Aoki & Bray 2006). This separation continues to this day.

In the United States, e-learning on the Internet was actively introduced by higher education institutions since the middle of the 1990's. In particular, with regard to distance education, the University of Phoenix introduced large-scale e-learning in a successful manner (Sperling 2000, Yoshida 2002). Japan's entrance into Internet-based education was delayed because Japanese law didn't allow universities to offer Internet-based education until 2001. Amendments to the standards for the establishment of universities by the Ministry of Education, Culture, Sports, Science and Technology in March 2001 specified that "a class utilizing the Internet" (i.e. a kind of e-learning) could be recognized as one form of "a class conducted by using media (remote teaching)." This allowed universities' correspondence courses to use the Internet as the primary means of delivering course content for all credits required for graduation (i.e. 124 credits) (Shimizu 2002).

Improved access to high-speed Internet connections also contributed to the development of Internet-based education in Japan. According to Japan's Ministry of Public Management, Home Affairs, Posts and Telecommunications, as of the end of March 2003, the accumulated number of subscribers of broadband Internet connections amounted to approximately 6.9 million (DSL: 6,589,867, FTTH: 305,387) (Economic Research Office 2004). The spread of broadband Internet connections made it easier to deliver dynamic picture images in high quality to the average home.

Various Japanese universities have created Internet-based educational programs. In Japan, national universities were given independent status in April 2004, and these universities were eager to highlight their school's assets, which created increasing interest in e-learning and distance learning (Shimizu 2004). Some universities, such as Yashima Gakuen University, Japan Cyber University, Nihon University Graduate School, Shinshu University, and Nagaoka University of Technology, started to offer e-learning-based curricula coordinated by each school. Yashima Gakuen University is a correspondence university established in April 2004. Students can graduate by using the Internet without the need to study on campus. The program's characteristic learning method is multiple simultaneous communications known as Media Schooling (Asai 2005). Nihon University Graduate School of Social and Cultural Studies was the first correspondence graduate school in Japan. Nihon University Graduate School of Social and Cultural Studies was established in 1999 and uses the Internet and various information and communication technologies to facilitate the communication among the teachers and the students. Shinshu University, Graduate School of Science and Technology on the Internet (SUGSI) was established in 2002, and the undergraduate course on the Internet (Shinshu University, School on the Internet; SUSI), was established in 2004. In particular, the Internet Graduate School of Shinshu University allows students to complete their master courses solely by taking classes over the Internet (Fuwa et al. 2004, Ueno 2004).

Following the establishment of e-schools by accredited Japanese universities, the Ministry of Education allowed companies to create online learning degree programs (Public Relations Office March, 2009). The first of these was Business Breakthrough University which has a singularly complex history. BBTU, as it is known, began teaching specialized, non-degree courses in 1998 (BBTU.com 2014). In 2005, an accredited graduate school was established (Ōmae 2012), followed by an undergraduate degree program in 2010 (Ōmae 2012). In the midst of this complex program development, Japan Cyber University's undergraduate program was established in 2007 in Fukuoka prefecture (Kawahara 2010). Cyber University maintains no face-to-face classes ("schooling" in Japanese) and all degree programs are conducted online (Kawahara 2010).

While other Japanese university programs offer Internet-based education, Waseda University was the first to offer a complete undergraduate degree program using the Internet graduating its first class in 2006. Through the activities carried out by the Digital Campus Consortium established in 1999 (Matsuoka 2001) and the active use of on-demand lectures that were started mainly by Waseda's School of Letters, Arts and Sciences in 2001 (lecture delivery using on-demand streaming), Waseda University had already accumulated considerable experience regarding classes utilizing the Internet and had established infrastructure such as a lecture transmission system (Matsuoka 2001). These programs were a valuable foundation upon which to build Waseda's e-School, Japan's first degree program the first university to offer correspondence courses enabling undergraduate students to graduate solely by taking classes using the Internet.

This online undergraduate degree program was developed by the faculty of the School of Human Sciences (established in 1987), an appropriate choice given the School's emphasis on a wide range of social concerns. The School of Human Sciences was established, in part, out of concern that humanity had been impaired by a number of social problems as it moved toward the 21st century. Waseda University advocated the broad study of human sciences with the lofty goals of correcting this situation, restoring humanity, and helping to cultivate people who are engaged in education and research with respect to a wide range of issues facing humans (Waseda University 2002). Initially, with the goal of solving various problems with modern society and establishing a sustainable society, the School of Human Sciences pursued education and research focused on comprehensive and academic perspectives as approaches that are different from deepening each segmented field of science. Later, the rapid change in the world and Japan society particularly in the last 10 years brought a significant change to the contents of the education and research at the School of Human Sciences of Waseda University. The School of Human Sciences, then, was reorganized in 2003 into three new departments that were developed based on the results of the education and research accumulated so far and set new targets for education and research. Specifically, the School of Human Sciences decided to address "environment," "health and welfare" and "information," to better address the urgent issues of the 21st century (Waseda University 2002).

Most members of society are conscious of problems in the environment, health and welfare, and information. When compared with students without work experience, people who are employed or supporting a family are considered to be more conscious of such problems more deeply and urgently concerned about such matters due to the various experiences they have accumulated in the real world. On the other hand, these working people often had limited opportunities to learn about different ways to approach and address such problems. The spread of broadband Internet access through ADSL and the amendments made to the standards for establishment of universities enabled such people to acquire their bachelor degrees by attending classes from home in their spare time.

Under these circumstances, it has become possible to provide a place for learning about the academic and technical approaches to working adults and other members of the society who are highly conscious about problems regarding the environment, health and welfare, and information. This article describes the correspondence courses of the School of Human Sciences, Waseda University (generally called "e-School of the School of Human Sciences, Waseda University" hereinafter referred to as "e-School"), the first ever university correspondence courses in Japan established in April 2003, enabling students to acquire their bachelor degrees solely by taking classes on the Internet. It also reports on the actual achievement in two years, and discusses e-learning as an educational method.

This paper will focus on the e-School's first 10 years of operation. The following sections of this paper outline the e-School's curriculum, management structure, and delivery system, and results of course evaluations and student engagement with the learning system.

ORGANIZATIONAL STRUCTURE

Faculty Organization and Administrative Structure

The e-School was launched in April 2003, at the same time of the reorganization of the School of Human Sciences and the integration of full-time faculties; all full-time faculty members (69 in 2003 which grew to 84 by 2012) teach classes for both e-School and on-campus courses. The burden on faculty members was adjusted to balance the classes for correspondence courses and on-campus courses, and the number of classes assigned to each faculty is almost the same as the average number of classes assigned to each faculty member overall at Waseda University (90 minutes per class, seven classes per week, for one academic year). In addition, an Associate Dean of Academic Affairs and an Associate Dean of Student Affairs are selected and assigned as executive members of the School of Human Sciences and they are engaged in the operation of the School.

With regard to the administrative work, the creation of lecture contents and the system's operation, aside from the two full-time staff members in charge of the e-School, are managed by professionals staff dispatched by a company funded by Waseda University (hereinafter referred to as the "University's affiliated company") as these tasks require know-how that is different from the on-campus courses. Creation of lecture contents, management and operation of the lecture delivery system, and Learning Management System (LMS), training of mentors (discussed below), personnel management, and publicity activities are mainly performed by such personnel.

For creating lecture videos, two directors, two camera operators, one editor, and one person in charge of copyright acquisition (including license acquisition for third parties' literary works) worked on a regular basis in the studio on the Tokorozawa Campus of Waseda University where the School of Human Sciences is located. The lecture delivery system and Learning Management System (LMS) are operated by three staff members of the University in charge of these systems in cooperation with staff members of the company that established the server and is hosting the same. In addition, three other staff members assisted with clerical work.

Academic Coaches

University faculty are assisted in their teaching of the e-School's courses by "Academic Coaches." The position of instructor under former university correspondence courses was reinterpreted as "Academic Coach" to match the system of the e-School that focuses on classes utilizing the Internet. During the semester, Academic Coaches, in cooperation with the professor of record, act as contact people to receive and answer questions posted by the students on the Bulletin Board System (BBS) or sent by e-mail as well as taking the role of mentors to provide other learning assistance, instruction, and advice. Academic Coaches are required to respond to questions from students within 48 hours, however, inquiries are usually answered within the same day.

Every semester, all Academic Coaches get together for a one-day training session on a variety of topics including the overall structure of the e-School, curriculum, coaching on the Internet, and how to utilize LMS. Then they take a two-week online training course using the training lecture contents placed on the system in a manner simulating actual class management. These training programs and recruitment are handled by the University's affiliated company under the supervision of the School of Human Sciences.

Ideally, Academic Coaches are researchers in a field closely related to the field of the professor of record, so most Coaches are Doctoral students in Waseda University (with the recommendation and approval of their academic advisor). As of December 2006 (the end of the Ministry of Education's mandatory four year supervisory period), 138 people have registered as Academic Coaches, of which 55 people belong to the Graduate School of Human Sciences of Waseda University, 37 people belong to other graduate schools of Waseda University, 22 people belong to graduate schools of other universities, and 24 people are homemakers who have a graduate degree or are active professionals in fields that are closely related to the topic area. By

2012, there were a total of 198 people registered as Academic Coaches, of which 44 belong to the Graduate School of Human Sciences at Waseda University, one person belongs to another graduate school in Waseda University, two people belong to graduate schools at other universities, and 152 people are homemakers or active professionals. From among these registrants, the Academic Coaches in charge are chosen for each subject/class after interviews with the faculty members in charge of the subject/class for each semester in consideration of the class schedule and the number of classes to be opened.

CURRICULUM

Allocation of Subjects

The e-School's curriculum is essentially the same as the curriculum for on-campus courses, and requires the same number of credits for graduation (124). One of the features of the School of Human Sciences' curriculum (both e-School and on-campus) is that students are allowed to freely choose classes regardless of whether they are offered by the department in which the students is enrolled or not (an unusual situation in Japan) and all courses passed count towards graduation. With regard to research methods and senior thesis s research courses, students can also take subjects taught by faculty members that belong to departments other than their own. However, as the maximum number of students for these subjects is limited, where the number of students wishing to take such subjects exceeds the maximum, students belonging to the same department as the professor will have priority. With regard to specialized lecture subjects, there is no enrollment limit and classes are opened in accordance with the number of students wishing to take them.

The number of subjects allocated for on-campus courses is 457, and 341 for the e-School. The reason for this difference is that there are time schedule and class size restrictions for the on-campus curriculum. In contrast, e-School students can register for subjects without being affected by the time schedule and class size, so fewer courses need to be available to accommodate full registration by all students.

The number of courses allocated for the e-School was determined based on an admission limit of 300 students. As the e-School allows students to take courses across departments, the following is a simplified estimation for the School as a whole. 84 courses are offered in the categories of Seminar I, II and Graduation Thesis Research, wherein one subject is taken by 3.6 students on average. In addition, the number of specialized lecture courses is 105 and students are required to take at least 100 credits (50 courses) by the time of their graduation. Based on the calculation of 300 (students) * 50 (courses) / 105 (courses) = 142.9, we have judged that where the enrollment limit per class is 30, we can secure the capacity by offering five classes per each subject on average.

The features of the allocation of courses are shared by both on-campus courses and correspondence courses: Students do not need to distinguish between the department to which they belong and other departments in selecting the subjects they take. In extreme cases, students can graduate by taking only subjects offered by other departments. However, with regard to research methodology courses, seminars and senior thesis research, there are enrollment limits for such course (research methodology is about 20 students, seminars and senior thesis research is about 10 students).

It was necessary to establish the curriculum for the e-School to respond to the needs of students based on the assumption of having various types of students with a wide variety of backgrounds. One of those changes was a subject selection step that is different from students in on-campus courses, most of whom graduate in four years. We introduced the concept of "levels" as a substitute for the concept of grades under on-campus courses. There are four levels and each level corresponds to the relevant year under on-campus courses, but, in order to advance to the upper level, students need to have earned a prescribed number of credits in the subject categories as designated by the current level. The definition of "levels" for e-School is shown in Table 1.

While on-campus courses require students to learn two foreign languages (eight credits in total) that are freely chosen by each student from German, French, Chinese, Spanish and English, the e-School only requires that the students take English courses (four credits). The methods for experiments, surveys, and research (subject group), which are the elective, required subjects (two subjects, eight credits), are

Table 1. Definition of e-School's "Levels"

Level 1 The required subjects of Level 1 are: Statistics I, II (two credits for each) English IA, IIA, IB, and IIB (one credit for each) and specialized subjects (13 courses, 26 credits). Upon earning sufficient credits for these courses (34 credits in total), students are allowed to take courses included in Level 2.
Level 2 The required subjects of Level 2 are: Research Methods (two subjects, eight credits) and specialized subjects (13 courses, 26 credits). Upon earning sufficient credits for these courses (34 credits in total), students are allowed to take courses included in Level 3.
Level 3 The required subjects of Level 3 are: Seminars (two subjects, eight credits) and specialized subjects (10 subjects, 20 credits). Upon earning sufficient credits for these courses (28 credits in total), students are allowed to take courses included in Level 4.
Level 4 The required subjects of Level 4 are: Senior Thesis Research (eight credits) and specialized subjects (10 subjects, 20 credits).

Note: Upon earning all credits for Levels 1-4 (124 credits in total), students will be eligible to graduate.

allocated over the first to third grades under on-campus courses, but are allocated to Level 2, which corresponds to the second grade, for the e-School courses.

Method of Conducting Classes

A class in the e-School mainly includes lectures and assignments given by faculty and discussions through the BBS. As this system is based on interaction among the faculty, Academic Coach and students, it is necessary for students to actively participate in the class. Classes with regard to specific subjects are conducted as below:

English Education

The only required foreign language course in the e-School is English. For the English subjects, four credits (two subjects) need to be taken in Level 1.

Classes are conducted by an outside language school company, and the students' performance is evaluated by the company's instructors under the supervision of the faculty group in charge of English education in the School of Human Sciences. Under the learning system provided by the language school company, native English speakers living all over the world serve as tutors and provide each student with reading/writing training by e-mail and listening/speaking training by telephone. All tutors are professional English teachers with a Master's degree or extensive experience teaching the English language to adults.

Statistics

For statistics, four credits (two classes) need to be taken in Level 1. Statistics are learned in Level 1 as the core methodology for experiments, tests and surveys and as basic literacy for understanding and processing quantitative or qualitative data. The subject is taught by using PSI (Personalized System of Instruction) (Kogo 2003) designed for online learning, and each question is separately answered by instructors online, through which it aims for students to be actively involved in learning the subject completely.

Specialized Lecture Subjects

Each specialized lecture class is taught for a half-year period and earns two credits. The total number of subjects is 105 (see Table 2). These courses are in the form of lectures which are allocated to each department. The volume of a lecture equivalent to one class under on-campus courses is divided into several segments of about 15 minutes (the length of a lecture for one week is 60 to 90 minutes) and new lecture

Table 2. List of Specialized Lecture Courses (2012 Academic Year)

Department of Human Behavior and Environment Sciences	Department of Health Sciences and Social Welfare	Department of Human Informatics and Cognitive Sciences
Studies on culture of representation	Basic Research Method of Behavior Therapy	Instructional Design
Ecological Science	Learning Research Methods and Technologies of Bioethics	Web Design
Regional/Global Environment	Health, Welfare, and Medical Policy	Measurement and Evaluation of Education
Environmental Information Science	Clinical Psychology	Human Information Processing
Geosphere-Biosphere System	Psychosomatic Medicine	Information and Man
Structure and Functions of the Brain	Behavior Therapy	Information of Colors
Environment Management Planning	Cognitive Behavior Therapy	Cognitive Psychology
Country Hills Conservation	Physiology	Teaching-Learning Process
Architectural Ergonomics	Health Sciences and Promotion	Sensory Information Processing
Safety and Disaster Prevention	Human Science of Lifestyle Related Disease	Basic Psychology
Environmental Psychology	Health Administration Medicine	Safety and Human Factors
Professional Sociology	Health and Welfare Industrial Technology	Response to Specific Environment
Life Course Theory	Bioethics	Biomedical Technology
Intercultural Education	Recreation	Media Production & Presentation
Motivation Theory	Welfare Date Processing	The Developing Adult
Ecological Anthropology	Social Work for the Aged	Intercultural Communication
Communication	Health and Welfare for Children	Information Society and Information Ethics
Cultural Anthropology	Welfare for Children and Families	Introduction to Computer Systems
German Society and Culture	Social Security I	Mathematics for Information Processing
French Culture	Social Security II	Programming I
Archaeology	Public Assistance	Programming II
Social Development	Environmental Physiology	Introduction to the Information System
Environmental Sociology	Sports Practice I	Database
Behavioral Development	Sports Practice II	Communication Network
Developmental Psychology	Clinical-cognitive Development	Multimedia
Constitution	Occupational counseling and consulting	Information and Profession
The History of Science	Neuromuscular control	Sports Practice III
Critiques of techniques, technologies and cultures	Independent Living of People with Disabilities	Ecological Psychology
Aquatic Environmental Science	Barrier-free Environment	Introduction to Artificial Intelligence
Architectural Environment Studies	Introduction of Clinical Thanatology	Instructional Design in Practice
Environment-Behavior Studies	Community Care I	Ecological Approach to Movement Science
Environmental Economics	Community Care II	Education with Information and Media Technology

continued on the following page

Table 2. Continued

Department of Human Behavior and Environment Sciences	Department of Health Sciences and Social Welfare	Department of Human Informatics and Cognitive Sciences
Regional Resource Management and Policy	Molecular Neurobiology	Internet Science
Theory of Environmental Design	School Community Psychology	Cognitive Science Approaches to Human Thinking and Learning
European Area Studies	Biomedical Instrumentation	Design of Learning Environment
Group and organizational psychology	Development of Medical and Assistive Product	Risk Psychology
Film Studies / Culture and Representation	Mind-Body Interaction in Clinical Psychology	e-Testing
Landscape Ecology	Sensory Physiology	Teaching Practice I
	Special Activities	Teaching Practice II
	School Counseling	Introduction to Teacher and Teaching
	Health Environment and Infectious Diseases	Principles of Education I
	Psychiatric Social Work	Principles of Education II
	Introduction to Palliative Medicine and Health Risk Communication	Guidance and Career Counseling
	Methods in Biodynamics	Educational Psychology
		Learning and Media
		Curriculum Theory
		Induction Program for Teaching Practice I
		Induction Program for Teaching Practice II

contents are delivered weekly. Lecture contents are accompanied by a Bulletin Board System (BBS), an assignment submission system, and a handout distribution system. Classes are formed for each subject on a 30-students-per-class basis. An Academic Coach is assigned to each class to coordinate BBS discussions and to give instructions to reports submitted by students. The Department of Human Informatics and Cognitive Sciences has slightly more subjects than other departments because it has a teacher-training course (information study for high school students).

Research Methods

Courses for students to learn basic research methodology are categorized in one subject group called "methods for experiments, surveys and research" which include preparatory training for seminars and writing senior theses. Each subject belonging to this group is taught for a half-year and provides four credits. Level 2 requires two classes to be taken. Methods for experiments, surveys and research have 59 courses in total, and half of them are offered once every two years and the other half are offered in the alternate years. From among these courses, students are required to choose two in Level 2.

In these classes, not only the methodology for each research field is studied, but also basic knowledge of the underlying theory is acquired. Limiting the number of students per class to 20 at maximum, these classes focus on discussions through BBS and the learning of research methods by working on surveys and assignments. Each class has an Academic Coach. Delivery of lectures, submission of assignments, etc., are all conducted online. However, with regard to subjects that include experiments using equipment or that are required to be conducted face-to-face, such intensive schooling is conducted using the university's Tokorozawa Campus, Oiwake Seminar House, etc. In such cases, the number of days for face-to-face schooling is limited to the minimum (about two days) and the required class hours are secured mainly through online classes.

Seminars I and II

The curriculum includes seminars in order to promote the determination by students of subject of their senior thesis research, the understanding of the current status of research in the research field as preferred by each student, and the effective implementation of research. Seminars are more than just small courses taken by upper-division students. Seminars at Waseda University are year-long courses that allow third year students to work intensively with one professor on a particular theme. After finishing their third-year seminar, fourth year students continue to work with their professor to write a senior thesis, a key graduation requirement for students in the School of Human Sciences. For seminar subjects, seminar I (half-year period, four credits) and seminar II (half-year period, four credits) are required to be taken in Level 3. The seminars have 84 subjects for seminar I and II respectively, which are assigned to all faculties each year. The methods of conducting the classes are the same as for the methods for experiments, surveys and research. Basically, one faculty member supervises two or three students wherein individual instructions are given which link to the research each student will conduct for their senior thesis, explained in the following section.

Senior Thesis Research

As mentioned previously, a senior thesis is a key graduation requirement. Senior thesis research is a full-year subject earning eight credits. Like seminars, the number of courses for senior thesis research is 84. The instructions for students' research are given by telephone and e-mail as well as through the video meeting system using the Internet. Upon successful completion of the senior thesis, all students are required to present their thesis.

Educational Considerations

In the e-School, in order to provide a strong motivation and more detailed instructions than those provided in face-to-face classes, class size is kept to 30 students on average (specialized lecture subjects) and one Academic Coach is assigned to each class. Where many students wish to take a certain subject, it is handled by increasing the number of classes not by increasing the number of students in a class. Class size is kept to 30 students because it was found that, based on the on-demand classes offered by Waseda University for the past three years (dozens of courses), the number of students that can be easily taken care of by one Academic Coach was 30. Based on the facts that, in the United States, the most advanced nation in online classes, online learning is easily discontinued unless there is strong motivation and that the dropout rate in correspondence courses is historically high (Priluck 2004), our e-School adopted the basic concept of promoting individual treatment and mutual learning between students: Academic Coaches provide mentoring mainly focusing on academic aspects.

In addition, in order to help students keep their motivation and to alleviate the sense of isolation, a BBS is utilized for communication not only between students and faculties but also among students to serve as a ground for interaction with faculties, other students and alumni. Furthermore, homerooms (30 students per homeroom at maximum) are established and a full-time faculty member is assigned to each such homeroom. An Academic Coach is also assigned to each homeroom to serve as a contact person for providing various types of support to students.

Additionally, student support, such as use of facilities including libraries, awarding of scholarships, and assistance to extracurricular activities, is provided to the extent possible.

CLASSES

E-Learning Based on a "Campus" Model

Traditional e-learning mainly uses self-learning materials (contents) based on the instructional design in high-quality finished form, and the focus is placed on independent learning by the learner rather than instruction by the teacher. This can be termed e-learning in the "desktop" model wherein learners study by opening "text books" at their desk (Nishimura, et al. 2004). The features of this desktop e-learning model are:

1. Teaching materials (contents) in high-quality finished form;
2. High degree of freedom with respect to study time (learners can learn at their own pace), and
3. Communication with faculty is supplementary (mainly for questions where it exists at all).

In contrast, e-learning that models a campus situation includes a virtual environment that includes:

1. Blackboard/platform (moving image contents).
2. Classroom (communication between faculty and students as well as among students through BBS, etc.).
3. Faculty room (Learning Management System).

This is called "campus model" e-learning here (Nishimura, et al. 2004). The features of this model are:

1. Teaching materials are prepared on the premise that communication between faculty and students exists (contents are not designed for independent use).
2. Reasonable degree of freedom with respect to study time (students are bound by semesters and required to study on a weekly basis.
3. Communication with instructors is essential.

The desktop model is highly effective for acquiring specific skills, such as in-company training, as learners can proceed with study at their own pace (Nishimura, et al. 2004). On the other hand, in a Japanese university curriculum, learners are required to take about 10 courses per semester in order to graduate in 4 years and learners need to take courses in a well-planned manner. Where general learners need to learn many subjects systematically, it is considered that they can pick up their study pace more easily and can learn more effectively with the campus model of e-learning which emulates the traditional on-campus educational situation and to which learners are accustomed. In addition, under this model, learners are given some sort of assignment for each course every week and learners can maintain the pace naturally by working on the assignment by the deadline. Furthermore, the campus model is desirable for Waseda's e-School as its curriculum has many subjects that are near-equivalents to on-campus courses.

Lecture Contents

As the e-School shares the curriculum with on-campus courses, basically lecture contents can be created by filming and editing classroom lessons. However, lectures are also filmed in a special studio for various reasons such as problems in arranging a camera crew.

Regardless of whether filming is conducted in the classroom or in a studio, lectures are filmed by the same professional camera crew and then edited and originally encoded for use with RealMedia at 400 x 300 pixels resolution and at 15 frames/second from 2003 until 2011. These contents were streamed at 384kbps until 2012 when RealMedia was replaced by Silverlight which steams at 1Mbps. Figure 1 shows one frame of a lecture in the resolution actually transmitted, the top image from 2003 and the bottom image from 2012. While it may be difficult to see in the printed photo, on a computer screen, the latter is clearer than the former although students were generally able to read notes written on the blackboard in both cases. Traditional e-learning contents used a narrower bandwidth (56 kbps), and in order to work within this limitation, materials needed to be treated as still images. Because of this restriction, it was necessary to integrate the images and audio of the faculty members and computerized teaching materials by using an authoring system which was a large obstacle in creating e-learning contents that simulated a classroom setting. Larger bandwidth allowances enable e-School courses contents to replicate the activities and contents used in the classroom or studio, anything that can be filmed by a video camera such as the lecturer, blackboards, OHP and images projected on the screen.

Once the lecture contents have been video taped, they must be processed and uploaded to the servers. Originally, this process took days or weeks to complete, but as the production staffs become more experienced, contents can now be published on the day after the lecture was filmed. This speedy processing increases the faculty members flexibility in amending or replacing online contents. It also provides the online students with the most up-to-date information available to on-campus students. This quick production and delivery system is one of Waseda's e-School's key elements. Although one-day processing is possible, most courses are completed in one academic year for use in the following academic year. However, for subjects that address current topics, the filming is conducted flexibly to suit speedy delivery.

Japanese on-campus courses tend to meet for 90 minutes once each week (one key exception is the seminar course described above). As part of the e-School's lecture processing, lecture contents corresponding to one day's lesson within an on-campus courses is divided into several files of about 15 minutes each which are placed on the server. The reasons behind such division of segments include

Figure 1. Lecture screenshots from 2003 (top) and 2012 (bottom)

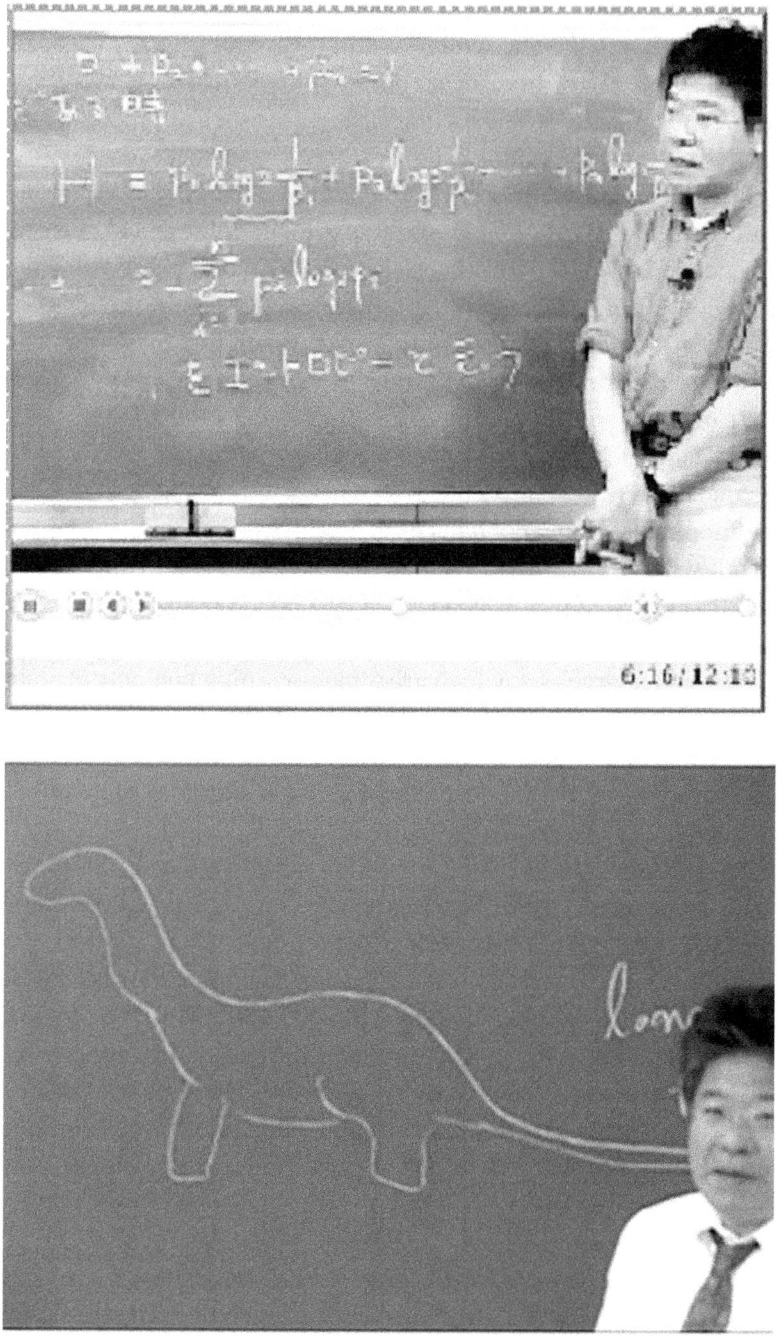

- Short lengths of about 15 minutes help to reduce the need for rebuffering if there is a network problem,
- Lecturers can more easily redo selected portions of a lecture, and
- It helps reduce student fatigue by giving them a break every 15 minutes similar to a TV program.

Course Evaluations

A student evaluation for all of the e-School's classes is conducted at the end of each semester. The following data were collected during the 2003-04 and 2012-13 academic years and are presented here to demonstrate the overall trajectory of student responses to the questionnaire. The questionnaire system is on the e-School Website and allows the students to respond voluntarily on an anonymous basis. The total number of responses was 661 (2003-04) and 2,810 (2012-13) out of a potential number of 1,123 (2003-04) and 3,885 (2012-13) students for the spring semester and 569 (2003-04) and 764 (2012-13) out of 1,094 (2003-04) and 3,257 (2012-13) for the fall semester, showing response rates of 58.8% (2003-04) and 72.3% (2012-13) and 52.0% (2003-04) and 20.0 (2012-13) respectively.

In addition to items regarding the quality of lecture contents, the survey included various items such as the BBS (43 items). Some of the characteristic survey items and answers included were, "Is the course generally well-planned?" and "Overall, was the course helpful?" For the first question (i.e. "Is the course well-planned?"), the mean score was 5.7 (2003-04) and 5.85 (2012-13) out of a high score of 7 and the results of a t-test showed this is a significant improvement ($p = 0.013$). The second question (i.e. "Is the course helpful?") averaged a score of 5.7 (2003-04) and 5.91 (2012-13) out of 7 also showing a significant improvement ($p < 0.01$). Thus, both questions received highly positive responses which was the tendency for the survey overall.

Table 3. Analysis of the results of lecture contents evaluations

Questionnaire items	Classroom	Studio	p-value
Could you comprehend the subject? (I could not – I could)	5 (2)/6	6 (1)/6	0.1672
Image quality (bad – good)	4 (2)/4	5 (2)/4	0.0309
Sound (bad – good)	5 (2)/4	5 (3)/4	0.8352
As your impression on the whole, was the lecture interesting? (Boring – Interesting)	6 (2)/7	6 (2)/7	0.9987

In order to check if there was any difference in the lecture contents filmed in the classrooms and those filmed in the studio, the data was analyzed in detail. Although 36 courses were offered in 2003 (the first year of operation), 25 subjects were covered by this analysis, excluding subjects that used Web materials only and that had both classroom-filmed lectures and studio-filmed lectures. The items that were analyzed included four items as shown in Table 3. Eight classes were filmed in classrooms (total number of responses was 270) and seventeen classes were filmed in the studio (total number of responses was 653).

The median values and mode values shown in Table 3 indicate that all four items covered by the analysis received a positive evaluation with scores of 4 through 6 out of 7. In addition, with regard to the comprehension of subjects, given the survey results that both classroom-filmed and studio-filmed lectures scored a mode value of 6, it is considered that the lecture contents were satisfactory for students to comprehend the subject matter.

In order to check if there was any difference in quality between classroom-filmed contents and studio-filmed contents, the two groups of lecture contents were examined based on the Mann-Whitney U test. As a result, a significant difference was recognized only with respect to the image quality at the 5% level. It is considered that where a lecture is filmed in a classroom with students present, due to the restrictions on the location of the camera and lighting, the image quality of the film tends to be lower than lecture contents filmed in a studio. On the other hand, no difference was indicated with regard to sound. The reason for this is attributed to the fact that the faculty members wear the same type of wireless pin microphone on the chest both in the classroom filming and studio filming.

For each questionnaire item, respondents were asked to answer by indicating any one score out of scores of 1-7, wherein the former answer in the brackets corresponds to score 1 and the latter correspond to score 7. X (Y)/Z in the table indicates the values of median value (X), quartile value (Y), and mode value (Z), respectively, and p-values are based on the Mann-Whitney U test.

With regard to the image quality, it was demonstrated that lecture contents filmed in classrooms have a slightly lower image quality than lecture contents filmed in a studio. On the other hand, with regard to the comprehension of a subject and the impression of the lecture as a whole, no significant difference was recognized between the classroom-filmed lectures and studio-filmed lectures. Based on these analyses, it is considered that the lecture contents of our e-School are of the quality needed for learning, although there is room for improvement with regard to lecture contents filmed in classrooms, in particular.

Figure 2. 2003 System Configuration

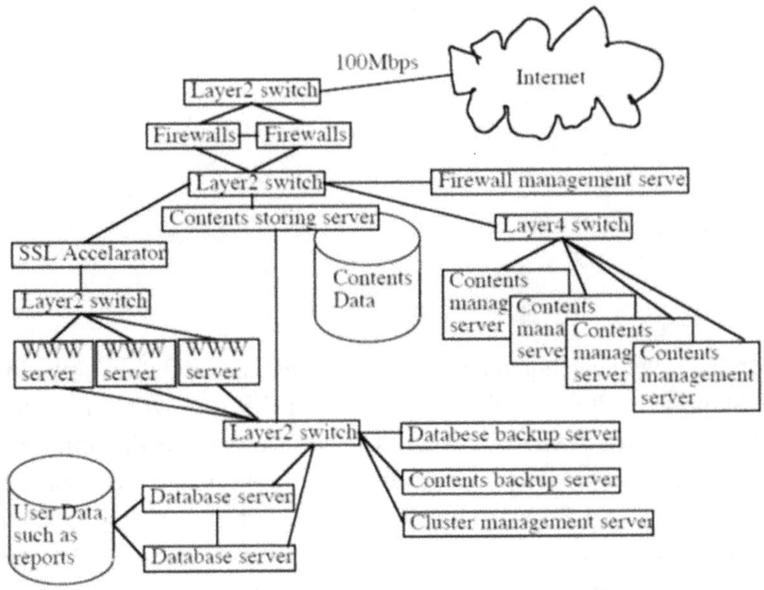

DELIVERY SYSTEM AND LEARNING MANAGEMENT SYSTEM (LMS)

Server Hardware

As the server hardware of the e-School system not only stores lecture contents but also records students' online activities, the hardware is configured by placing importance on stability and security. The hardware is designed in such a manner that the devices are basically duplicated and the entry is protected by firewalls (see Figure 2). In addition, in order to deliver streaming contents of 384 kbps without any delay, the bandwidth for connection to the Internet backbone is 100 Mbps which has proven to be more than sufficient to handle daily traffic: A test with 300 people accessing the system at the same time was conducted and favorable results were obtained.

Actual loads were analyzed during the first and second academic years to confirm that the system was operating as designed. Access records from the middle of April 2004 to the middle of May 2004—a period just after the start of classes having a relatively high amount of traffic—were examined and showed that the number of access attempts peaked at 77 per hour (April 25, 2004, 22:00-23:00), and no processing delays were experienced during that time period. In addition, the bandwidth used for streaming peaked at 10.78 Mbps throughout 2004. This system ran until

Figure 3. 2011 System Configuration

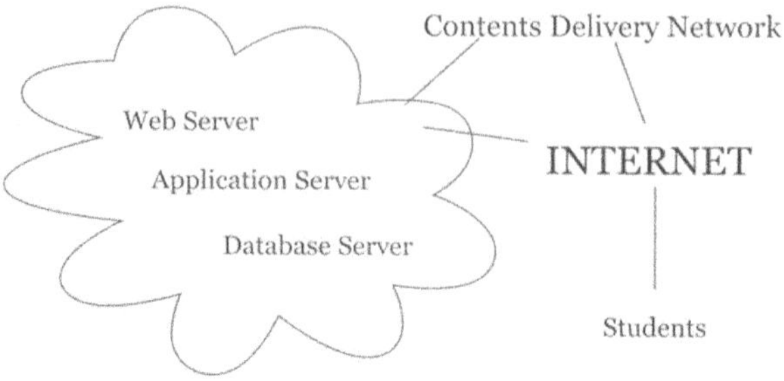

2011 when the severe earthquake and tsunami that damaged the Fukushima Nuclear Power Station resulted in rolling blackouts in the area where the servers were kept. Concern about unexpected power outages compelled the administration to move the course contents from a centralized server to a new cloud-based delivery network operated by J-Stream, Inc. (http://www.stream.co.jp/english/about_us/overview.html). As the course contents are in the cloud, there is no concern over a central server malfunction or server-side power outage. Using this system, the e-School's system operation has run uninterrupted since its creation (see Figure 3).

Learning Management System (LMS)

The LMS used in the e-School is unique to Waseda University and started in 2003 as the On-demand Internet Class (OIC). The OIC has functions that are equipped with general LMS, including lecture contents references, handout distribution, attendance management, report submissions, quizzes, Bulletin Board System (BBS), learning history management and questionnaires. In April 2007, the OIC system was renamed "CourseN@vi" and is described in greater detail below. Despite the name change, the appearance and function of the two systems was largely identical, with periodic minor improvements added.

Front Page of the On-Demand Lecture System

Figure 4. shows the screen that appears after login. The screen shows the menu shared by the whole system (on left, under the OIC logo), information and a list of registered subjects, etc.

1. Information: Indicates important information from faculty members in charge or system administrators. In order to ensure all pieces of information have been checked, any unread information is marked "unread."

Figure 4. Front page screen

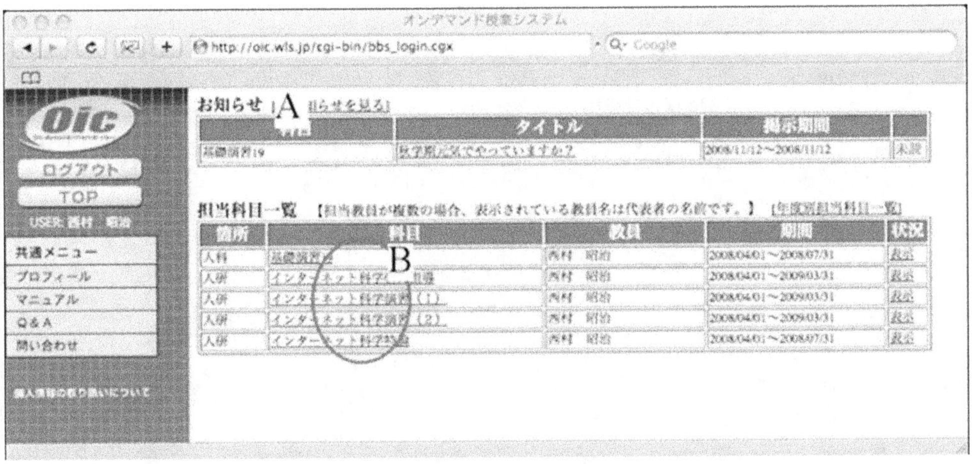

a. When the title is clicked, the details of the information are displayed.

b. The details of the information may be sent to the e-mail address registered as profile information if it is so arranged by the author of the information.

c. The front page displays unread information only. To check all pieces of information within the posting period, "See all information" option needs to be clicked.

2. List of registered subjects: Subjects for which the student is registered are listed. By clicking the name of a subject, a screen to take a class (list of lectures) is displayed. From this screen, students can refer to assignments and the syllabus, use the BBS, confirm and submit report assignments, answer questionnaires and work on quizzes.

Weekly Course Content Page

For each subject, the class contents are divided by week, similar to their face-to-face counterpart. The lecture contents for the week are about 60 to 90 minutes in total length although the week's contents are divided into several chapters, usually 10 to 15 minutes in length, enabling students to view each segment when it is convenient for them, at different times or different locations. Figure 5 shows the original Japanese version and Figure 6 shows similar content with the system's language setting on "English."

Assignments: assignments, reference materials, etc., are displayed. To see the details, the "reference" button needs to be clicked.

Figure 5. Weekly course content screen shot

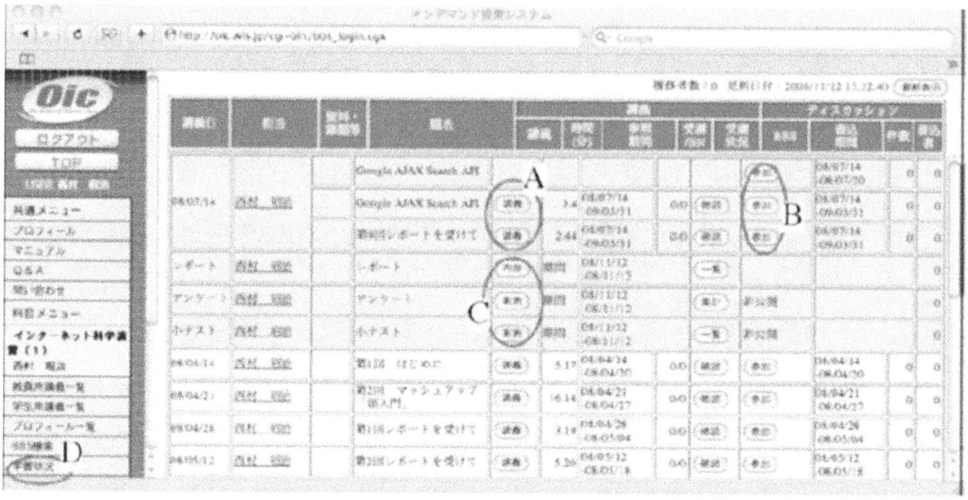

Figure 6. Weekly course content screen shot in English

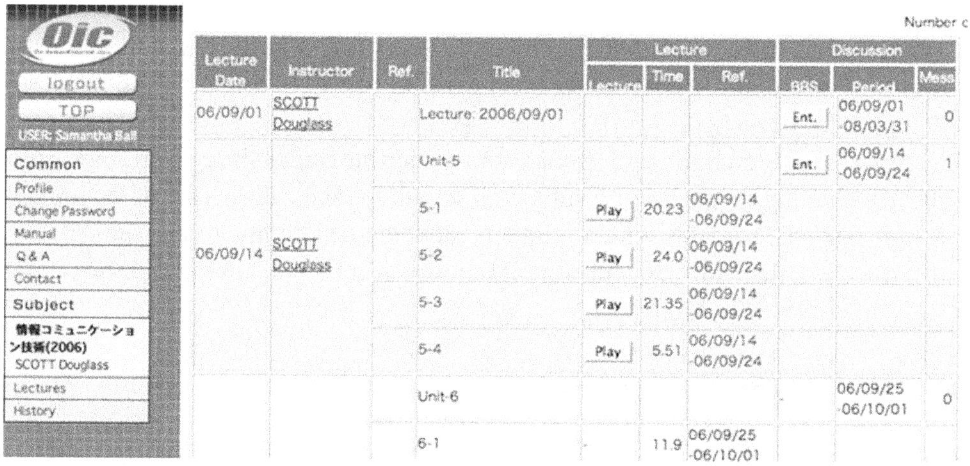

1. Lecture contents: When the "lecture" button is clicked, the video of the lecture for the chapter is replayed.
2. BBS: When the "reference" button is clicked, the BBS is displayed. The BBS can only be accessed in the week in which the lectures are running, after that, the discussion for the week is closed and the following week's discussion is opened.
3. Report functions, etc.: Reports, questionnaires and quizzes are also dealt with on the website.

4. Learning history: Status of attendance at the lectures and submission of reports can be confirmed.

STUDENTS

Selection

Student application and admissions processes are different for the e-School and the on-campus academic programs. e-School applicant screening is conducted based on a statement of purpose no longer than 3,000 Japanese characters and a study plan of up to 1,000 words submitted by each applicant. In the second stage of selection, face-to-face interviews are conducted by committees of three faculty members. The ratio of successful applicants is shown in Table 4.

Student Enrollment

The number of undergraduate students enrolled in 2003 was 169 in total consisting of 40 for the Department of Human Behavior and Environment Science, 85 for the Department of Health Science and Social Welfare, and 44 for the Department of Human Informatics and Cognitive Sciences, of which 164 were on the register as of April 2004 and 152 were on the register as of February 2005. These totals fluctuated by year—including a high of 246 in 2008—and while total enrollment in 2012 was similar to the first year, there was a noticeable shift of students away

Table 4. e-School Acceptance ratios by department

Year	Human Behavior & Environmental Science	Health Science & Social Welfare	Human Informatics & Cognitive Sciences
2003	1:1.33	1:1.22	1:1.38
2004	1:1.38	1:1.36	1:1.32
2005	1:1.71	1:1.48	1:1.51
2006	1:1.57	1:1.26	1:1.42
2007	1:2.02	1:1.77	1:1.53
2008	1:2.10	1:2.23	1:1.74
2009	1:2.13	1:1.80	1:1.87
2010	1:1.80	1:1.63	1:1.37
2011	1:1.95	1:1.62	1:1.70
2012	1:1.98	1:1.58	1:1.85

from Informatics and Cognitive Sciences and Health Sciences and Social Welfare departments toward Behavior and Environmental Sciences department (see Table 5).

Area of Residence, Age, and Occupation

According to the results of a survey conducted in the spring of 2004, 80% of the students on the registry lived in the Kanto region (in and around Tokyo) with 108 out of 292 living in Tokyo itself. However, students from nearly all of Japanese 47

Table 5. Undergraduate enrollment data for the three departments

Year	Human Behavior & Environmental Science	Health Science & Social Welfare	Human Informatics & Cognitive Sciences	Total Enrollment
2003	40	85	44	169
2004	35	64	44	143
2005	44	83	41	168
2006	34	79	30	143
2007	49 (17)	109 (75)	68 (33)	226 (125)
2008	59 (29)	111 (72)	76 (35)	246 (136)
2009	52 (23)	93 (55)	53 (20)	198 (98)
2010	54 (26)	79 (43)	43 (24)	176 (93)
2011	39 (18)	76 (50)	47 (24)	162 (92)
2012	53 (25)	69 (42)	39 (18)	161 (85)

* Total (transferred in with sophomore status)

Graduate student enrollment began in 2007 and the number of students enrolling in the program has more than doubled in six years as shown in Table 6.

Table 6. Graduate enrollment data for the three departments

Year	Human Behavior & Environmental Science	Health Science & Social Welfare	Human Informatics & Cognitive Sciences	Total Enrollment
2007	14	28	11	53
2008	20	30	21	71
2009	18	52	18	88
2010	26	67	28	129
2011	30	68	27	125
2012	28	60	39	127

Figure 7. Countries where students (marked by numbers) and Coaches (marked by dots) has participated in the e-School (2003-2012)

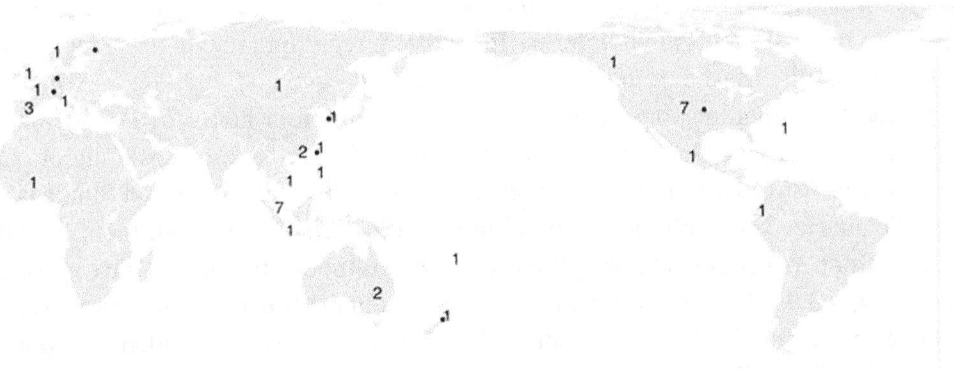

prefectures were enrolled, although in most cases by only a couple of students. All e-School students are Japanese, but some of them lived and studied in other countries. e-School students have taken classes while in 22 countries outside of Japan (see Figure 7) and currently four students are living abroad: One each in Morocco, England, United States and Australia.

Educational Coaches have taught while in seven countries outside of Japan: One each in the United States, Switzerland, Germany, South Korea, Finland, New Zealand, and Taiwan (see Figure 7). About 62% of the total students were 30 years old or older at the time of their enrollment and about 80% of them were employed. The male-female ratio is almost 1:1. It is notable that about 27% of the students on the registry have already graduated from a four-year university.

Indonesia (1), Singapore (7), Philippines (1), Vietnam (1), Mongolia (1), South Korea (1), Taiwan (1), Hong Kong (2), Australia (2), New Zealand (1), Fiji (1), USA (7), Canada (1), El Salvador (1), Bermuda (1), Mexico (1), Italy (1), Great Britain (3), Spain (3), Norway (1), France (1), Burkina Faso (1)

Questionnaire on Learning Conditions

In the beginning of July 2003, a questionnaire survey of the students was conducted with regard to the number of courses for which they had registered and the length of time they had spent studying[1]. The number of respondents was 83 out of the 164 total students on the registry at that time. The most common answer was nine courses, the second most common was 10 followed by eight. This number of courses is roughly equal to the total courses taken by on-campus students.

Regarding the day of the week on which they study, there is not much difference according to the day of the week except that slightly more time is spent for studying on the weekends. The peak time for their study was between 22:00~24:00 probably because many students are employed. In addition, regarding the hours spent studying per day, the most common answer was between two and three hours with the next most common response being between three and four hours. From the above results, it was found that typical students of the e-School study an average of one or two classes for two to three hours everyday including Saturdays and Sundays.

We analyzed the volume of outgoing video lecture signals from the e-School servers for two weeks in October 2004. The total volume of traffics for the two week period was 3.95Tbits. The total number of course hours (i.e. total students enrolled classes) was about 2,039, so the amount of the packets received per student per course was about 1.94Gbits during the two week period. In one week, one student had received approximately 970Mbits. The bitrate of the streaming video was 385Kbps, so one student watched video lecture clips for about 42 minutes (2,536 seconds) per course per week. The average weekly lecture for e-School courses is about one hour so on average students were watching somewhat less than a full lecture each week.

A breakdown of the network traffic is provided for weekends (Figure 8) and weekdays (Figure 9).

We analyzed the record of the volume of outgoing video lecture signals from the e-School servers for two weekends in October 2004 (i.e. October 16, 17 and 23, 24) as shown in Figure 8. The figure shows that the heaviest access was during the evenings starting at 9:00 p.m. (2100 hours in the Figure).

Figure 9. shows the volume of outgoing video lecture signals during the weekdays for the two-week sample period in October 2004. The figure shows that the heaviest access was during the evenings starting at 9:00 p.m. the same as on the weekends, however, total access was higher than on the weekends.

Figure 8. Transmission volume of lecture videos—weekends

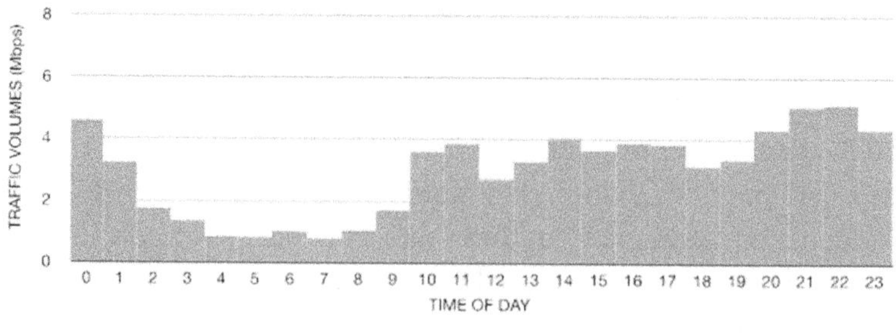

Figure 9. Transmission volume of lecture videos—weekdays

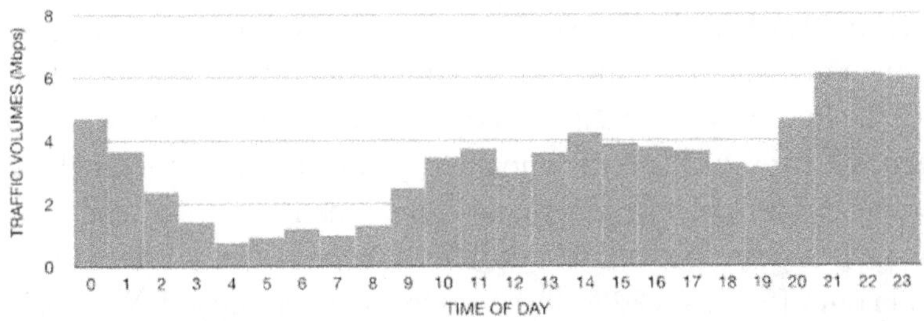

Registration and Graduation

The average number of credits earned by e-School students is similar to those earned by on-campus students. From among the new entrants in 2003, the number of students who registered for subjects in both the spring semester and autumn semester was 150. The total number of credits for which they registered was 5,514 credits (about 36.8 credits per one student). On the other hand, the total number of credits acquired in the same period was 4,484 credits (about 29.9 credits per one student). This means that the ratio of acquired credits to registered credits was 81%. In addition, 82 students (which accounts for about 55% of the total students) acquired 30 credits or more in one year. From among students who enrolled in 2003, 53 students (about 31% of the total enrollment) graduated in four years and the accumulated rate of graduation is 57% by the end of March 2010. From among those who graduated in March 2007, 20 people advanced to graduate school (mainly the Graduate School of Human Sciences, Waseda University). For comparison purposes, students who entered on-campus courses in 2003, the number of students in the registry was 745 and the number of total credits registered was 26,481 credits (about 35.5 credits per student), of which 21,995 credits were acquired (about 29.5 credits per student). This ratio of acquired credits to registered credits is almost the same as the ratio for the e-School courses. In addition, from among the 646 new entrants in 1999, 512 (about 79%) graduated in four years although this data refers to a previous course.

DISCUSSION AND CONCLUSION

With the improved information infrastructure and changes to relevant educational laws, the environment was conducive to creating Japan's first undergraduate degree-awarding e-learning course back in 2003. We were hopeful that our on-campus curriculum (which focuses on the environment, health and welfare, and information sciences) would appeal to working adults and other members of society as these topics are currently of great interest. Through this new online learning environment, Waseda University would be able to offer unique opportunities for lifelong learning in the era of the Internet. At the same time, however, we were anxious about whether we would be able to provide an education that would be satisfactory to those enrolled. Our experiences over the last ten years—confirmed in part by the answers from the questionnaires described above—lead us to believe that we have been generally successful in our efforts. As 82% of the students are employed, Waseda's e-School is meeting a larger need for lifelong education in Japan. Some people argue that an online education program that forces learners to follow a relatively strict schedule (i.e. not self-paced learning) is not suitable for lifelong learning targeting working adults. However, many students of our program are in their 30's and 40's and are able to manage to work and study at the same time.

As previously explained, Waseda's e-School enables students to graduate without taking on-campus classes (i.e. "schooling") and we stress this point as a key feature of our program. However, in our experience, many students want to visit the campus and meet with their classmates and instructors face-to-face if they had the chance. One example from the programs first year, 2003, was that about 60% of registered students took physical education classes that required attending intensive, two-day, on-campus classes held on the weekend. Intensively conducted over two days after taking online lectures and completing physical exercise assignments for about 10 weeks for the teacher-training course. 30 students in a teacher certification course were asked why they came all the way to attend on-campus schooling, many students replied that they wanted to meet their friends with whom they normally communicate only on the BBS. In addition, many students stated that the education system of the e-School is perfect for those who want to come to school and learn every day if possible but cannot do so due to their occupation and who seek a learning style that is similar to on-campus courses.

Interest in distance learning, coupled with a desire for more personal contact, is an ongoing challenge for the e-School faculty. It seems that many students joined the e-School because they were attracted to the relatively small class size and the importance put on person-to-person communication between both students and faculty and students and their peers. In order to better meet these needs, we are trying different media to enhance the communicative experience. For instance, we now allow the uploading of video clips taken by cell phones or digital cameras to the BBS (up to 1MB) in order to express themselves and exchange opinions. These efforts have been met with positive feedback from many students. In another example, seminars with one teacher supervising one or two students, we plan to utilize not only e-mails and BBS but also video chat and telephone. Of course, we continue to work to improve the lecture contents, but at the same time, we need to provide a communication means for more personal exchanges.

The acquisition of credits by students in the e-School courses is about the same level as students in on-campus courses. While the rate of graduation within four years for e-School students—at 31%—falls short of the four-year graduation rate for on-campus students (most e-School students need six years to graduate), is remarkably high for a university distance-learning program (the rate climbs to 43% when the 19 students who graduated in September 2007 are included). Our original goal was for the graduation rate to exceed 70%; while we haven't quite reached this level, the class of 2005 graduated 64.3% which is extremely good for a Japanese e-learning program.

We asked many students and found they generally have a strong sense of purpose for learning in the e-School. As noted above, e-School students typically study from around 21:00 to around 24:00 after work and dinner at home, and study intensively on weekends to make up for any delay during weekdays. It is true that for one course, it takes about 60-90 minutes to view the lecture contents (many students take notes) plus about one hour to work on the quizzes and assignments which are given to students in standard classes. As the average student takes nine classes, they must make considerable effort just to keep up. In addition, it is notable that the quality of their reports submitted compares favorably with that of students in on-campus courses. We think it is probably because students are not just viewing lecture contents passively, but also actively exchanging opinions and deepening their ideas on the BBS, etc.

Following the e-School's 10th anniversary celebrations, thoughts turned to the goals for the next 10 years. While students and Coaches have participated in classes from over 20 different countries, it is hoped that that number will increase greatly over the next few years. e-learning is uniquely suited to support education from any location although several challenges must be addressed to realize this goal. The first of these is the creation of multilingual course materials and lectures. Adding subtitles or dubbing are two obvious methods, but increasing the number of bilingual/multilingual instructors and Coaches could provide real-time multilingual educational opportunities for e-School students.

A related second goal for the future of our program is the establishment of Massive Open Online Courses (MOOCs). The e-School currently supports about 400 courses but nearly all of the course contents are in Japanese. Adapting current course contents with other languages and adding the support of bilingual Coaches, part or all of the curriculum could be opened to anyone regardless of their location or native language.

While some technological elements have improved—as noted above e.g. updating RealMedia streaming with Silverlight—there is still ample room for improvement. Thus, our third future goal is for the developments in bandwidth and display technologies to enable the presentation of more lifelike lecture videos to more closely mimic face-to-face environments. Fourth, students are able to view short introduction videos of both their instructors and Academic Coaches, however, neither student profile pictures nor introductory videos are currently available. It is planned to develop this system in the near future to increase familiarity in the virtual classroom. It is hoped such a system will improve communications and enhance camaraderie between students. Finally, while students can participate in the online discussion using their mobile devices, the current content delivery system does not support lecture videos on such devices. Enabling students to access the e-School's courses on any device may increase their interest in, and engagement with, the online classes. These are some of the challenges the e-School faculty and administration look forward to tackling over the next few years.

The e-School's first 10 years went by quickly and there is much work left to do. The high degree of satisfaction students feel (reflected in the results of the learning conditions questionnaire, credit acquisition, and graduation rates) supports the conclusion that the current status of the e-School is on the right track, and we look forward to the next 10 years.

ACKNOWLEDGMENT

The authors would like to thank Dr. Shogo Kato (Tokyo Woman's Christian University, Japan) for his contribution to an earlier version of this chapter. Thanks, also to the e-School staff who have supported the operation of the e-School, the Academic Coaches who have made great efforts in managing classes, and to the faculty members who have worked hard to create the highest-level courses possible. We also want to thank our students; As educators, we feel very fortunate to have such excellent students as you.

REFERENCES

Aoki, K., & Bray, E. H. (2006). Learning styles of distance learners in Japan: Cultural considerations. *Proceedings of the 11th Annual Conference of the European Learning Styles Information Network.*

Asai, K. (2005). Yashimagakuendaigaku Ni Okeru E-Learning Sisutemu No Genjou To Kadai [The Current Situation and Issues of e-Learning System at Yashima Gakuen University]. *Media Research, 1*(2), 59-71.

BBTU.com. (2014). *What's BBT University?* Retrieved from http://bbt.ac/about/

Economic Research Office, General Policy Division, Information and Communications Policy Bureau, Ministry of Public Management, Home Affairs, Posts and Telecommunications. (2004). WHITE PAPER Information and Communications in Japan.

Fuwa, Y., Kunimune, H., Niimura, M., Wasaki, K., Shidama, Y., & Nakamura, Y. (2004). Shinshu-Daigaku Internet Daigakuin No Genjyo To Shorai-Keikaku [Current Status and Future Plan of the Graduate School on the Internet, Shinshu University]. *Media Research, 1*, 11–18.

Kawahara, H. (2010). Student Authentication for Course Credit in Distance Learning. *Journal of Multimedia Education Research.*, *7*(1), 57–63.

Kogo, C. (2003). Daigaku Ni Okeru Web Base Kobetsu-Ka Kyojyu Shisutemu [Conducting Classes through Web-based Personalized System of Instruction (PSI) in Universities]. *Annual Journal of Educational Psychology*, *42*, 182–192. doi:10.5926/arepj1962.42.0_182

Matsuoka, I. (2001). *Dejitaru Kyanpasu* [Digital Campus]. Tokyo: Toyo Keizai Inc.

Nishimura, S., Asada, T., Kogo, C., Kikuchi, H., Jin, Q., Matsui, T., & Nojima, E. (2004). *Kyampus Moderu e-Learning No Jissen: Waseda Daigaku Ningen Kagakubu e-School No Torikumi* [The "Campus Model" of e-Learning in Practice: A Case Study of Waseda University's School of Human Sciences' "e-School."]. Paper presented at Japan Society for Educational Technology Annual Conferenc.

Ōmae, K. (2012). *Shinka Suru Kyōiku: Anata No Nōryoku Wa Shinka Suru* [Evolving education: Evolve your brainpower]. Tokyo: Business Breakthrough Publishing.

Public Relations Office, Government of Japan. (2009). *Flexible Education, 20*(11). Retrieved from https://www.gov-online.go.jp/pdf/hlj_ar/vol_0020e/14-15.pdf

Randi, P. (2004). Web-Assisted Courses for Business Education: An Examination of Two Sections of Principles of Marketing. *Journal of Marketing Education*, *26*(2), 161–173. doi:10.1177/0273475304265635

Shimizu, Y. (2002). E-Learning Wo Sasaeru Seisaku To Kongo No Tembo [Polices to Support e-Learning and Foresight Thereof]. *Information Processing*, *43*, 421–426.

Shimizu, Y. (2004). Koto-Kyoiku Ni Okeru E-Learning No Shien To Kyoiku Kontentsu No Kyoyu [Support by e-Learning in Higher Education and Sharing of Educational Contents]. *Media Research, 1*, 1-10.

Sperling, J. (2000). *Rebel with a Cause: The Entrepreneur Who Created the University of Phoenix and the For-Profit Revolution in Higher Education*. New York: John Wiley & Sons.

Ueno, M. (2004). Kompakuto Na E-Learning Keiei [Small Scaled e-Learning Management]. *Articles Compiled for* the *29th National Conference of* the *Japanese Society for Information and Systems in Education.*

Waseda Daigaku. (1972). *Kōhon Waseda Daigaku Hyakunenshi* (Vol. 1). Waseda University Press.

Waseda Daigaku. (2007). 早稲田大学 125年 [Waseda 125: 1882-2007]. Waseda University Press.

Waseda University. (2002). Waseda-Daigaku Ningenkagakbu Setsurisu Shui Oyobi Tokuni Secchiwo Hituyou To Sururiyu [Intent and purpose of Establishing the School of Human Sciences, Waseda University]. Unpublished application submitted to the Ministry of Education, Culture, Sports, Science, and Technology, Government of Japan.

Yoshida, A. (2002). Koto-Kyoiku Ni Okeru E-Learning - Virtual University No Tojyo [e-Learning in Higher Education - the Advent of the Virtual University]. *Information Processing*, *43*, 407–413.

ENDNOTES

1 The online system was changed in 2007 and it is no longer possible to track e-School student system usage separate from the rest of the network traffic.

Chapter 7
From Healthcare Services to E-Health Applications: A Delivery System-Based Taxonomy

Riccardo Spinelli
University of Genoa, Italy

Clara Benevolo
University of Genoa, Italy

ABSTRACT

The increasing adoption of ICT – and especially Internet-based technologies – in healthcare has been very fruitful and has led to the innovative approach to healthcare practice commonly known as e-health. However, the boundaries of this new approach to healthcare are not clear, as it is reflected by the various properties and taxonomies of e-health applications which have been proposed. In this chapter, we first review the definition of e-health and the main taxonomies for its constituents. Then we propose an original taxonomy for e-health applications, based on the structural features of the delivery system of the services which are digitalized: the need for a physical interaction between the subjects involved in the service provisioning and the possibility of delivering the services through Internet-based technology.

DOI: 10.4018/978-1-4666-9870-3.ch007

INTRODUCTION

The advent of the so-called "ICT revolution" can be undoubtedly considered a turning point in economic history, due to the strong impact it has had on the structure of the economic system and on the way business is done. Many authors – see, among others, Castells (2000), Porter (2001) and Burman (2003) – have theorized the progression from the traditional industrial economic paradigm to the so-called "digital economy", stressing the central role that digital technologies and ICT play in this progression. Underlying this shift in paradigms has been the increasing digitalization of information – that is the process of representing any kind of information as a sequence of *bit,* that is *binary digits* – which has come into conflict with real world processes that remained substantially analog-based (Tocci, 1988) and not always reducible to binary storage. However, modern digital technologies allow for an accurate digitalization of information from many different sources (words, sounds, images, etc.), with minimum loss of the processed information. In other words, more and more typologies of data and information can be properly turned to the digital format or, in short, "digitalized" (Aldrich & Masera, 1999). If digital technologies have enhanced the possibility of processing information more efficiently and effectively, it is thanks to ICT – and especially to Internet-based technologies – that digital information can be transmitted and shared, dramatically increasing its value and its contribution to economic activities.

This process has certainly involved healthcare services too; in fact, the increasing adoption of ICT and Internet-based technologies in that industry has been very fruitful and has led to the innovative approach to healthcare services commonly known as e-health. With respect to this concept, literature is not consistent, as several definitions have been proposed together with just as many taxonomies and classification schemes. Taxonomy studies does not only help to better understand phenomena, but also provide tools to categorize concepts in a field: indeed a taxonomic tool is one of the basic tools in the development of scientific knowledge, as such systems aid in research by helping to identify unexplored phenomena and providing a context for their relationship with other aspects of the environment (Tulu et al., 2007). At present, proposed taxonomies for e-health activities are quite heterogeneous and allow for just a partial view on such a complex phenomenon. As a consequence, to fully appreciate the origins, the structure and the great potential of e-health applications we propose to trace them back to a more general phenomenon, that is the Internet-driven digitalization of services. Healthcare activities, in fact, are part of the wider area of service industries, which have been deeply changed and redesigned by the possibility of performing their delivery through Internet-based technologies.

The main objective of this chapter is therefore to propose an original taxonomy for e-health activities, built around the characteristics of the delivery system of healthcare services; by doing so, it is possible to understand the way in which healthcare activities evolved towards a new digital configuration and to speculate about their potential future development.

To this purpose, we first place the healthcare industry within a wider framework of the digital economy; then we move to a closer analysis of the e-health construct and components. Afterwards we introduce a classification model for services in accordance with their characteristics and their delivery modes. This scheme is then applied to the healthcare industry, to get to a classification scheme which gathers e-health applications into homogeneous groups built around the features of their delivery systems and, consequently, to the way in which they have evolved towards their new digital structure. Finally, we propose some reflections on future technology-driven trends which could affect the healthcare industry.

BACKGROUND

In this section we first present some considerations on the role of healthcare industry within the new economic paradigm of the digital economy, useful to encompass the e-health development within a more comprehensive framework. A definition for e-health is later proposed, which embraces the most relevant elements of this phenomenon; then, the main objectives associated with the development of e-health are illustrated, to show its great potential in terms of efficiency, effectiveness, innovation and relationships. Finally, the issue of e-health taxonomies is introduced.

Healthcare Industry and the Digital Economy

Atkinson and McKay (2007) state that the digital economy "represents the pervasive use of ICT (hardware, software, applications and telecommunications) in all aspects of the economy, including internal operations of organizations (business, government and non-profit); transactions between organizations; and transactions between individuals, acting both as consumers and citizens, and organizations" (p. 7). We certainly recognize the value of this technology-focused definition; nevertheless, the advent of the digital economy has not only a technological origin, but is the result of complex dynamics in the economic system, both on the supply and demand side (Spinelli, 2008), which – together with the innovation in ICT – contribute to shape the new economic paradigm. Consider, in particular, the increasing dematerialization of the economy, namely the complex evolution from material to immaterial, from the preeminence of physical transformation to the prominence of information and knowledge creation; this trend dates back to much earlier than the advent of the ICT revolution: the progressive digitalization of goods and services has historical roots, even if it gained new momentum when ICT made it much easier their transmission and communication. Furthermore, digital technologies – thanks to automation – made information available to manage and govern business processes.

The consequences of the evolution from the traditional to the digital economy are deep and involve almost every aspect of economic activities. In this chapter, the attention is focused on how the development of the digital economy influences one of the most important service sectors that is the healthcare industry.

Over the last decades, the economic scenario and the structural and operative conditions of service firms have deeply changed. First, deregulation, liberalization and globalization processes have had an impact on the general environment; the healthcare industry has been certainly involved in this processes, even if the industry has been "partially protected" by some structural peculiarities (in particular the significant presence of national public operators along with national public policies and regulations) which have kept it somewhat protected from the new and more intense forms of competition. Then, industrialization, digitalization, IT networks, evolution in communication and transport, virtualization and demand-side changes have strongly modified the way of conceiving, producing and delivering services (Javalgi, Martin, & Todd, 2004; Rahman, 2004). In particular, "the industrialization of at least some processes and the digitalization of information [have changed] the options about 'how' to produce and deliver services (e.g. reducing the contact with the consumer) and 'where' (from a distance or across the borders of a country)" (Benevolo & Spinelli, 2011, p. 252).

Figure 1. The pyramid of the digital economy
Source: Adapted from Malecki and Moriset (2008, p. 6).

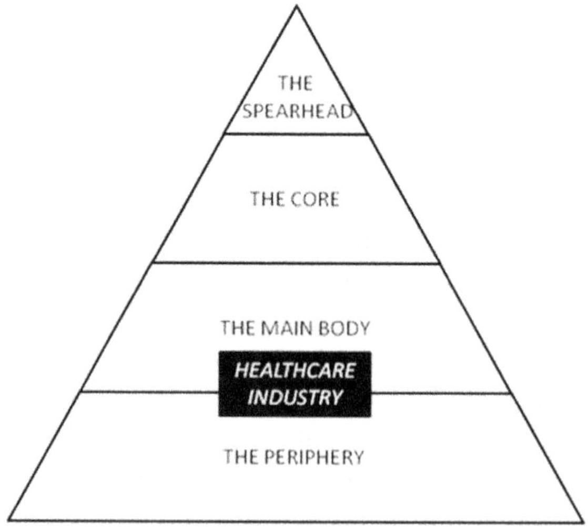

Given this overall trend of development of the digital economy, its extent is still rather uneven on an industry basis. On industry specificities, Malecki and Moriset (2008, p. 6) use the metaphor of the "pyramid of the digital economy" (see Figure 1) to help identify four distinct groups of industries, that vary in terms of ICT diffusion.

Malecki and Moriset first consider what they call the "spearhead" of the pyramid, that is, the chips and processors industries which produce the basic components of all digital technologies. Below this lies the "core", including the computer and telecommunication industries, which we define as ICT in a narrow sense. The third level, the "main body", includes all fully ICT-enabled industries, that is, those manufacturing and service industries which rely heavily on ICT; we can cite here the great majority of the most relevant industries in the contemporary economy: automotive, high-tech mechanics, media and entertainment, business and financial services, and so on. The last group – at the base of the pyramid – is the "periphery", which comprises those sectors not yet or only partially, ICT-enabled or, in other words, where the use of ICT is still limited and not critical. Sectors traditionally included in this group are usually "old economy" ones, such as farming, fishing, mining, forestry or basic consumer and public services. However, examples of intense ICT use are present in these sectors as well, forerunners of a more widespread adoption still in progress. This explains why the boundary between the "main body" and the "periphery" is continuously moving down, as more and more industries reconfigure themselves through greater use of ICT in processes and in organizations.

Those industries belonging to the "spearhead" and the "core" are part of the "engine" of the ICT revolution, as they are the "main actors" of the revolution and drive the process. On the contrary, industries in the "main body" and the "periphery" perceive the ICT revolution as an exogenous factor influencing their general and competitive environment, being, in a way, "victims" of these forces.

In our opinion, the healthcare industry, is progressively entering the "main body" of the pyramid, due to the great changes caused by the pervasive application of ICT: as we are going to analyze in detail in the next sections, the structure of the organizations in this industry is being fundamentally re-shaped; new ways of taking care of the patients are becoming possible; public and private institutions are looking for new and more efficient ways to cooperate; the "consumer" (the patient or a friend or relative) is becoming more and more informed and therefore more active and demanding – in terms of convenience, control and choice (Ball & Lillis, 2001) – in the relationship with the healthcare system. The more innovative components of the industry have already been experiencing such a process, towards the so-called e-health: "ICT has already modified medical practice patterns extensively while facilitating coordination and close cooperation between health care professionals to improve patient management; it is already providing some solutions to the growing need for information and knowledge sharing" (Fieschi, 2002, p. 87). However, the more traditional components too – which are still in the "periphery" of the pyramid – will get soon to a new, more ICT-based, configuration.

Definition, Objectives and Contents of E-Health

Despite the frequency of use of the term, there does not appear to be a general consensus about the meaning of e-health. Many definitions have been proposed, but so far there has not been any universal agreement about what things might be excluded or included within the scope of the term (Showell & Nohr, 2012). Furthermore, terms such as e-health, telemedicine, and telehealth are quite often used interchangeably, although e-health is quickly becoming the most adopted (Fatehi & Wootton, 2012).

In general terms, e-health can be defined as "the use of emerging information and communications technology, especially the Internet, to improve or enable health and healthcare" (Eng, 2001). A more complex and widely accepted definition is provided by Eysenbach (2001), who defines e-health as:

an emerging field in the intersection of medical informatics, public health and business, referring to health services and information delivered or enhanced through the Internet and related technologies. In a broader sense, the term characterizes not only a technical development, but also a state-of-mind, a way of thinking, an attitude, and a commitment for networked, global thinking, to improve health care locally, regionally, and worldwide by using information and communication technology. (p. e20)

The core elements of Eysenbach (2001)'s definition are consistent with the four common perspectives that Sood et al. (2007) find in all 104 definitions of the term "telemedicine" they analyze:

- Medical perspective, which results into mentioning the provision of healthcare services;
- Technological perspective, when the role of ICT is stressed;
- Spatial perspective, which underlines the geographical separation between provider and recipient of medical information;
- Benefits perspective, when the positive repercussions on patients' quality of life are highlighted.

Several more definitions of e-health have been proposed in literature, as Oh et al. (2005) report. Their analysis of 51 definitions confirms that the term e-health encompasses a wide set of concepts, including health, technology, and commerce.

A very important conclusion they come to is that "most commonly, the word health [is] used in relation to health services delivery which suggests that eHealth may refer more to services and systems rather than to the health of people"; furthermore, "health, as used in these definitions, usually [refers] explicitly to health care as a process, rather than to health as an outcome".

Moreover, a major importance is given to the communication between the subjects involved in healthcare processes: patients and relatives/friends, hospitals, practitioners, local and central public authorities, private corporations, etc. With respect to this topic, we make reference to Pagliari et al. (2005), who – in another review of e-health definitions – find that:

the majority of definitions [...] specify the use of networked information and communications technologies, primarily the Internet, and digital data, thus differentiating eHealth from the broader field of medical informatics, which incorporates 'harder' technologies, such as scanning equipment, and bioinformatics research which tends to take place in isolation and is less directly applicable to health care service delivery. (p. 83)

Our interest in this topic – and the relevance of the study too – is justified by the great potential associated with the adoption of ICT in healthcare services (Commission of the European Communities, 2004; Stroetmann, Jones, Dobrev, & Stroetmann, 2006; WHO, 2006a & 2006b). Healthcare costs are growing at an unsustainable rate throughout much of the world, due to factors such as the aging process of population, the request for better and more effective healthcare services, the introduction of more sophisticated technologies in caretaking processes (Haux et al., 2002). In response, "many governments are taking steps to prod the health care industry to aggressively expand its use of IT" (Kennedy & Berk, 2011, p. 1).

In fact, an increasing number of studies show the potential benefits and limitations of multifunctional clinical ICT systems (Shekelle & Goldzweig, 2009; Buntin et al., 2011); even if data on cost and cost-effectiveness remains limited and a large gap between the postulated and empirically demonstrated benefits of e-health technologies is still present (Black et al., 2011), there is a general consensus that health ICT has the potential to dramatically transform healthcare.

According to the OECD (2010), the use of health information technology can improve the efficiency, cost-effectiveness, quality and safety of medical care delivery. Similarly, Osservatorio ICT in Sanità (2008) proposes another classification of e-health benefits for healthcare organizations, where four main drivers (divided into sub-drivers) of benefit from ICT application to healthcare processes are proposed (p. 19):

- Efficiency, declined into staff productivity, equipment usage, cost control;
- Quality, with respect to diagnosis, cure, clinical risk and processing time;
- Relationship, with both the patient (in terms of service personalization and access) and other organizations;
- Monitoring and control of the healthcare organization, which includes regulations accomplishment and the monitoring of performance and processes.

In our view, five broad inter-related categories of objectives for ICT implementation in healthcare industry arise from the wide literature on e-health (see Figure 2):

1. Reducing operating costs of clinical services;
2. Reducing administrative costs;
3. Increasing efficiency and quality of care;
4. Achieving wider interoperability and integration of health services
5. Enabling entirely new modes of care;

Objective 1 and 2 focus mainly on the efficiency gain obtainable through ICT application to core and ancillary healthcare activities. Nevertheless, this view alone would be quite reductive: "if greater investment in health IT simply automates a broken health care system, vital opportunities for transformation will be missed" (Frisse, 2009, p. w380). Objective 3, on the contrary, is centered on cost-effectiveness, quality

Figure 2. The main objectives of e-health
Source: Constructed by the authors.

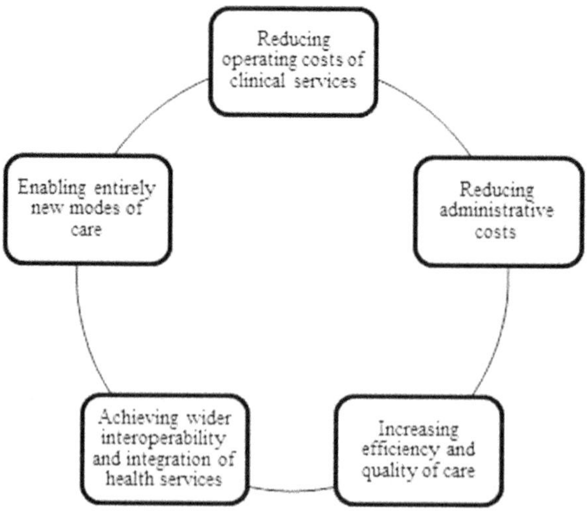

and safety and is consequently more demanding than simply cutting expenses. It is worth underlying that this objective jointly focuses on two complementing elements: on the one side, the direct savings and quality improvements obtainable through a new ICT-intensive way of performing health-related activities; on the other side, the equally important indirect savings which derive from the more intensive and effective prevention initiatives which ICT make possible, for example the reduction of the incidence of chronic disease attributable to prevention. Indeed, the payoff of some types of preventive care, such as for diabetes and heart failure, can be very high, as they reduce the need for very expensive and long-term treatments. As regards Objective 4, the coordination and integration of the many subjects involved in the provisioning of healthcare services (patients and relatives, clinicians, hospitals, public administrations, etc.) could guarantee a further increase in both efficiency and effectiveness of the whole process, as "poor care coordination negatively affects patients — particularly those with multiple chronic conditions who account for an overwhelming proportion of [...] health care expenditures (O'Malley, 2011, p. 1090). As Safran (2003) highlights, "the next stage of collaborative business (for healthcare) is where cooperation among customers (individuals, families, and communities), suppliers (pharmaceutical, device manufacturers and medical supply companies), partners (national health systems, insurance companies and payers), and colleagues (physicians, nurses, other care providers, and support personnel) lets companies (health systems) do business in different and better ways" (p. 186). Of particular interest is the possibility of a shift of focus from the hospital to the patient's house as primary place of treatment, through patient empowerment and home monitoring techniques (Alpay et al., 2010). Finally, objective 5 casts light on the most innovative scenario, which is the development of new ways of taking care of people's health – again, with respect to both patient treatment and prevention – thanks to the comprehensive application of ICT to the whole care process, from the administrative side to the clinical one.

The limited consensus on the definition of e-health is reflected in a similarly limited consensus about its constituents: indeed several taxonomies are provided in literature, with the aim of classifying the many applications of ICT to healthcare. Usually the focus is twofold, because – together with actual applications – also potential ones are introduced, which could be consequence of the continuous technology innovation and the gradual overcoming of context-related limitations on the economic, managerial, organizational, legal and social side.

One of the first and more cited taxonomies of e-health applications was created in 2005 by the World Health Organization for the surveys of the *WHO Global Observatory for eHealth*. The list includes the following tools (WHO, 2006a, p. 15):

- Electronic health records, including patient's clinical history, test results, medication, etc.;
- Patient information systems, which contain information about a hospitalized patient and are used to support both the administrative and clinical activities in a hospital;
- Hospital information systems, that support information processing within a hospital in areas such as administration, appointments, billing, planning, budgeting and personnel;
- General practitioner information systems, that support the work of a general practitioner and often link to other health care systems such as billing, GP reimbursement or laboratory results reporting systems;
- National electronic registries, which contain data on specific medical subjects such as births, mortality, cancer, diabetes or other subjects of medical or epidemiological interest;
- National drug registries, containing national pharmaceutical information;
- Directories of healthcare professional and institutions;
- Decision support systems, that is automated or semi-automated systems that support decision-making in a clinical environment;
- Telehealth, which relate with the use of ICT to either support the provision of health care or as an alternative to direct professional care and encompasses telemedicine and the use of remote medical expertise;
- Geographical information systems, which capture, integrate, analyze and display data related to geographic coordinates.

The list does not pretend to be exhaustive but provides a general overview of the various areas in which the application of ICT to healthcare can contribute. Its main limit, in our view, is that tools are listed without a clear classification criterion and the resulting groups are very heterogeneous in width and potentially overlapping.

An alternative proposal is provided by Vincent et al. (2007), who suggest classifying what they call "telehealth technologies" according to the following features:

- The type of telehealth interaction, which indicates whether the patient is with a medical provider and how the communication is structured;
- The location of the controlling medical authority, which distinguishes whether the provider in charge of the patient care is with the patient or away from the patient;
- The urgency of care, which addresses whether the communication is for an emergent or non-emergent health issue;
- The timing of communication, which considers whether the communication is real-time (synchronous) or store-and-forward (asynchronous).

We find the proposed taxonomy quite promising, as it does not simply list applications but provides higher-level classification criteria which make reference to structural features of the adopted technologies and the provided service; by doing this, they introduce a tool that is potentially able to classify new applications which have not been developed yet. However, the chosen criteria seem to suffer from a lack of clarity – especially as regards the differences between the first two of the list – and risk to be only partially effective when trying to classify the wide variety of e-health applications.

Tulu et al. (2005, 2007) adopt a similar methodological approach in their proposed taxonomy for telemedicine activities. Their tool considers three main dimensions, which in turn include several classification criteria:

- Medical dimension, which includes two classification criteria
    - Application purpose (clinical and non-clinical applications)
    - Application area (among the main domains in the medical field such as cardiology, ophthalmology, home care, etc.)
- Delivery dimension, with three criteria
    - Environmental settings (the physical environment that the physician or the patient will be using during the telemedicine event, e.g. hospital, outreach clinic, health center, home, mobile, etc.)
    - Communication infrastructure (wired or wireless, with different technologies and bandwidth)
    - Delivery options (audio, video or data, in a synchronous or asynchronous way)
- Organizational dimension, focused on four areas of interest
    - Human resources
    - IT management
    - Cost, budget and financial issues
    - Legal, procedural and regulations issues

The proposed taxonomy – partially consistent with Vincent et al. (2007)'s one – certainly identifies critical dimensions for classifying e-health applications, but is in our view quite difficult to adopt due to its high level of granularity. Nine criteria are very difficult to jointly manage, so much that the Authors themselves do not consider the organizational dimension in the pilot applications they propose. More generally, the three dimensions are viewed in a hierarchical way, as the classification process should first consider application purpose and area, then move to the delivery dimension and finally focus on the organizational one. From our point of view, such an approach do not provide solution to one of the main aim a taxonomy should have, that is the creation of a finite number of categories into which it should be possible to encompass all the objects we want to classify. Indeed, in the examples the Authors list e-health applications providing a classification on a single criterion at a time, without crossing them.

A different and simpler approach is proposed in the process-centered taxonomy of the Polytechnic of Milan (Osservatorio ICT in Sanità, 2008); according to this classification, three major healthcare macro-processes can be identified, which are increasingly supported by ICT applications:

- Primary processes, directly related to the main steps in the process of caretaking of the patient: admission, diagnosis, treatment and discharge;
- Support processes to caretaking activities, such as quality and risk management, public relations, facility management, programming and controlling, human resource management, etc.;
- Network processes, associated with the whole assistance process in a broad sense; the perspective is the "continuing assistance" view, which goes beyond the moment of hospitalization or of the treatment for acute disease and includes a continuing relation between the individual and the healthcare system, to exchange information, monitor the patient's health, prevent future disease, support healthier behavior, etc..

Even if conceptually distinct, in practice the three processes are deeply connected and mutually crossing, to such an extent that it would be reductive to identify e-health applications specific for each process, as a great part of the value added by these applications lie exactly in their cross-process nature.

A more recent attempt is made by Bashshur et al. (2011), who talk about "telemedicine" as the wider concept for all ICT application in healthcare. In their taxonomy they distinguish between:

- Telehealth, whose components are health behavior/health education, health & disease epidemiology, environmental/industrial health, health management & policy;
- E-Health, which comprises electronic health record, health information, clinical decision support systems, physician order entry;
- M-Health, which is centered on mobile technologies and encompasses clinical support, health worker support, remote data collection, helpline.

The criterion at the basis of this structure is in our opinion not clearly defined and, furthermore, the classification seems to be by no means exhaustive. On the contrary, the proposed dimensions of the telemedicine concept look quite interesting;

the Authors, in fact, find three criteria which can be adopted to distinguish between telemedicine applications:

- **Functionality:** consultation, diagnosis, mentoring, monitoring;
- **Applications:** specialty, disease, site, treatment;
- **Technology:** synchronicity, network, connectivity.

We agree on the value of these criteria which, however, could again result in an excess of granularity when trying to classifying specific applications; furthermore, they could be subject to overlapping, as some complex applications could fall into more categories; finally, they seem to exclude those applications related to support processes in healthcare, which do not correspond to any of the proposed functionalities.

A NEW TAXONOMY FOR E-HEALTH APPLICATIONS

After presenting e-health and the most common categorizations of its activities, we introduce our original taxonomy for e-health applications. Our aim is to overcome the limitations of the proposed classifications, by offering a new one built around the characteristics of the delivery system of the services which are digitalized.

In comparison with its antecedents, our tool shows two strengths. First, it does not simply list and group e-applications but finds classification criteria. Second, while other taxonomies propose a wide set of criteria – very difficult to jointly consider – our choice is to concentrate on just two criteria: they are much simpler to handle and more focused on those aspects we consider critical to achieve the strategic goals of healthcare delivery. Furthermore, these criteria are of "high-level", being related to the characteristics of the provided service and not to very specific technical features of a given application. By doing so, the tool is able to potentially classify not yet developed applications and to trace them back to the more general framework of the digitalization of services; the latter, in particular, is in our view quite relevant, as encompassing e-health development into a more general economic trend – such as service digitalization – can allow for a deeper understanding of its origins, dynamics and potentialities than simply looking at it as the adoption of IT in the health industry.

To this purpose, as aforementioned, we are going to trace e-health back to a more general phenomenon, that is the Internet-driven digitalization of services. To support our taxonomy with a strong knowledge basis, we have consequently performed a deep analysis of the literature on service management and service science (Thomas, 1978; Lovelock, 1983; Lovelock & Wirtz, 2004; Chesbrough H., 2005; Spohrer &

Maglio, 2008), which can support us in building a conceptual framework of analysis for the digitalization of services.

First of all, we note that a service is not a physical good, but the output of an economic activity which is characterized by a high degree of intangibility. The distinctive characteristics of services are: intangibility; simultaneous delivery and consumption; contact and interaction between producer and user; perishability; variability; social innovation (Chase, 1978; Normann, 1984; Eiglier & Langeard, 1987; Grönroos, 1990; Lovelock, 1996; Zeithaml & Bitner, 2000). These characteristics are common to all services, but appear with differing intensity according to the kind of service and delivery mode adopted. In the healthcare industry, for instance, public hospitals adopt a different mode of managing and delivering service compared to private hospitals.

Furthermore, every service shows a high degree of complexity, as it is composed by a set of core and additional services: when a customer purchases a service, she actually buys a "package" of core and peripheral attributes (Normann, 1984). The service components may vary in number and be combined in different ways; as a consequence, the service package may be very complex: depending on the pursued strategy and the target customer, every firm offers one or more core services, to which it adds a set of ancillary services which complete the "package". As a consequence service firms, even within the same industry, may differ for several reasons: the service package they offer; the balance between core service and ancillary services; the degree of standardization; the degree of externalization; the delivery mode; the extent of the contact during the delivery, etc. A home-care service, for example, can present various degrees of completeness and personalization, according to the services which are provided, the frequency of the interventions, the kind of staff involved, etc.

Nowadays the role of information and the customer involvement in the delivery system have acquired a crucial role in many services: "today, the more knowledge-intensive and customized the service, the more it depends on client participation and input, whether through clients providing labor, property, or information via organizational or technological value chains" (Maglio & Spohrer, 2008, p. 18). Within this framework, service science aims to respond to the emerging issues related with the intrinsic features of services, to support the search for maximization of service quality and productivity, and to enhance the exploitation of technological and organizational innovation in services (Bitner et al., 2008).

In particular, customer is increasingly considered a resource in action, a co-producer of the service. In healthcare activities this approach is as more relevant as the service delivery system is built around the individual, not only as the receiver of the service but also as co-creator of the value. From this point of view, the customer becomes a part of the service system, defined as "value-co-creation configurations of people, technology, value propositions connecting internal and external service systems, and shared information (e.g., language, laws, measures, and methods)" (Maglio & Spohrer, 2008, p. 18). ICT heavily accelerate this process and sustain such a customer-centered approach.

Posed these premises, we need to focus our attention on those service features which most contribute in identifying different kinds of healthcare services, which have been differently impacted by the advent of the digital economy.

To this purpose, we refer to a model developed by Benevolo and Spinelli (2011). The model was primarily intended to support the analysis of service firms' internationalization according to the characteristics of the services they offer and the supply system they set up, and with a specific focus on the impact on the internationalization processes of the application of internet-based technologies to service delivery systems. Regardless of any reference to those parts of the model more strictly related to the internationalization processes, we consider it useful to adopt the service taxonomy proposed by the Authors when evaluating the impact of ICT on the service delivery; in fact, this part of the model can contribute to casting light on those features of healthcare services which most influenced their evolution towards a new digital configuration in a framework of e-health and which constitute the foundation for our taxonomy.

The aim of Benevolo and Spinelli (2011)'s model is to show the relationship between the characteristics of the service and of its delivery modes, and the way in which the application of Internet-related technologies impacts on the service delivery itself. The Authors focus their attention on a specific group of ICT, which includes those informatics solutions and application platforms based on network technologies: EDI and databases via the Internet, intranet and extranet, website and blogs, marketplaces and e-commerce, live chat, computer reservation systems, etc. Part of the Internet-based technologies (for example, corporate websites or marketplaces) are also Web-based – as they are supported by the system of interlinked hypertext documents which constitutes the World Wide Web – while others (for instance Voice Over IP systems or machine-to-machine communication systems) can do without the Web interface.

Internet-based technologies overcome the limitations, develop the potential and re-define the applicability of the service delivery, reshaping the way in which many services are actually performed and made available to the recepients.Thanks to these technologies it is feasible to create and manage in a more functional way the business processes involving customers, providers, employees, etc.

In the model, services are divided into clusters, designed around two key dimensions. The first dimension is the need of physical co-presence or interaction between producer and user in service delivery. As regards this dimension, the aim is to identify those services in which delivery requires co-presence and interaction (even if from a distance) or a high degree of personalization, which necessarily implies a level of relationship directly related to the need for co-presence (Cho, 2005). Some services require the physical presence of both producer and consumer, such as most personal services. Some others do not: consider, for instance, long-distance services where the contact is not present (such as in telecommunications) or is virtual; or service-embodied goods, where the delivery is mediated by a good (for instance a movie in a DVD) (Bhagwati, 1987). As regards healthcare services, most medical and nurse treatments belong to the first group of services, while other information-intensive services – such as communication, education, and administrative services – belong to the latter group.

The second dimension evaluates the possibility, opportunity and convenience of performing the service delivery through the Internet, that is, replacing the traditional service delivery with Internet-based technologies. The service production and delivery system, as commonly known, consists of two parts: front office and back office, divided by the so-called 'line of visibility' (Eiglier & Langeard, 1987). The front office is the part of the system visible to the customer and where the encounter of customer and personnel/physical support of the service firm takes place, while the back office supports and integrates the front office (Silvestro et al., 1992; Zeithaml & Bitner, 2000). Unlike manufacturing firms – where product and production are conceptually and physically separated – in service firms it is quite difficult to separate the service from its delivery system: the production process of a service partially coincides with its delivery, which in turn becomes a part of the service itself. As a consequence, the transportability of the delivery system is evaluated in terms of replacing the traditional delivery system with an Internet-based one.

When jointly considered, these two dimensions generate four groups of services, as in Table 1, which are now briefly described.

Table 1. Service delivery and Internet-based technologies

Physical Co-Presence or Interaction/ Personalization	**Service Delivery**	
	Can be Performed through the Internet	*Cannot be Performed through the Internet*
Necessary	Virtual relationship or reality [C]	Unavoidable "physical-ness" or humanization [D]
Unnecessary	Digital goods and services [A] On-line delivery [B]	

Source: Adapted from Benevolo and Spinelli (2011) © 2011, Inderscience Publishers. Used with permission.

Digital Goods and Services [A]

Digital goods and services are services where the physical co-presence is not required and the service delivery can be performed through the Internet.

They often represent the evolution from service-embodied goods, or services which used to need the support of a physical good to be delivered. Here, technological innovation has acted in two seemingly conflicting ways: firstly, it has supported the "materialization" of services into transferable and tradable goods (for example, recording music on a digital device); later, it has increased the immateriality of services, separating them from physical evidence through digitalization and new Internet-based transferability (Evans & Wurster, 2000; Cho, 2005). In this sense, transferability has been made more pervasive by the possibility of digitalizing and transmitting data, archives, sounds, images, codified knowledge and anything that can be considered "information" (Shapiro & Varian, 1999). Consequently, information-based services are separated from their physical evidence and their delivery can be easily processed through Internet-based technologies. The production of service-embodied goods tends to adopt 'manufacturing' models, exploits new technologies and consequently increases the overall efficiency of sale and delivery. At the same time, consumers are no longer bound to the producer's location and time, as they can buy, receive and consume the service wherever and whenever they like to. Even in these services, however, some sort of interaction with the deliverer or the Internet-based technology may be possible and useful, for ICT allow an unprecedented level of personalization, based on the contact with consumers.

On-Line Delivery [B]

The second group too includes services where the delivery can be performed through the Internet and co-presence is not necessary. In this case, we focus on the evolution of long-distance services, where delivery system is non-transportable but can work from a distance, and the co-presence of both producer and consumer is unnecessary (such as in telecommunications); these services can be delivered via remote communication and strongly benefit from Internet-based technologies.

Some of these services originated as digital services to satisfy on-line market needs, which were not, or not fully, satisfied by existing firms (on-line search engines, "wiki" encyclopedias or on-line tourist guides). Others have fundamentally changed their core service and delivery system (on-line insurance companies and banks, live chat services, on-line news and trading). Others have taken advantage of the greater transmission and communication capability and pervasiveness of the new technologies, their lower usage costs, and the opportunity to enrich the service offer with new additional services (digital TV, Web radio, multimedia dictionaries, VOIP) (Benevolo & Spinelli, 2011).

The services presented so far are those where physical presence was unnecessary and delivery was consequently more easily performable through the Internet. Now we are going to introduce the other groups, where co-presence – or at least interaction – is necessary and the need for a greater personalization usually follows.

Virtual Relationship or Reality [C]

In this third group of services, the co-presence and interaction of the producer and the consumer of the service is necessary, but this co-presence can be made virtual by performing the service delivery through Internet-related technologies. The contact degree required for the delivery and how much this can be replaced by a simulation or an Internet-based relationship is crucial. The feasibility of this process is a consequence of the degree of contact required for delivery and of how much this can be replaced by a simulation or an Internet-based relationship. In personal services, a partial replacement for a physical presence and a Web contact is sometimes possible, where a relationship is unnecessary or not critical for service quality.

Unavoidable "Physical-Ness" or Humanization [D]

In this last group, services are included which need co-presence and whose delivery cannot be performed through the Internet. As a consequence, for these services it is not possible to substitute an Internet-based delivery for a traditional one and the direct impact of the digital economy on them is thus indirect. Nevertheless, ICT can play a major role in the delivery of the additional services which precede, follow or accompany the delivery of the core service, thus enriching the traditional service and generating more value for the user (Benevolo & Spinelli, 2011). Consider, for instance, those services assisting the potential consumer in the information-gathering process or in the evaluation of possible options (pre-delivery); those services supporting the sale, the assistance and customer services (post-delivery); those additional services helping the customer during off-line delivery.

Once defined the structure of the matrix, it is possible to place e-health applications on it, in accordance with the features of their delivery system; by doing so, we create various groups of e-health applications which share common structural features and which lead to our proposed taxonomy. The value of this taxonomy is that applications are not grouped on the basis of technological features – which are also exposed to the risk of quick obsolescence – but with respect to the structural characteristics of the services to be digitalized. In other words, we do not gather applications together only because they are delivered through mobile technologies (like the so-called m-health applications); we prefer to put together applications which share a common nature in terms of kind of processes and activities involved. However, as we are going to discuss in the "Future trends" section, it is likely that many services and groups will move on the matrix, because innovation will make available new ways to deliver healthcare services and redefine the borders between necessary and unnecessary co-presence and – even more – between the possibility or not to perform a given service through the Internet.

Moreover, those groups are "open", in the sense that new services could enter them due to important technological innovation which makes it possible their digitalization.

Given the present level of technological development, our classification exercise returns the following four groups of e-health applications:

1. Health information digitalization, transmission and sharing through the Internet;
2. Distance or virtual relationship in the delivery of medical care;
3. Support services to the management of healthcare facilities;
4. Online retrieval of medical data and information for clinicians, patients and the general public.

Figure 3 shows the position on the model matrix of each group, which is later discussed.

Figure 3. Healthcare service delivery and e-health applications
Source: Constructed by the authors.

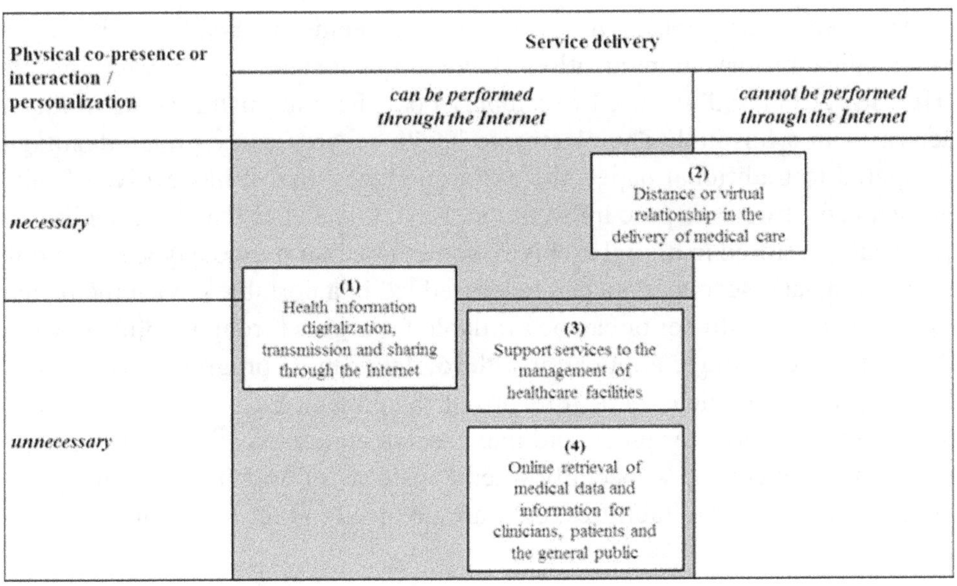

Health Information Digitalization, Transmission and Sharing through the Internet [1]

In health care systems, a widely recognized source of inefficiencies is the fragmentation of the care delivery process and the poor transfer of information along the various steps (OECD, 2010, p. 32). The efficient sharing of health information is, however, indispensable for the effective delivery of care (IOM, 2001). "Before the advent of Internet technology, there was no way to escape the inefficiencies of a paper-based system: the piles of prescriptions, forms, and charts, the frustration associated with registering and filling in medical histories more than once, the high cost of such inefficiencies" (Ball & Lillis, 2001, p. 5). In group 1 we gather information-centered applications which focus on processes and activities directly related with care provisioning and based on the collection and sharing of information about the patient, her pathologies and therapies. They allow to transfer and share digital data and information via the Internet among doctors and clinicians, within a single healthcare structure or between the several entities involved in the delivery of healthcare services in complex healthcare systems.

In Figure 4 the position of group 1 partially overlaps the border line between necessary and unnecessary physical co-presence of the subjects involved; in our opinion, in fact, the collection of the information to digitalize usually requires a certain physical interaction with the patient, while its transmission and sharing can be generally performed through the Internet without relevant problems.

Among the applications included in this group, the most relevant are patient information systems and electronic health records. These electronic records include patient demographics, progress notes, problems, medications, vital signs, past medical history, immunizations, laboratory data and radiology reports, etc. (HIMSS, 2011) and are used to support both the administrative and clinical activities in a hospital. The electronic health records carry great advantages compared to traditional paper, the main one being that it has evolved from a physical construct into pure information. First, this means that multimedia data can easily be stored in digital archives, something that previously was true only for written data; second, data can be embedded in a portable device the patient can easily carry with her or can be available for access through mobile devices, thanks to cloud storage applications; third, data can be progressively updated, allowing for a complete clinical record of the patient. Furthermore, electronic health records allow for quick and inexpensive communications between doctors or medical centers, especially when a wide set of organizations (hospitals, clinics, long-term care facilities, etc.) are involved in the treatment.

Exploiting the same principle, the results of an exam – for instance an ECG or a radiograph – can be remotely transmitted for analysis by a doctor who is not physically present with the patient. Picture archiving and communication systems (PACS), for example, are computer systems that "replace conventional x-ray film, and greatly improves access to patient information by making it possible for referring clinicians to review their patient's images on PCs from their own offices" (OECD, 2010, p. 36).

Further applications which exploit the digitalization of medical information are the so called e-Prescriptions, that is the computer-based electronic generation, transmission and filling of a medical prescription, and the electronic fit/sick notes, for sick leaves and insurance purposes. In both cases, the information flows becomes quicker, cheaper and more error-free than the traditional paper-equivalent; moreover, these applications allow for a better monitoring of the medical expense by the spender, usually the public entity responsible for the sanitary system.

Distance or Virtual Relationship in the Delivery of Medical Care [2]

In this group, applications are included which focus on the core process of care delivering and consequently require interaction between clinicians and patients. This is the case of those healthcare services, such as diagnostics and treatment, which have traditionally meant local services with high levels of contact and interaction between supplier (the doctor and her team) and consumer (the patient and her family).

Thanks to the advent of the digital economy, the delivery of many of these services can be significantly redesigned and supported by Internet-based technologies. We have especially in mind, for instance, the ubiquitous biometric data measurement and the remote patient monitoring and compliance, that is the mobile real time monitoring of patient vital signs, when patients are continually monitored on health-related parameters with wireless sensors, irrespective of where they happen to be (Van Halteren et al., 2004). Sensors can be embedded on the patient – for instance, in small monitoring devices or in her clothes (Castillejo et al., 2013) – and mobile phones or personal digital assistants (PDAs) with wireless networking capabilities may serve as gateways that process, store, and transfer data to clinicians for further analysis or diagnosis (Bardram et al., 2006). The monitoring device could have multimedia capabilities – allowing for the transmission of audio and video too – or even be coupled with an operating device (for example an insulin pump) which performs a remotely controlled therapy on the patient (Haux et al., 2002, p. 13).

These solutions offer great benefits because they free the patient from the need of being always "within reach" of the doctor, making it possible to remotely monitor a person's health without hospitalization; by doing so they allow for early detection and prevention of diseases by reporting events or changes which could require an intervention by the patient herself, e.g. by taking a medication or ceasing a dangerous behavior, or by a third person, such as a nurse or a doctor. Finally, they represent a tremendous innovation in situations of limited mobility of the patients, such as with remote communities, or in developing countries, since they lack both expert practitioners and health structures on the territory and distances can be significant between patients and hospitals. In this case, patients can be monitored by doctors who are very far away, with a great benefit to the population of disadvantaged countries (Gerber, 2009). Similar considerations could be made as regards specific situations in which continuous monitoring is needed but the presence of a doctor or nurse is unfeasible: we have in mind, for instance, post-partum home recovery, post-discharge home treatments, long-term and chronic home care, etc. In general, these applications could support the development of a more home-based approach to care delivery, with a shift of focus from the hospital to the patient's house as care-delivery place. An example is given by the EU-funded project "GiraffPlus" (www.giraffplus.eu), which has led to the creation of a complex system which can monitor activities in the house using a network of sensors, both in and around the house as well as on the body (Coradeschi et al. 2013). The sensors can measure blood pressure or detect whether somebody falls down. Different services, depending on the individual needs, can be pre-selected and tailored to the requirements of both older adults and health care professionals. At the heart of the system is a unique telepresence robot – Giraff, which lends its name to the project – that uses a Skype-like interface to allow, for instance, relatives or caregivers to virtually visit an elderly person in the home (Frennert & Östlund, 2014).

The last frontier in this virtual relationship regards the treatment step and is represented by tele-surgery via virtual reality 3D systems: in fact, they allow the surgeon to perform the operation from a distance, through an Internet connection by means of a robot-surgeon (Slack, 2007; Zhijiang et al. 2006). As the information flow is bidirectional, the surgeon receives back all the information about the patient (data, images, simulation of the response of the patient's body to the surgeon's actions), without being close to her. This opens the way to a virtual relationship between doctor and patient, with promising consequences for the development of long-distance surgery, which can now be performed regardless of geographical separation; some visionary authors are even imaging space surgery, to support quality of life and medical care in human outposts on the Moon or Mars (Haidegger et al., 2011)!

Nevertheless, the transition to a fully Internet-based delivery is still unfeasible, as some healthcare services require such an intense and personal contact between clinicians and patients which cannot be – and quite often does not even need to be – completely substituted by a virtual surrogate; for this reason, the corresponding box on the matrix overlaps the line between service which can and cannot be delivered through the Internet. In those cases as well when Internet delivery is not possible, Internet technologies can however play a major role in the delivery of the additional services which precede, follow or accompany the delivery of the core service, thus enriching the traditional service and generating more value for the user (Benevolo & Spinelli, 2008). A great part of the medical and nursing activity, in particular, is subject to these limitations: even though part of the traditional set of medical and surgical activities has moved to the Internet in some pioneering experiences, in the vast majority of cases it still has to face the need of a real physical contact with the patient who is going to receive the service. This is certainly relevant for medical activity but may be even more significant for nursing, which in some cases requires a closer contact between the nurse and the patient than the doctor-patient relationship. So long as technological development does not introduce really break-through innovations, it is quite difficult to imagine an Internet-based delivery for nursing services which support the patient in her everyday activities – such as cleaning or feeding – or which relate to applying a medication or dressing a wound. Nevertheless, the development of the digital economy can have a strong indirect impact on this group of healthcare activities as well, if we consider the additional services which always complement the physical performance of the core service. Electronic health records are for instance a powerful tool for constantly accessing and updating the patient's history, so ensuring that the most effective therapy is determined and provided. Similarly, mobile real time monitoring of the patient can limit physical contact to circumstances where it is strictly needed, so allowing the medical staff to concentrate on higher-value creating activities. A doctor who does not have to look for medical examination results but finds them always available on a portable device, can concentrate on diagnosis without losing time; similarly, a nurse who always has access to the prescribed therapies in the patient's file is much less likely to make mistakes or to misinterpret the doctor's instructions (Bates et al, 2001).

Support Services to the Management of Healthcare Facilities [3]

In this third group we gather those applications which aim to support the non-core administrative processes in healthcare facilities. These services do not require a specific interaction of the subjects involved and can consequently be shifted to the Internet to a significant extent. A proper example is given by hospital information systems, enterprise resource planning (ERP) systems that support information processing within a hospital in areas such as administration, appointments, billing, planning, budgeting and personnel; similarly, we can cite LIS (Laboratory Information Systems) and RIS (Radiology Information Systems), which support the management of specific departments. Other areas supported by such applications are, for instance, order management, medication management, disaster recovery, business intelligence, quality management and assessment, etc. Even if not strictly related with the "main" caretaking process, these services are crucial for health organizations, especially in terms of administrative costs and service quality; their impact on the overall efficiency and effectiveness is consequently very strong, as witnessed by the fact that they have long been the main target of investment in IT by healthcare institutions (Osservatorio ICT in Sanità, 2013).

Online Retrieval of Medical Data and Information for Clinicians, Patients and the General Public [4]

In this final group we include those processes and activities which are information-based (as in group 1) but are not directly related with the information generated during the care delivery. In other words, these information-based processes concern ancillary activities such as education, training, knowledge dissemination etc.

A first example is given by online registries, such as national electronic registries (which contain data on specific medical subjects such as births, mortality, cancer, diabetes or other subjects of medical or epidemiological interest), national drug registries (containing national pharmaceutical information) or directories of healthcare professional and institutions (which can support patients and the general public when choosing a clinician or an institution for treatment).

With a closer focus on e-learning and support to clinicians training and education, we can cite Internet-based on-demand clinical case analysis services, such as those developed by MEDgle©. MEDgle is a case analysis engine with a wide range of real-time, predictive health uses. The MEDgle platform is built on top of a large database of relationships between symptoms, diagnoses, drugs, tests, procedures and associated statistical information (MEDgle Inc., 2014). Even if still at the experimental stage, this service could potentially bring valuable support to the medical staff in decision-taking. The user is even excused from the need of acquiring any ICT device or advance infrastructure, as the service is totally web-based and can be accessed from everywhere and by using any kind of Internet-capable device. This last feature is particularly interesting, because it allows for the use of the platform even in extreme situations, such as in a rescue service, when the medical staff is outside the hospital facilities but can access the Internet with portable tools such as an IPad or similar. MEDgle belongs to the family of the Clinical Decision Support Systems (CDSS), a large group of stand-alone or Web-based systems which aim to support the decision-making process of medical staff with inference engines or artificial intelligence software (Garg et al, 2005). The reliability of CDSS is still questioned by the medical community, due to the limit that these technologies face in properly interpreting the whole clinical picture of a patient; nevertheless, the value of the business idea is certainly high and it is probable that, once refined and completely implemented, MEDgle and its competitors will become a useful and reliable support tool for medical staff.

A further research and diagnostic service which is delivered though the Web are bibliographic databases such as MEDLINE© (Medical Literature Analysis and Retrieval System Online), which includes bibliographic information for articles from academic journals covering most of medical science fields. The value added of such a service does not lie only in that the articles are digitalized; more important is the aspect related to the accurate ways in which this knowledge base can be explored, thanks to the connections which are created between the single piece of information and all the rest.

Finally, Internet-based technology can support the development of online professional communities, allowing for virtual consultation and collaboration among doctors, to enhance research and improve healthcare quality through the sharing of best-practices and the opportunities for all the subjects involved to exchange views and disseminate knowledge. This can be particularly useful, for example, in case of public health emergencies, such as epidemics or pandemics like Ebola, that require a strong global sharing of information on how the virus is spreading but also on what cures are being provided and with what results, to improve the treatments and their effectiveness.

FUTURE TRENDS: OPPORTUNITIES AND CRITICAL ISSUES

In this chapter, we have tried to propose a new taxonomy of e-health applications, based on the structural features of the delivery system associated with the services which are digitalized. To this purpose, we have traced back the development of e-health applications to a wider framework of digitalization for services; structural differences among services categories then result into different forms of digitalization and delivery through Internet-based technologies.

As previously stated, our taxonomy presents several advantages over other alternatives, because it is not based on specific technological features but on:

- The structural characteristics of the services to be digitalized;
- The subjects involved and the relationships which are activated in the service delivery;
- The operational potentiality of Internet-based technologies.

However, it is important to speculate on the major trends in the development of e-health, as they could influence the position of the groups on the matrix, moving the borders between necessary and unnecessary co-presence and between possibility or not to perform a given service through the Internet. Hitherto, e-health has not yet revealed all its potential; as reported by Kennedy and Berk (2011), the health care industry "despite being arguably the most information-intensive industry in the world, has been slow to join the digital revolution" and "the transition will be a sea change" (p. 1). Nevertheless the innumerable cases of innovative adoption of ICT – both in the intangible and tangible components of healthcare activities – suggest that the evolution of healthcare activities towards new digital configurations is a structural process already in progress, even if still far from reaching full deployment. On the one side, the adoption, diffusion and pervasiveness of e-health applications could be boosted by technological innovation but also by social and cultural evolution in regards to health services; on the other side, e-health could be restrained by obstacles and limitations of various origins which could even get worse in the future.

In this section, we aim to point out both opportunities and critical issues, trying to highlight the repercussions on our taxonomy.

A significant part of healthcare services are by their nature "high-touch services", due to the need for physical contact and relation, and they are consequently slow in evolving from "low-tech" to "high-tech" configurations, where the use of automatic systems, ICT and other physical supports is more and more significant (Salomann et al., 2006). The progress is therefore not easy, due to cultural, organizational and budget constraints, but the results already achieved suggest that innovation horizons in healthcare are broad and promising. Coming back to the Malecki and Moriset (2008) classification which was presented in the "Background" section, we confirm that the healthcare industry is going to increasingly join the pyramid's "main body", as more and more of its activities will require extensive use of ICT to be performed in innovative and more effective ways, with great benefits for patients, medical staff and national budgets too. More broadly, this trend is stronger when we consider that medical activities in the strict sense of the word are only a part of the complex healthcare industry. Indeed, it includes several service-providing and manufacturing sectors – such as research companies, information providers and diagnostic equipment manufacturers – which are already heavily ICT-enabled and consequently push the "medical core" of the industry towards new digital configurations. While at the beginning of the century the Institute of Medicine (IOM, 2001) could state that the healthcare service delivery remained "relatively untouched by the revolution in information technology that [had] swept nearly every other aspect of society" (p. 15), nowadays the situation has radically evolved and the "revolution" is absolutely in progress.

This is especially true for the "Distance or virtual relationship in the delivery of medical care" group, which will certainly shift leftwards due innovative solutions to substitute a virtual relationship for a physical one in healthcare delivery. The main emerging trend is the shift from a model where the patient "moves towards the cure" (being it at the doctor or at the hospital) to a new one where is the cure to "move towards the patient", thanks to all those technologies which allow to share and transfer health information. As Mukhopadhyay (2015) reports, "the advancement of sensing technologies, embedded systems, wireless communication technologies, nano technologies, and miniaturization makes it possible to develop smart systems to monitor activities of human beings continuously", (p. 1321). In the perspective of the so-called Internet-of-Things, we have especially in mind the further evolution of the aforementioned wearable medical devices, where the interconnection is on a machine-to-machine basis; this means that the first recipient of the transmitted information is not a person but another device, which is programmed to react in a certain way when receiving specific data, such as alarm systems which start other devices up.

These sensors forward their collected data to an M2M device (e.g., a patient's cell phone) that acts as an information aggregator and forwards the data to the M2M application server [...]. The M2M server responds to the collected data by sending alerts and appropriate medical records to medical providers. In emergency situations, an M2M device can directly provide the medical status of a patient en route to the hospital (e.g., in the ambulance), allowing physicians to prepare for treatment in advance of the patient's arrival. (Geng et al., 2011, p. 38)

The device could even be "inside" the patient: this is the case, for instance, of sensors in pills that are swallowed and could automatically send patient information to doctors and nurses; this would allow a sick or elderly person to manage her healthcare from home, rather than in a hospital or nursing home, getting automatic reminders to take medicines or immediate preventive care for changes in health status.

Furthermore, enhanced devices could collect, elaborate and transfer information in real time, enabling faster communications and decision making. and allowing to access information not otherwise available, in terms of width, depth, updating and precision (Safavi, 2014)

This new approach to healthcare delivery would benefit from innovation in georeferencing too: with respect to the objectives of e-health we previously cited, georeference could increase the quality of the assistance and make it feasible to provide healthcare services more integrated and less bounded to physical location.

Big Data is another field of innovation which is certainly going to have a strong impact on healthcare (Srinivasan & Arunasalam, 2013; Liu & Park, 2014; Mancini, 2014; MeriTalk, 2014); as previously mentioned, all the subjects involved in healthcare delivery generate large amount of data, which could be effectively used to reduce the cost of healthcare while improving quality, and supporting prevention and personalization. So far it has been quite difficult to explore them and turn them into valuable information; Big Data solutions now make it possible to exploit the mass of available data in unexperienced manners, offering the potential to improve trial safety, disease surveillance, prescribed treatments, and patient outcomes. Big Data adoption in healthcare is still in its initial stages, but its potential is already beyond doubt.

Nevertheless, the process towards a widespread implementation of e-health practices has to face several obstacles, most of which do not strictly relate to technical matters (Karsh et al. 2010). With respect to technical difficulties, in fact, it is very often just "a matter of time", as continuous innovation is able to progressively overcome them. We are more interested in non-technical questions and – even though a full examination of them is beyond the aim of this chapter – some references cannot be omitted.

A first major barrier concerns the financing of e-health initiatives; purchasing and implementation costs for these projects usually require a significant amount of financing with an uncertain (at least in the short term) assessment of the extent of the achievable benefits and of who is actually benefitting from the gains in efficiency and effectiveness:

one significant barrier to investment in ICTs is the widely recognized fact that any resulting cost savings may not always accrue to the implementer, but may be passed on to a third party. Benefits may appear at one site and in one budget, while a large share of the cost commitments appear at another site and in another budget. (OECD, 2010, p. 46)

Furthermore, there may be lags between ICT investments and benefit realization (Devaraj & Kohli, 2000); quite commonly, the financial benefits are not realized until a level of functionality is reached – a kind of "critical mass" – that allows systems to truly serve the needs of clinicians and system planners. "Until IT investment reaches a threshold, total operating expenses increase in hospitals that have little IT" (PricewaterhouseCoopers, 2007, p. 18). In addition, there are no incentives, and may even be disincentives for care providers to be the first to adopt ICT (Taylor et al., 2005), as commonly happens with radical innovations. At the same, the development of a strong business case is crucial, because – as in Dixon (2007) – it "lowers the risk of adoption, implementation, and use of e-health" (p. 11) and is the first step of an effective roadmap for e-health adoption.

The situation is however extremely varied worldwide. Western countries are certainly dealing with an increase in the elderly share of population and in the diffusion of diseases related to lifestyle and physical inactivity, which result in rapid rises in healthcare costs; furthermore, they have long-established health services and structures, that need deep changes to be converted to ICT adoption; finally, they often face shrinking public budget for healthcare, which make it much more difficult to respond to the challenges that those trends pose. Poorer countries, instead, still have big issues to solve: endemic health problems, undersized structures compared to the needs, chronical lack of resources; as a consequence, they could be excluded from the innovation process for a long time yet. Finally, emerging country are probably those with the greatest potential of adoption: on the one hand, they can count on vast resources, which allow for large budget for healthcare; on the other hand, they are still building their health services and structures: not having to face path dependencies and resistance to change – as we are going to better detail later on – they may be the quickest to efficiently adopt new e-health technologies pervasively.

A second important barrier is associated with organizational factors, both between and within healthcare organizations.

As regards the first aspect, we have to keep in mind that several e-health services involve a plurality of organizations: healthcare systems, indeed, are usually very fragmented, with a multiplicity of public and private providers and payers. This constitutes a significant barrier to the adoption of e-health services, as it implies connecting systems managed by different organizations and with relevant differences as regards the standard and content of the collected data, the transmission protocol, etc. (Kaye et al., 2010). For this reason, a crucial role is played by the organizations for standardization – such as the International Organization for Standardization (ISO) or the Comité Européen de Normalisation (CEN) – which are working, in particular, for the definition of common standards for the Electronic Health Records (Chávez et al., 2009; Moruzzi, 2009). Kennedy and Berk (2011) report about the US experience, where "a host of standards – Including Logical Observation Identifiers Names and Codes (LOINC), Digital Imaging and Communications in Medicine (DICOM), Health Level Seven International (HL7), and Systematized Nomenclature of Medicine Clinical Terms (SNOMED CT) – are allowing for rich information interchange across care settings and are being used by regional health-information organizations [...] to coordinate care across regions, with impressive results" (p.5). The development work on standards is surely critical, but when standards are refined and become more commonplace, the ability to exchange, aggregate, and analyze health care data will increase dramatically. With respect to our taxonomy, this could increase the scope for both the "Support services to the management of healthcare facilities" and the "Health information digitalization, transmission and sharing through the Internet", which strongly rely on shared standards and communication protocols between and within healthcare institutions.

The barrier associated with organizational factors internal to the healthcare organization represents an aspect not yet adequately studied in the literature (Shekelle & Goldzweig, 2009); nevertheless, as previously cited, this topic is crucial and impacts all the categories of e-applications we identified: in particular, the implementation of health information systems (group 3) represents a strong organizational discontinuity and questions consolidated procedures, routines and habits (Gagnon et al., 2005). This opens the door to a vast discussion about leadership and governance for ICT projects (Bernstein, McCreless, & Cötè, 2007; Fickenscher & Bakerman, 2011); about technical education and training for doctors and nurses who are asked to use new technologies (Masys, 1998; Ball & Lillis, 2001; Anderson, 2007; Moghaddasi et al., 2012); about how to increase the actual adoption of new systems and overcome the organizational and individual inertia (England, Stewart & Walker, 2000; Gaggioli et al., 2005). Furthermore, we should not forget that high technology cannot do without human skills and capabilities, which must remain absolutely central in the service delivery (Demattè et al., 2007; Freema et al., 2010).

Another big problem is related to privacy, security and legal issues in sharing sensitive patient data in a large and heterogeneous environment through the use of web-based and mobile applications (Berner, 2008; Moruzzi, 2009; Lateef, 2011; Safavi, 2014), as in group 1 ("Health information digitalization, transmission and sharing through the Internet") and in group 4 ("Online retrieval of medical data and information for clinicians, patients and the general public"). Several surveys and studies highlight the concern about the privacy of patients' health information. This concern is well motivated because, "as the contents of electronic health records are shared more widely, the risk increases that stigmatizing disclosures could affect areas such as employment status, access to health insurance and other forms of insurance, and participation in community activities" (OECD, 2010, p. 106). This is certainly a major issue, which is becoming even more important with the advent of Big Data solutions and which needs to be addressed from both the legal and the technical side: from the legal side, to build a regulatory framework (better if on an international scale) for information gathering, storing and sharing; from the technical side, to develop those standards and applications which make possible to match the adoption of e-health practices with the protection of individual rights.

Finally, another issue is also the degree of acceptance of e-health practices by the recipients, that is, the patients and their family. With respect to this topic – crucial in particular for applications in the "Distance or virtual relationship in the delivery of medical care" group – both cultural predisposition and technology acceptance are relevant, especially in older patients (see, among others, Eikelboom & Atlas, 2005; Whitten & Love, 2005); patients have to accept the substitution of a technology-mediated relationship with the medical staff for physical contact and also have to develop such minimum skills which allow them to interact with the devices, such as in the mobile real time monitoring of vital signs. This is a subject that deserves much more attention and could be of major interest not only for medical practitioners but also for engineers and software developers, who have to design those devices.

Nevertheless, some studies return quite surprising results, as both patients and their relatives seem to be prepared to take on semi-autonomous telepresence robots but health care providers are not (Frennert & Östlund, 2014). Again, deficiencies in the organization of the introduction of the new approach pose an obstacle and a challenge for the development of modern medical care.

CONCLUSION

Our reflection about e-health applications has tried to trace them back to the more general trend of services digitalization. An original taxonomy has been proposed, which is actually based on the structural characteristics of the delivery systems of the services that are impacted by the Internet technologies. The resulting framework returns an exhaustive picture of e-health applications and allows for some reflections about the evolution of the digital healthcare industry. We believe e-health should not be considered simply a technological innovation, but a paradigm shift which results in a radical redesign of the whole industry. In essence, the adoption of ICT – and especially of Internet-based technologies – triggers a virtuous cycle of innovation: the new opportunities enabled by digital technologies stimulate the creation of original practices and the reconfiguration of the processes; this, in turn, supports the research for latest technologies to apply to healthcare, and so on. Physical limitations – mostly due to the undoubted importance of the physical co-presence of producer (healthcare staff) and user (patient) in many healthcare services – are still present and central. In spite of these obstacles, the future of e-health is nevertheless very promising and will lead to an efficiency gain, together with an increase in the quality of healthcare delivery and practice. As commonly known, health is, in turn, a strong driver of well-being and quality of life (Stiglitz, Sen, & Fitoussi, 2009): as a consequence, the possibility and hope of improving people standards of life strongly rely on e-health applications to turn into reality. This certainly leads to interesting developments in research. New applications are constantly developed and the adoption of ICT in healthcare is increasingly pervasive, rich and deep. It is consequently of undoubted interest to keep on monitoring these innovative activities to track their evolution and to assess the drivers and impediments of e-health development worldwide.

However, a final consideration is worth mentioning: how does the pervasive adoption of ICT in healthcare change the doctor-patient relationship? What remains of non-technological and closely tied to the encounter between people? In our view, empathy remains together with the motivation leading health personnel to take care of patients and, finally, the recognition of the sanctity of the human life. These elements are still, if you will, out of the control and management of technology.

REFERENCES

Aldrich, D., & Masera, P. (1999). *Mastering the Digital Market Place*. New York, NY: John Wiley & Sons.

Alpay, L. L., Henkemans, O. B., Otten, W., Rövekamp, T. A., & Dumay, A. C. (2010). E-health applications and services for patient empowerment: Directions for best practices in The Netherlands. *Telemedicine Journal and e-Health*, *16*(7), 787–791. doi:10.1089/tmj.2009.0156 PMID:20815745

Anderson, J. G. (2007). Social, ethical and legal barriers to e-health. *International Journal of Medical Informatics*, *76*(5), 480–483. doi:10.1016/j.ijmedinf.2006.09.016 PMID:17064955

Atkinson, R. D., & McKay, A. S. (2014). *Digital Prosperity – Understanding the Economic Benefits of the Information Technology Revolution*. Retrieved May 7, 2014 from http://www.itif.org/index.php?id=34

Ball, M. J., & Lillis, J. (2001). E-health: Transforming the physician-patient relationship. *International Journal of Medical Informatics*, *61*(1), 1–10. doi:10.1016/S1386-5056(00)00130-1 PMID:11248599

Bardram, J. E., Mihailidis, A., & Wan, D. (Eds.). (2006). *Pervasive Computing in Healthcare*. Boca Raton, FL: CRC.

Bashshur, R., Shannon, G., Krupinski, E., & Grigsby, J. (2011). The taxonomy of telemedicine. *Telemedicine Journal and e-Health*, *17*(6), 484–494. doi:10.1089/tmj.2011.0103 PMID:21718114

Bates, D. W., Cohen, M., Leape, L. L., Overhage, J. M., Shabot, M. M., & Sheridan, T. (2001). Reducing the frequency of errors in medicine using information technology. *Journal of the American Medical Informatics*, *8*(4), 299–308. doi:10.1136/jamia.2001.0080299 PMID:11418536

Benevolo, C., & Spinelli, R. (2011). International service delivery and Internet-based technologies. *International Journal of Services. Economics and Management*, *3*(3), 251–266.

Berner, E. S. (2008). Ethical and legal issues in the use of Health Information Technology to improve patient safety. *HEC Forum*, *20*(39), 243–258. doi:10.1007/s10730-008-9074-5 PMID:18803020

Bernstein, M. L., McCreless, T., & Côté, M. J. (2007). Five constants of Information technology Adoption in Healthcare. *Hospital Topics*, *85*(1), 17–25. doi:10.3200/HTPS.85.1.17-26 PMID:17405421

Bhagwati, J. (1987). International trade in services and its relevance for economic development. In O. Giarini (Ed.), *The Emerging Service Economy* (pp. 3–57). Oxford, UK: Pergamon Press.

Bitner, M. J., Brown, S. W., Goul, M., & Urban, S. (2008). Services science journey: foundations, progress, and challenges. In B. Hefley & W. Murphy (Eds.), *Service science, management and engineering education for the 21st century* (pp. 227–233). Springer; doi:10.1007/978-0-387-76578-5_35

Black, A. D., Car, J., Pagliari, C., Anandan, C., Cresswell, K., Bokun, T., & Sheikh, A. et al. (2011). The impact of eHealth on the quality and safety of health care: A systematic overview. *PLoS Medicine*, *8*(1), e1000387. PMID:21267058

Buntin, M. B., Burke, M. F., Hoaglin, M. C., & Blumenthal, D. (2011). The benefits of health information technology: A review of the recent literature shows predominantly positive results. *Health Affairs*, *30*(3), 464–471. doi:10.1377/hlthaff.2011.0178 PMID:21383365

Burman, E. (2003). *Shift!: The Unfolding Internet: Hype, Hope and History*. Chichester, UK: John Wiley & Sons.

Castells, M. (2000). *The Rise of the Network Society*. Oxford, UK: Blackwell Publishers.

Castillejo, P., Martínez, J. F., Rodríguez-Molina, J., & Cuerva, A. (2013). Integration of wearable devices in a wireless sensor network for an E-health application. *IEEE Wireless Communicatons*, *20*(4), 38–49. doi:10.1109/MWC.2013.6590049

Chase, R. B. (1978). Where does the customer fit in a service operation? *Harvard Business Review*, *56*(5), 137–142. PMID:10239167

Chávez, E., Krishnan, P., & Finnie, G. (2010). A taxonomy of e-health standards to assist system developers. In G. A. Papadopulos et al. (Eds.), *Information Systems Development. Towards a Service Provision Society* (pp. 737–745). New York, NY: Springer US.

Chesbrough, H. (2005). Toward a science of services. *Harvard Business Review*, *83*(2), 16–17.

Cho, S.-E. (2005). Developing new frameworks for operations strategy and service system design in electronic commerce. *International Journal of Service Industry Management*, *16*(3), 294–314. doi:10.1108/09564230510601413

Commission of the European Communities. (2004). e-Health - making healthcare better for European citizens: An action plan for a European e-Health Area. Luxembourg: Commission of the European Communities.

Coradeschi, S., Cesta, A., Cortellessa, G., Coraci, L., Gonzalez, J., Karlsson, L., . . . Otslund, B. (2013). Giraffplus: Combining social interaction and long term monitoring for promoting independent living. In *Human System Interaction (HSI), 2013 The 6th International Conference on*. IEEE.

Demattè, C., Biffi, A., Mandelli, A., & Parolini, C. (2007). Firms and the Digital Technology in Italy: The Network Moves Forward. In U. Apte & U. Karmarkar (Eds.), *Managing in the Information Economy* (pp. 429–471). New York, NY: Springer. doi:10.1007/978-0-387-36892-4_18

Devaraj, S., & Kohli, R. (2000). Information Technology payoff in the healthcare industry: A longitudinal study. *Journal of Management Information Systems*, *16*(4), 41–67. doi:10.1080/07421222.2000.11518265

Dixon, B. E. (2007). A roadmap for the adoption of e-Health. *e-Service Journal*, *5*(3), 3–13. doi:10.2979/ESJ.2007.5.3.3

Eiglier, P., & Langeard, E. (1987). *Servuction. Le marketing des services*. Paris, France: McGraw-Hill.

Eikelboom, R. H., & Atlas, M. D. (2005). Attitude to telemedicine, and willingness to use it, in audiology patients. *Journal of Telemedicine and Telecare*, *11*(8), S22–S25. doi:10.1258/135763305775124920 PMID:16375788

Eng, T. (2001). *The e-Health Landscape – a terrain map of emerging information and communication technologies in health and health care*. Princeton NJ: The Robert Wood Johnson Foundation. Retrieved May 23, 2014 from http://www.hetinitiative.org/media/pdf/eHealth.pdf

England, I., Steward, D., & Walker, S. (2000). Information technology adoption in health care: When organizations and technology collide. *Australian Health Review*, *23*(3), 176–185. doi:10.1071/AH000176 PMID:11186051

Evans, P., & Wurster, T. S. (2000). *Blown to bits. How the new economics of information transforms strategy*. Boston, MA: Harvard Business School Press.

Eysenbach, G. (2001). What is e-health? *Journal of Medical Internet Research*, *3*(2), e20. doi:10.2196/jmir.3.2.e20 PMID:11720962

Fatehi, F., & Wootton, R. (2012). Telemedicine, telehealth or e-health? A bibliometric analysis of the trends in the use of these terms. *Journal of Telemedicine and Telecare*, *18*(8), 460–464. doi:10.1258/jtt.2012.GTH108 PMID:23209265

Fickenscher, K., & Bakerman, M. (2011). Leadership and governance for IT projects. *Physician Executive*, *37*(1), 72–76. PMID:21302752

Fieschi, M. (2002). Information technology is changing the way society sees health care delivery. *International Journal of Medical Informatics*, *66*(1-3), 85–93. doi:10.1016/S1386-5056(02)00040-0 PMID:12453562

Freema, W. D., Vatz, K. A., & Demaerschalk, B. M. (2010). Telemedicine in 2010: Robotic caveats. *Lancet Neurology*, *9*(11), 1046. doi:10.1016/S1474-4422(10)70261-1 PMID:20965432

Frennert, S., & Östlund, B. (2014). Domestication of a telehealthcare system. *Gerontechnology (Valkenswaard)*, *13*(2), 197. doi:10.4017/gt.2014.13.02.105.00

Frisse, M. E. (2009). Health Information Technology: One step at a time. *Health Affairs*, *28*(2), 379–w384. doi:10.1377/hlthaff.28.2.w379 PMID:19273814

Gaggioli, A., Di Carlo, S., Mantovani, F., Castelnuovo, G., & Riva, G. (2005). A telemedicine survey among Milan doctors. *Journal of Telemedicine and Telecare*, *11*(1), 29–34. doi:10.1258/1357633053430476 PMID:15829041

Gagnon, M.-P., Lamothe, L., Fortin, J.-P., Cloutier, A., Godin, G., Gagné, C., & Reinharz, D. (2005). Telehealth adoption in hospitals: An organisational perspective. *Journal of Health Organization and Management*, *19*(1), 32–56. doi:10.1108/14777260510592121 PMID:15938601

Gantz, J., & Reinsel, D. (2011). Extracting value from chaos. *IDC iview*, 1-12.

Garg, A. X., Adhikari, N. K. J., McDonald, H., Rosas-Arellano, M. P., Devereaux, P. J., Beyene, J., & Haynes, R. B. et al. (2005). Effects of Computerized Clinical Decision Support Systems on practitioner performance and patient outcomes: A systematic review. *Journal of the American Medical Association*, *293*(10), 1223–1238. doi:10.1001/jama.293.10.1223 PMID:15755945

Geng, W., Talwar, S., Johnsson, K., Himayat, N., & Johnson, K. D. (2011). M2M: From mobile to embedded internet. *IEEE Communications Magazine*, *49*(4), 36–43. doi:10.1109/MCOM.2011.5741144

Gerber, T. (2009). Health Information Technology: Dispatches from the revolution. *Health Affairs*, *28*(2), 390–w391. doi:10.1377/hlthaff.28.2.w390 PMID:19273816

Grönroos, C. (1990). *Service Management and Marketing: Managing the Moments of Truth in Service Competition*. New Britian, CT: Lexington Books.

Gunter, T. D., & Terry, N. P. (2005). The emergence of national electronic health record architectures in the United States and Australia: Models, costs, and questions. *Journal of Medical Internet Research*, *7*(1), e3. doi:10.2196/jmir.7.1.e3 PMID:15829475

Haidegger, T., Sándor, J., & Benyo, Z. (2011). Surgery in space: The future of robotic telesurgery. *Surgical Endoscopy*, *25*(3), 681–690. doi:10.1007/s00464-010-1243-3 PMID:20652320

Haux, R., Ammenwerth, E., Herzog, W., & Knaup, P. (2002). Health care in the information society. A prognosis for the year 2013. *International Journal of Medical Informatics*, *66*(1-3), 3–21. doi:10.1016/S1386-5056(02)00030-8 PMID:12453552

HIMSS – Healthcare Information and Management Systems Society. (2014). *Electronic health record (HER)*. Retrieved on May 16, 2014 from http://www.himss.org/ASP/topics_ehr.asp

Holler, J., Tsiatsis, V., Mulligan, C., Avesand, S., Karnouskos, S., & Boyle, D. (2014). *From Machine-to-machine to the Internet of Things: Introduction to a New Age of Intelligence*. Oxford, UK: Academic Press.

IOM – Institute of Medicine. (2001). *Crossing the Quality Chasm: A New Health System for the 21st Century*. Washington, DC: National Academy Press.

Javalgi, R. G., Martin, C. L., & Todd, P. R. (2004). The export of e-services in the age of technology transformation: Challenges and implications for international service providers. *Journal of Services Marketing*, *18*(7), 560–573. doi:10.1108/08876040410561884

Karsh, B. T., Weinger, M. B., Abbott, P. A., & Wears, R. L. (2010). Health information technology: Fallacies and sober realities. *Journal of the American Medical Informatics Association*, *17*(6), 617–623. doi:10.1136/jamia.2010.005637 PMID:20962121

Kaye, R., Kokia, E., Shalev, V., Idar, D., & Chinitz, D. (2010). Barriers and success factors in health information technology: A practitioner's perspective. *Journal of Management & Marketing in Healthcare.*, *3*(2), 163–175. doi:10.1179/175330310X12736577732764

Kennedy, S., & Berk, B. (2011), Enabling E-Health: A revolution for informatics in health care. *BCG Perspectives*. Retrieved on June 17, 2011 from www.bcgperspectives.com

Lateef, F. (2011). The practice of telemedicine: Medicolegal and ethical issues. *Ethics & Medicine*, *27*(1), 17–25.

Liu, W., & Park, E. K. (2014). Big Data as an e-Health Service. In *Computing, Networking and Communications (ICNC), 2014 International Conference on*. IEEE. doi:10.1109/ICCNC.2014.6785471

Lovelock, C. H. (1983). Classifying services to gain strategic marketing insights. *Journal of Marketing*, *3*(47), 9–20. doi:10.2307/1251193

Lovelock, C. H. (1996). *Service Marketing* (3rd ed.). London: Prentice Hall International.

Lovelock, C. H., & Wirtz, J. (2004). *Services Marketing: People, Technology, Strategy* (5th ed.). Upper Saddle River, NJ: Prentice Hall.

Maglio, P. P., & Spohrer, J. (2008). Fundamentals of service science. *Journal of the Academy of Marketing Science*, *36*(1), 18–20. doi:10.1007/s11747-007-0058-9

Malecki, E. J., & Moriset, B. (2008). *The Digital Economy: Business Organization, Production Processes, and Regional Developments*. Oxon, UK: Routledge.

Mancini, M. (2014). Exploiting big data for improving healthcare services. *Journal of e-Learning and Knowledge Society, 10*(2), 23-33.

Masys, D. (1998). Advances in Information Technology. Implications for medical education. *The Western Journal of Medicine*, *168*(5), 341–347. PMID:9614791

MEDgle Inc. (2014). *The details*. Retrieved on May 15, 2014 from http://www.medgle.com/front.jsp?task=technology&section=details

MeriTalk. (2014). *The Big Data Cure*. Retrieved on January 25, 2015 from http://www.meritalk.com/bigdatacure

Moghaddasi, H., Asadi, F., Hosseini, A., & Ebnehoseini, Z. (2012). E-health: A global approach with extensive semantic variation. *Journal of Medical Systems*, *36*(5), 3173–3176. doi:10.1007/s10916-011-9805-z PMID:22113437

Moruzzi, M. (2009). *E-health e fascicolo sanitario elettronico*. Milano, Italy: Il Sole 24 Ore.

Mukhopadhyay, S. (2015). Wearable sensors for human activity monitoring: A review. *IEEE Sensors Journal*, *15*(3), 1321–1330. doi:10.1109/JSEN.2014.2370945

Normann, R. (1984). *Service Management Strategy and Leadership in Service Business*. Chichester, UK: John Wiley & Sons.

O'Malley, A. S. (2011). Tapping the unmet potential of health information technology. *The New England Journal of Medicine, 364*(12), 1090–1091. doi:10.1056/NEJMp1011227 PMID:21428764

OECD – Organisation for Economic Co-operation and Development. (2010). *Improving Health Sector Efficiency. The Role of Information and Communication Technologies*. Paris, France: OECD.

Oh, H., Rizo, C., Enkin, M., Jadad, A., Powell, J., & Pagliari, C. (2005). What is eHealth (3): A systematic review of published definitions. *Journal of Medical Internet Research, 7*(1), e1. doi:10.2196/jmir.7.1.e1 PMID:15829471

Osservatorio ICT in Sanità – School of Management of the Politecnico di Milano. (2008). *ICT e innovazione in sanità: nuove sfide e opportunità per i CIO*. Milano: Politecnico di Milano, Dipartimento di Ingegneria gestionale.

Osservatorio ICT in Sanità – School of Management of the Politecnico di Milano. (2013). *ICT in sanità: perché il digitale non rimanga solo in agenda*. Milano: Politecnico di Milano, Dipartimento di Ingegneria gestionale.

Pagliari, C., Sloan, D., Gregor, P., Sullivan, F., Detmer, D., Kahan, J. P., & Mac Gillivray, S. et al. (2005). What is eHealth (4): A scoping exercise to map the field. *Journal of Medical Internet Research, 7*(1), e9. doi:10.2196/jmir.7.1.e9 PMID:15829481

Porter, M. (2001). Strategy and the Internet. *Harvard Business Review, 79*(2), 63–78. PMID:11246925

PricewaterhouseCoopers. (2007). *The Economics of IT and Hospital Performance*. Retrieved July 14, 2011 from http://www.pwc.com/us/en/healthcare/publications/the-economics-of-it-and-hospital-performance.jhtml

Rahman, Z. (2004). E-commerce solution for services. *European Business Review, 16*(6), 564–576. doi:10.1108/09555340410565396

Safavi, S., & Shukur, Z. (2014). Conceptual privacy framework for health information on wearable device. *PLoS ONE, 9*(12), e114306. doi:10.1371/journal.pone.0114306 PMID:25478915

Safran, C. (2003). The collaborative edge: Patient empowerment for vulnerable populations. *International Journal of Medical Informatics, 69*(2), 185–190. doi:10.1016/S1386-5056(02)00130-2 PMID:12810122

Salomann, H., Kolbe, L., & Brenner, W. (2006). Self-services in customer relationships: Balancing high-tech and high-touch today and tomorrow. *E-Service Journal, 4*(2), 65–84. doi:10.2979/ESJ.2006.4.2.65

Shapiro, C., & Varian, H. R. (1999). *Information Rules: A Strategic Guide to the Network Economy*. Boston, MA: Harvard Business School Press.

Shekelle, P., & Goldzweig, C. L. (2009). *Costs and Benefits of Health Information Technology: An Updated Systematic Review*. London, UK: The Health Foundation.

Showell, C., & Nohr, C. (2012). How should we define eHealth, and does the definition matter?. *Quality of Life through Quality of Information, 180*, 881-884.

Silvestro, R., Fitzgerald, L., Johnston, R., & Voss, C. (1992). Towards a classification of service processes. *International Journal of Service Industry Management, 3*(3), 62–75. doi:10.1108/09564239210015175

Slack, C. (2007). The robot surgeon. *Proto Magazine*. Retrieved May 17, 2014 from: http://www.protomag.com/assets/the-robot-surgeon?page=1

Sood, S., Mbarika, V., Jugoo, S., Dookhy, R., Doarn, C. R., Prakash, N., & Merrell, R. C. (2007). What is telemedicine? A collection of 104 peer-reviewed perspectives and theoretical underpinnings. *Telemedicine Journal and e-Health, 13*(5), 573–590. doi:10.1089/tmj.2006.0073 PMID:17999619

Spinelli, R. (2008). The digital economy: A conceptual framework for a new economic paradigm. *The Journal of Business, 8*(1/2), 53–59.

Spohrer, J., & Maglio, P. P. (2008). The emergence of service science: Toward systematic service innovations to accelerate co-creation of value. *Production and Operations Management, 17*(3), 238–246. doi:10.3401/poms.1080.0027

Srinivasan, U., & Arunasalam, B. (2013). Leveraging big data analytics to reduce healthcare costs. *IT Professional, 15*(6), 21–28. doi:10.1109/MITP.2013.55

Stiglitz, J. E., Sen, A., & Fitoussi, J.-P. (2009). *Report by the Commission on the Measurement of Economic Performance and Social Progress*. Retrieved on January 25, 2015 from http://www.stiglitz-sen-fitoussi.fr/en/index.htm

Stroetmann, K. A., Jones, T., Dobrev, A., & Stroetmann, V. N. (2006). eHealth is Worth it. The Economic Benefits of Implemented eHealth Solutions at Ten European Sites. Luxembourg: Commission of the European Communities.

Taylor, R., Bower, A., Girosi, F., Bigelow, J., Fonkych, K., & Hillestad, R. (2005). Promoting Health Information Technology: Is there a case for more-aggressive government action? *Health Affairs, 24*(5), 1234–1345. doi:10.1377/hlthaff.24.5.1234 PMID:16162568

Thomas, D. R. E. (1978). Strategy is different in service businesses. *Harvard Business Review*, *56*(4), 158–165.

Tocci, R. (1988). *Digital System- Principles and Applications* (4th ed.). Englewood Cliffs, NJ: Prentice-Hall International.

Tulu, B., Chatterjee, S., & Laxminarayan, S. (2005). A taxonomy of telemedicine efforts with respect to applications, infrastructure, delivery tools, type of setting and purpose. In *Proceedings of the 38th Hawaii International Conference on System Sciences*. IEEE. doi:10.1109/HICSS.2005.56

Tulu, B., Chatterjee, S., & Maheshwari, M. (2007). Telemedicine taxonomy: A classification tool. *Telemedicine Journal and e-Health*, *13*(3), 349–358. doi:10.1089/tmj.2006.0055 PMID:17603838

Van Halteren, A., Bults, R., Wac, K., Konstantas, D., Widya, I., Dokovsky, N., & Herzog, R. et al. (2004). Mobile patient monitoring: The MobiHealth system. *The Journal on Information Technology in Healthcare*, *2*(5), 365–373.

Vincent, A., Cusack, C. M., Pan, E., Hook, J. M., Kaelber, D. C., & Middleton, B. (2007). A new taxonomy for telehealth technologies. In *AMIA Annual Symposium Proceedings*.

Whitmore, A., Agarwal, A., & Da Xu, L. (2014). The Internet of Things—A survey of topics and trends. *Information Systems Frontiers*, 1–14.

Whitten, P., & Love, B. (2005). Patient and provider satisfaction with the use of telemedicine: Overview and rationale for cautious enthusiasm. *Journal of Postgraduate Medicine*, *51*(4), 294–299. PMID:16388172

WHO – World Health Organisation. (2006a). eHealth Tools and Services. Needs of the Member States. Geneva, Switzerland: WHO.

WHO – World Health Organisation. (2006b). *Building Foundations for eHealth. Progress of Member States*. Geneva, Switzerland: WHO.

Zeithaml, V. A., & Bitner, M. J. (2000). *Service Marketing: Integrating Customer Focus across the Firm*. New York, NY: McGraw Hill.

Zhijiang, D., Zhiheng, J., & Minxiu, K. (2006). Virtual reality-based telesurgery via teleprogramming scheme combined with semi-autonomous control. *Proceedings of the 27th Annual International Conference*. Engineering in Medicine and Biology Society.

KEY TERMS AND DEFINITIONS

Big Data: A new generation of technologies and architectures, designed to economically extract value from very large volumes of a wide variety of data, by enabling the high velocity capture, discovery, and/or analysis (Ganz & Reinsel, 2011).

Digital Economy: The pervasive use of ICT in all aspects of the economy, including internal operations of organizations; transactions between organizations; and transactions between individuals and organizations (Atkinson & McKay, 2007).

E-Health: The use of emerging information and communications technology, especially the Internet, to improve or enable health and healthcare (Eng, 2001).

Electronic Health Records: A systematic collection in digital format of health information about an individual patient (Gunter & Terry, 2005).

E-Prescriptions: Computer-based electronic generation, transmission and filling of a medical prescription, and the electronic fit/sick notes, for sick leaves and insurance purposes.

Georeferencing: The act of assigning locations to pieces of information, objects or individuals.

Internet of Things: A paradigm where everyday objects can be equipped with identifying, sensing, networking and processing capabilities that allow them to communicate with one another and with other devices and services over the Internet to accomplish some objective (Whitmore et al. 2014).

M2M: Solutions that allow communication between devices of the same type and specific application, all via wired or wireless communication networks (Holler et al., 2014)

RFID (Radio Frequency Identification): A technology that uses electronic tags placed on objects, people, or animals to relay identifying information to an electronic reader by means of radio wave.

Wearable Technology: A category of technology devices that can be worn by a consumer and that incorporates computer and advanced electronic technologies.

Chapter 8
Semantic Interoperability-Enabled Architecture for Connected Health Services

Adel Taweel
King's College London, UK & Birzeit University, Palestine

ABSTRACT

With the increasing availability of connected health organisations, key medical information is expected to be accessible at the point of care. However, the high sensitivity of the clinical data and the large heterogeneity in health information systems pose a great interoperability challenge, including solutions that rely solely on the use of data exchange standards. Due to low adoption of these standards, such solutions will not sufficiently scale to achieve this objective. This chapter presents a service-based approach that utilises domain models combined with extensible problem models, enriched with domain terminology and knowledge services to enable autonomous data governance and semantic interoperability. The chapter addresses the resulting requirements, describes the proposed a solution and reports the results from the prototype of the approach.

DOI: 10.4018/978-1-4666-9870-3.ch008

INTRODUCTION

The increasing availability of connected health, demand on healthcare to be present at each point of care has become a normal expectation. To achieve, it requires health institutions to share medical data for both delivering and improving healthcare, and facilitating clinical research [Stead W. et al (2000), Garde, S. et al (2007), Taweel, A. et al (2006), Taweel, A. et al (2004)]. The need for integrated systems that can provide up-to-date information about patients and their healthcare is not only critical to the day-to-day running and delivery of health functions but also potentially means saving lives. It is increasingly expected that patient health information is available at the point of care irrespective of its location. This expectation is driven by rapid developments in information technology, alongside their increasing dominance at the heart of individual healthcare institutions, through the use of data-intensive electronic health records systems (EHRs) that drive the health care process. One of the primary visions of eHealth has been to achieve a technology supported, seamlessly integrated health service that ensures the delivery of the right information about the right individual to the right person at the right time (Stead et al., 2000; Taweel, et al., 2006). This vision, however, present many challenges, including:

- The heterogeneity of health systems and their data representations across health institutions, not just across the health domain as whole but even within individual clinical domains, e.g. secondary care, primary care etc.
- Delivery of complete clinical information at the point of care, potentially requires health information exchange across geographically distributed health centres, thus creating a massive scalability challenge that puts demands on networking and distributed system architectures.
- Legacy and proprietary systems and the lack of, or at best, slow pace adoption of standards make exchanging clinical data more difficult and hampers the chances of integrated healthcare. This puts demands on knowledge representation methodologies that must cope with the complexity of (heterogeneous) health information, whilst remaining easy to deploy and use by system providers.
- The requirements of patient privacy and confidentiality that require strict data governance policies. These policies vary across institutions to include a variation of access constraints that observe strict ethical rules to maintain patient confidentiality at all times. This requires secure yet configurable independent data sharing policies that reflect the needs of the participating organizations within the domain.

The large number of system providers and their business models and variations in ethical and regulations for accessing clinical information across health organisations implies an exponential explosion in the number and type of stakeholders that need to be involved in achieving the seamless interoperability required to achieve the above vision. To achieve the need is to enable interoperation between data centres not just at the system or data levels but also at the governance level. However, consider the complexity involved in reaching agreements on or enforcing conformance to interoperability standards at these different levels within a single enterprise let alone multiple enterprises or countries. Therefore, the approach taken here is motivated by the practical implications of not being able to completely rely on the use of common interoperability standards (Orguna, et al 2006; Naml, et al., 2009) to address this issue. Instead, this needs to be addressed at the granularity of the application, data and/or centre levels, in which an interoperability framework should overcome heterogeneity and adapt at run-time and dynamically interoperate with data providers. Heterogeneity between health information systems and data, however, takes several dimensions; the most challenging of which is the semantic one, which the approach proposed in this paper attempt to address.

In this chapter, we focus on health data sharing in the context of clinical research, in the context of health organisations that use electronic health records systems (EHRs) through which patient health data is managed and stored. The stores that hold patient health data are referred to in this chapter as data sources. We present an approach based on the use of domain ontologies (Musen, 1998) combined with rich terminology and knowledge driven *problem* models used at the heart of a service-based framework to enhance semantic interoperability in eHealth services. An example of an eHealth service is EHRs or data sources that in this service-based framework become (for example web or grid) services (thus referred to below as eHealth services or services). The chapter proposes the use of extensible problem models enriched with well-defined domain concepts that can be dynamically translated into individual data sources (or services). Data sources or services themselves are semantically described in terms of the domain ontology, which is dynamically discovered and bound to at run-time. A data governance ontology is also used to define data access constraints, that enable enacting the defined ethical rules and constraints on accessing the clinical data and maintaining patient confidentiality, thus enabling what is usually referred to as 'local ownership, local control'.

The following sections first outline service interoperability and heterogeneity challenges in eHealth systems, describing related semantic web and ontology-based approaches to addressing semantic interoperability. Then the chapter presents our approach to the auto-generation of rich domain concepts and problem models and their translation across the architecture to individual data sources. An outline of a prototype (IIA) is then presented as an implementation of the approach reflecting on our experiences using the prototype and identifying requirements and limitations.

CHALLENGES OF SERVICE INTEROPERABILITY AND COMPOSITION IN EHEALTH

The vision of eHealth as enabling flexible and dynamic connectivity and data integration shares many of the challenges that are being addressed in the arena of service-oriented architectures. However, the focus in eHealth is on the data itself and less on the functionality, but in principle these challenges are similar and include:

- Using common interoperability mechanisms to dynamically discover and integrate services from a potentially large number of disparate health data sources, in this case electronic health record systems located in health institutions.
- Separating the interoperability of service functionality from that of communication mechanisms, in this case the main element is the heterogeneity of the data that is being served through the services.
- Enabling dynamic run-time binding to services without prior detailed knowledge of how it will be used that can be computationally interpreted at run time.

We therefore propose a domain focussed interoperability representation that utilises service-oriented architecture technologies. In other words, to define the service-oriented interoperability mechanism based on the clinical data that constitutes the heart of the services. In a complex and closed domain, such as eHealth, where the purpose of function of services is defined, the interoperability mechanism is enabled through a domain-specific semantic representation or ontology that provides the required richness and accuracy. While services provide the uniform abstract interfaces for communication, their functional focus include specific definition of a semantic representation of the data and its access constraints that can be controlled and supported by the clinical data providers themselves. This does not just enable semantic-awareness in services but also propagates it through the architecture.

Basing the interoperability mechanism within services, using a domain-specific representation provides the required extensible richness and complexity needed in the domain, opposed to having one for all or incorporating it in the functional interface, thus over-complicating or limiting its extensibility respectively. Instead, this approach makes the architecture potentially re-usable across other domains that require such requirements. However, for the purposes of this paper, we will be focusing on interoperable semantic composition in the health domain. In particular, we aim to address service interoperability and the pressures placed on the service engineering process through the use of semantic representation in data-intensive services in complex, sensitive and closed domains, focusing on health. To do so, we propose that the service-oriented approach must be supplemented by a (run-time) computationally interpretable domain-based semantic representation, for both the data and its access constraints.

SEMANTIC SERVICE INTEGRATION

Several approaches have been proposed to enable dynamic composition of web services based on the semantic expression of their functionality (Ankolekar, et al 2002; Martin, et al 2007; Martin, et al 2004; Akkiraju, et al 2005). The more recent are the efforts from the semantic web community (Liu et al 2013; Garcia et al 2013; Martin, et al 2007; Martin, et al 2004) and W3C (Akkiraju, et al 2005). OWL-S is based on the earlier work on DAML-S, which uses ontologies to define the requirements and capabilities of web services that can be reasoned about at run-time to dynamically discover appropriate services and bind to them. WSDL-S proposes an extension to the widely used WSDL standard to enable semantic expressivity. It defines a mechanism to associate semantic annotations with web services that are described using WSDL. WSDL-S assumes that service semantics are described in formal models, referred to as *semantic models*, which have link annotations into WSDL documents. However, both OWL-S and WSDL-S are bound to WSDL and only include semantic information that describes the service specific elements, such as the definition of preconditions, inputs, outputs and operations. More recent approaches on semantic models have improved on enriching representation of web services functional descriptions to include non-functional features (Lin J. et al 2013; Liu et al 2013; Garcia et al 2013). These are aimed to enable service discovery, composition and binding on some of its key quality of service attributes. Although address some of the key aspects of quality, they remain limited on direct applicability and not meaningful to some domains. These definitions remain oriented towards function-intensive services and lack the needed richness in expressivity for data-intensive services, especially in complex domains, where the focus is on defining or representing the data itself. The key need is to assess the meaningfulness use of the data itself for the “use purpose”. This will require including semantic description not just of the service, but also the data it serves, in terms of purpose, meaning and context.

Further, because these approaches' focus has been on creating autonomous, self-describing web services that exist independently in the market place, more suited to application-oriented or function intensive web services that provide concrete services to other consumers. However, for data-intensive web services that cover specific domain needs, these approaches can be expensive and less suitable. For data-intensive web services, the main effort in creating semantic interoperability between them will be focused on, describing the heterogeneity, access policies etc. of the underlying data itself in computer-interpretable formats, rather than the functions of the web services themselves. Within well-defined and potentially closed and sensitive domains, such as health, the actual importance and the value is associated with the data itself and the mechanisms of its access. But also these required semantic descriptions are often more comprehensible and compatible within the domain and thus the need is to find a domain-dependent mechanism to facilitate their interoperability and management.

SEMANTIC INTEROPERABILITY AND ONTOLOGIES

Healthcare systems are typical information systems. Due to the large and complex nature of the Health Service (the word Service here refers to the overall provided health and medical services to the patient, thus HS will be used to remove confusion) in various countries and the ways they are provided, a typical health organization can have several different information systems, ranging from diagnostic medical devices to electronic health record systems (EHRs), the focus of this paper. EHRs hold patient health record information and support the delivery of day-to-day care in hospitals in speciality clinics and primary care clinics.

The concern for the project upon which this paper is based (ePCRN: electronic Primary Care Research Network) was to leverage the use of EHRs, from primary care clinics, to support clinical research. Due to various historic reasons, such clinics use many different EHR systems with varying degrees of complexity. This heterogeneity has resulted in significant differences across EHRs in terms of their data representations, let alone communication and interoperability between them.

This heterogeneity (and/or interoperability) occurs in several ways (Sheth, 1998; Jakobovits, 1997; El-Khatib, et al 2002):

- **System:** e.g. numerous heterogeneous hardware platforms and operating systems;
- **Syntactic:** e.g. different data formats or query languages; differences in systems programmable interfaces or the way data is accessed; differences in transaction mechanisms.

- **Structural:** e.g. different model representations, composite structures of attributes.
- **Semantic:** Differences in the meaning of the terms used, different terms used for the same concept and differences in the context in which the data has been captured.
- **Chronology:** Differences in the representation of attributes and the way values may change over time.
- **Security:** Differences in data access controls and data governance policies.

Various methods have been suggested to resolve system and syntactic interoperability problems, which are often easier to resolve (Sheth, 1998; Jakobovits, 1997). However, achieving Structural and Semantic interoperability, for example, in information interrogation or interchange between information systems continues to be a difficult problem. In order to achieve semantic interoperability in a heterogeneous environment, the meaning of the information that is interrogated (or communicated) has to have the same semantics or meaning across the systems. In clinical systems, the complexity is in the ways that different systems represent their medical information. For example, references to clinical procedures, problems or diagnosis and they way each system records or code each concept. Equally, different systems use different codings to refer to or represent their data, such as SNOMED-CT, Read Codes, ICD9 etc.

Therefore the requirements for the clinical research domain and linkage to EHRs require the following capabilities:

- Provide a coherent view of the data from different autonomous heterogeneous systems or data sources.
- Access data securely.
- Enable independent and different data access and sharing policies.
- Maintain data and patient privacy at all times, observing strict ethical rules.
- Enable data source or system changes independently.
- Enable transparent or seamless integration or interrogation of data sources.

These capabilities require a flexible framework that enables dynamic binding or access-on-demand to the data sources or systems through an interoperable integration framework. The need is not only to enable configurable yet rich semantic descriptions of these systems, but also the underlying data that they serve. Such descriptions are not currently supported in current web services standards or approaches.

Ontologies can be used to describe the semantics of health systems or resources and make the content explicit, and thus can be used to discover semantic equivalence between information concepts. The use of shared or standard ontologies as a possible solution to the semantic interoperability problem has been studied for over a decade. They have also been found to provide reasonable results for semantic interoperability (Wache, et al 2001; Cruz, et al 2009; Wu, et al 2009). Several approaches have emerged recently to address the semantic heterogeneity in the ehealth domain (Martin, 2011; Ethier, et al 2013; Bache, et al 2013). These can be seen to fall into two general approaches: ETL (extract-transform-load) based or mediation solutions (Lee, et al 2013; Issarny, 2013). The former use the concept of extracting the data from data sources and transform them into a homogenous format into often a centralised repository. However, this approach is obviously not useful for situations where live feed or connection to health institutions is required. The mediation approach overcomes this limitation by using domain ontologies to enable data translation at run-time. This approach is similar to the approach proposed here, however, some of these approaches assume the use of standard representation of data in sources to maintain consistent meaning of data across different sources. Others assume the creation a comprehensive ontology for data representation and mapping which can be an expensive effort not easily possibly by all sources. This creates a limitation on the scalability of such solutions. The second issue that web semantic approaches may encounter is the need to provide users with a freedom of choice in terms of how they structure their concepts or semantics and their preferred representation language. This is may be essential or at least difficult to enforce for the wide use of web services in the market place. This, however, will in turn lead to what is often referred to as the ontology heterogeneity problem (Visser, et al 1997; Farooq, et al 2010). Several recent approaches have been proposed to address this issue (Kandpal, et al 2014; Shvaikko, 2013), however these approaches are focusing on addressing the discovery of mismatches between ontologies, less on actually resolving mismatches or creating converged ontologies from sources. This may make it difficult to achieve semantic interoperability as intended. However, given the closed domain need, this can be avoided by standardizing the ontology that can be used to describe data as well as the service. Equally, this domain ontology needs to be clear enough and to employ an agreed format to be used by data providers to describe their data in a meaningful way. To resolve this issue, in our approach we built our ontology based on the CCR (a variation of the widely adopted HL7) standard to represent the core medical domain concepts for primary care, thus maintaining consistency of interpretation of concepts, values, units and their context between different sources.

OUR APPROACH

The HSs in many countries are often made up of independent organizations and institutions providing health care services to its patients or customers, forming often isolated yet loosely interconnected organizations within the enterprise – Health Service (HS). Across the domain, they have their own rich and complex data representations, terminologies, acronyms that are represented in real terms by the health systems that support these organizations. While services provide a potential solution to enable interoperability between the organizations and their systems, the focus needs to be on sufficiently describing the data, and to a lesser extent the systems themselves, opposed to the functional services that enable access to them.

This is the approach taken in the ePCRN project. The proposed services composition architecture includes a rich semantically annotated representation of the 'problem' or the 'user data requirement' model and an enactment broker that interoperates with health systems using information from a meta registry that holds the domain ontology and mapping to health systems. As illustrated in ***Figure 1***, the architecture, referred to as IIA (Interoperable Integration Architecture), includes five main semantic elements to achieve this objective: 'Problem' models referred to as *Extensible Query Abstraction Model* (EQAM); terminology and knowledge services that provide rich domain terminologies, referred to as *Knowledge Services*; domain and data governance ontologies referred to as *Extensible Domain Data Abstraction Ontology* (EDAO) and *Extensible Data Governance Abstraction Ontology* (EDGAO) and mapping between them; and a *Meta Registry* that holds rich metadata descriptions of services (i.e. physical resources or health systems). The general approach is to capture the 'problem' in a semantically annotated extensible model, which can be passed across the infrastructure and translated to or by individual services or EHRs using the domain and mapping ontology while respecting individual data governance policies, thus creating a semantically-aware architecture. The function of each of these elements is described below in more details.

The *EQAM* is a model representation that allows end users to capture their data needs in simple or reasonably complex logical constructs based on vocabulary controlled clinical concepts enriched by the terminology knowledge resources. Each EQAM instance represents a semantically annotated set of logically combined clinical concepts that can be translated into other more specific formats. We refer to this as the problem model, in which users specify their specific data requirements or characteristics. For example, for clinical trials, this model can represent the eligibility criteria of a trial; for clinical care, it can represent the combination of data elements that need to be retrieved. An example of an eligible criteria model to support clinical trials in primary care is illustrated in Figure 2.

The use of the *domain ontology* stems from the growing recognition of the importance of semantic differences in application areas and the use of models to represent them and the value of making these models more explicit, configurable and maintainable (Musen, 1998; Cruz, et al 2009; Farooq, et al 2010). These models are referred to as *domain models*. For EHRs, the domain model is one of patients,

Figure 1. Overall Architecture of IIA

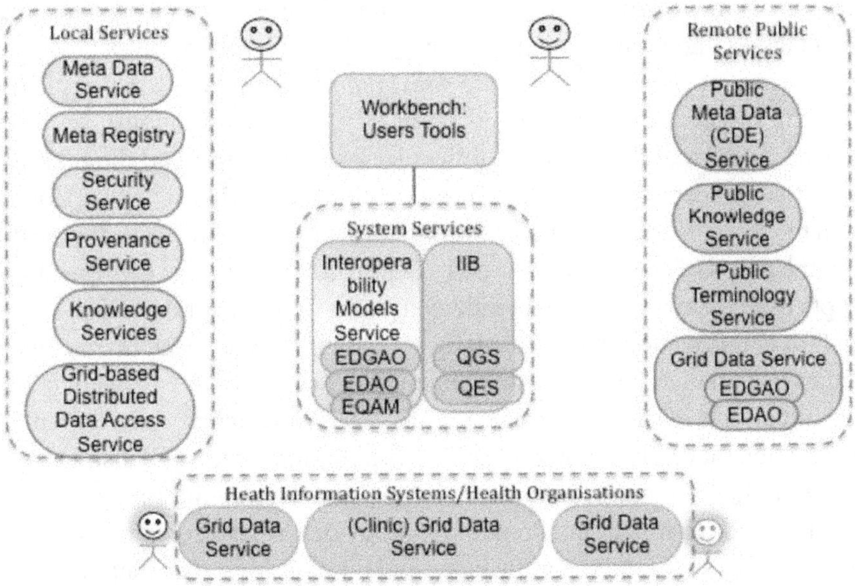

Figure 2. EQAM - an example of a generic eligibility criteria model

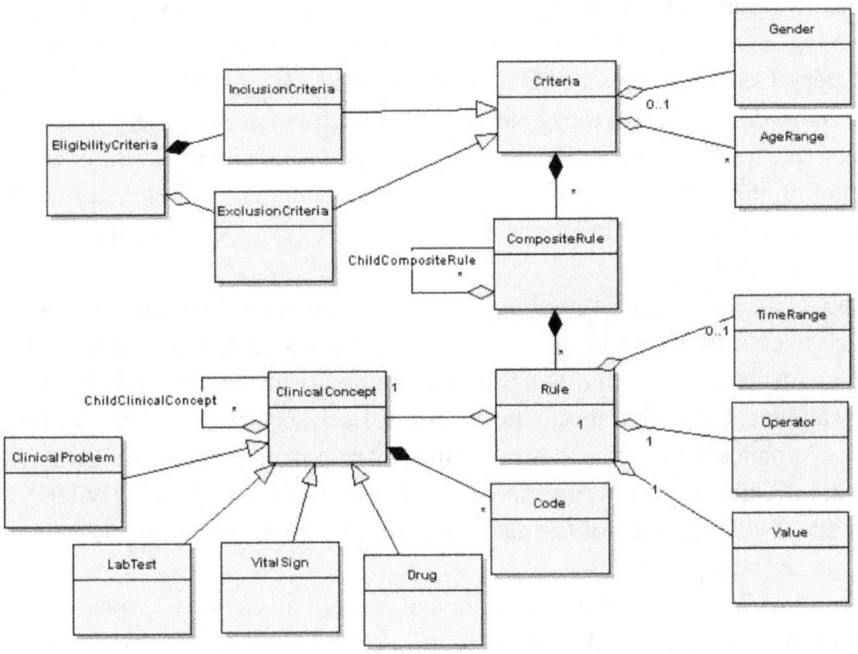

of their medical problems and the interventions that health practitioners may make in the management of patients. However, domain models represent instances of domain classes and their relationships, which if used by themselves create system dependencies. However, the *domain (data) ontology* provides a representation of the domain respective main concepts, their attributes and relationships. They can be viewed as 'formal descriptions of the classes of concepts and the relationships among those concepts that describe an application area' (Musen, 1998), from which domain models can be generated. In the proposed approach, the focus for the domain was on the needs of the primary care as a health domain, but the expressed medical concepts can be expanded or generalized to other domains. It describes the data in a standard classification, based on HL7 or CCR, specifying each main concept, its attributes and relationships. The domain ontology concepts are mapped to the local health system service data using a mapping ontology, which is a configurable XML representation that can be edited by the users as systems evolve. It also includes the used terminology for each class, their versions and the way they are used in coding their values. For example, the domain ontology describes Problems, Medications, Tests, Procedures etc. and their attributes and relationships. The mapping ontology describes the corresponding concepts or attributes in the local health system. The attributes that correspond to each class may come from different locations, or tables in the local health system. Each class may be described by a different terminology, medical vocabulary or coding system, such as SNOMED-CT, Read Codes etc. This ontology is used by the IIB (Interoperable Integration Broker) services, in this case the Query Generator Service (QGS), to translate the EQAM into one or several queries that correspond to the respective local health system to query or retrieve the respective data. The Query Enactor Service (QES) is responsible for enacting and assembling the output. In our recent work, an example of this domain model has been developed and used in another recent project to expand to include genetic data (Ethier, et al 2013).

The *Data Governance ontology* describes the rules that the service should enforce to control access to the data in the health systems. This enables a flexible mechanism that allows individual health institutions to specify their data governance policy and the way their data can be accessed. Each service includes a configurable data governance policy that can be changed or updated by the data owner. These rules are defined as policy rules in terms of roles and their access privileges. They allow specifying the type of the data, or specific data elements and associate them with the selected privileges.

The *Meta Registry* combines the knowledge about services (i.e. physical resources or health systems and their descriptions), the domain ontology capturing the relevant domain concepts (focusing on primary care) and the mappings between the two. It also holds the services' corresponding data governance policies. It acts as a central (domain) description service that holds functional descriptions of the data services themselves, and descriptions of the underlying health data that they provide access to, alongside a description of the access mechanism or rules that governs access to the data. The Meta Registry is updated by two mechanisms: self-registration of services and on-request update of service descriptions. The *self-registration* occurs when a new service is deployed at an organization and the service registers itself with the meta-registry, declaring its intention to participate in the architecture, describing its physical resources, data and data access rules. For services already in the network, the registry can request updates of the service descriptions. Each data service also holds a copy of its data description and its access rules to enable local configuration of changes in the system.

Knowledge Services provide access to custom-built or publicly available domain support ontologies or terminologies. In the IIA, these represent the available clinical terminologies and vocabularies, some of which are tailored to the primary care domain. These resources are facilitated by intuitive interfaces that enable users to search and find relevant clinical concepts. These interfaces are linked to the EQAM to enable vocabulary controlled capture of a semantically annotated 'problem model' or ' user data needs'. Figure 3 illustrates an interface to capture the eligibility criteria EQAM. Terminology and knowledge resources are key to the capture of individual user needs in a computer-interpretable format and their translation to individual health systems. For our approach to scale, several knowledge services are used, including the Enterprise Vocabulary Service (NCI 2014) inclusive of the UMLS MetaThesaurus, and a local Vocabulary Service inclusive of UK Read Codes and some specific EHRs' codes. These services have been brought together by a common service and interface to enable as rich as possible definitions of clinical concepts. The definition of concepts includes annotating each requested concept in as many as possible available terminologies, creating rich multi-mappings. These mappings are then stored in the EQAM at the point of definition for each instance. The QGS service uses these mappings and domain data ontology mappings to create a tailored data request or query format specific to the designed health system. The richer the knowledge services, the richer and often more accurate is the outcome, and the greater is the number of health systems that can be supported in the network. In the few cases that we came across where the health systems uses own-custom terminologies, for specific part of its data, that are not supported or provided by the knowledge services, the outcome of the queried or retrieved data or its quality end up being limited to the supported data.

Figure 3. EQAM Capture Interface

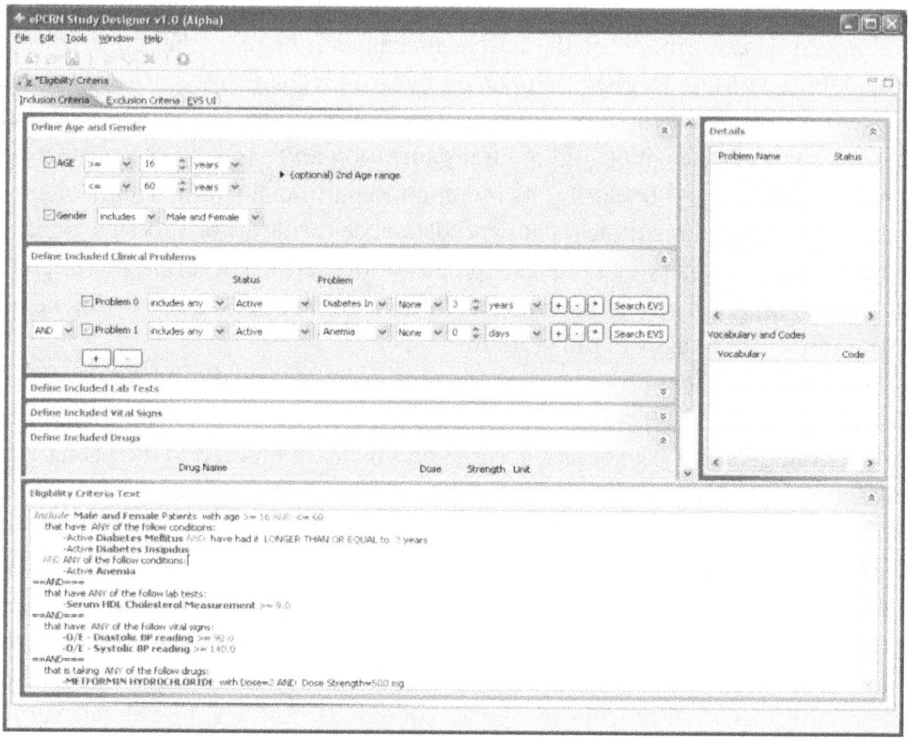

DYNAMIC GENERATION OF SEMANTIC INTEROPERABLE DOMAIN CONCEPTS AND DEFINITIONS

To enable semantic translations between services (or data sources) and the defined problem models, a mechanism for bridging between the two is needed. This bridging mechanism includes translations at two levels: at the problem models level, definition annotated by the knowledge services' terminologies, and at the services' levels translated through the Query Generation Service. Figure 4 illustrates the process of the problem model definitions through bridging between models and the services.

The Domain Concept Mapping (DCM) service works across different ontologies (or concept definitions returned from each knowledge service) and aims to dynamically produce the richest possible definition for each requested domain concept. Each clinical concept definition returned from each knowledge service is analysed for a possible mapping route from the returned definition. If a mapping route is found, as illustrated in *Figure 5* the respective knowledge services that contain extra mappings or definitions are accessed and the returned data is added to the problem model, i.e. EQAM. These additional mappings are annotated separately for the user and the QG Service exclusion if needed.

Figure 4. Dynamic Generation of semantically interoperable defined domain conceptsh

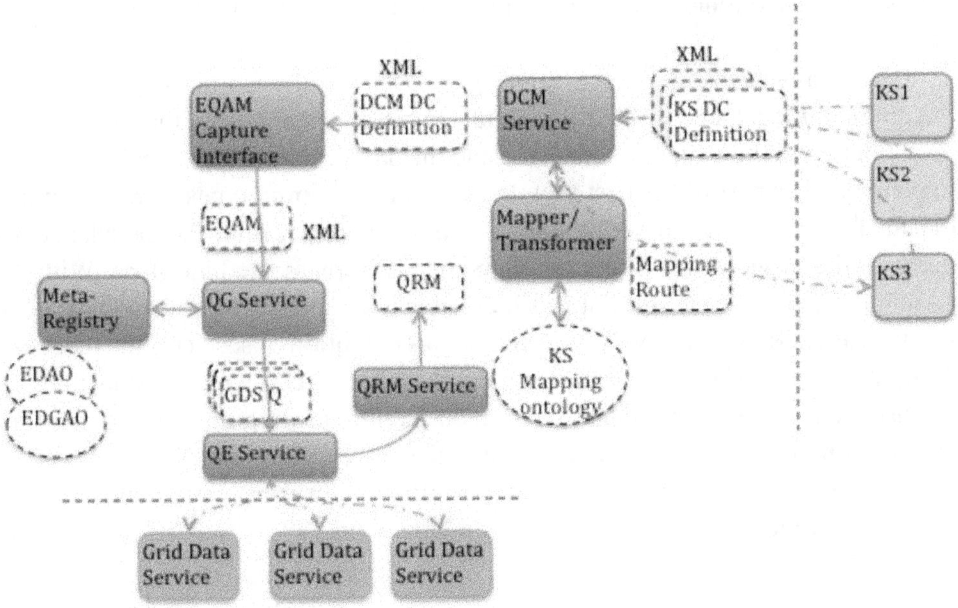

Figure 5. Route Mapping (Example)

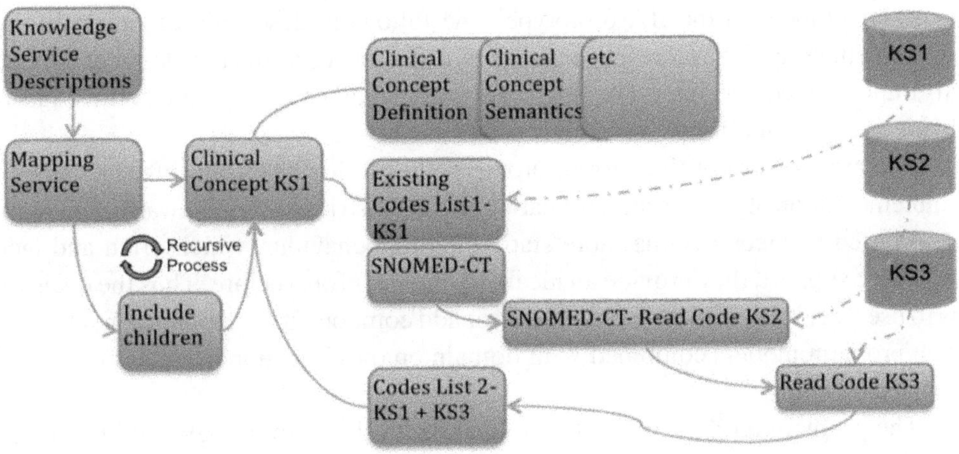

The QG service performs the second bridging or translation function between the captured EQAM instances and the data services using service metadata, domain and data governance ontologies of the respective services from the meta-registry.

The exact format of the QG service output depends on several factors, including the data schema representation, terminologies used, data storage mechanism and the data service functional interface definition, defined by the QRM (Query Result Model) service.

This approach maintains the semantic-awareness of each domain concept in the problem model across the different layers of the system, from the top end user level through to the system middleware and the data services. This mechanism was implemented as part of the first prototype. In the early prototypes, it was assumed that data services would have the same functional interface, thus the metadata definition of the services was limited in scope by the implemented interface. With the addition of more data sources, it was inevitable that data services would change in versions as EHR systems evolve. To enable this evolution of services, the metadata definition model of the services was redeveloped to become more extensible. As a consequence, this enabled the used transformation or bridging mechanism to interface with different types of data services that have different functional interface or data representations, thus potentially enabling the broker to communicate with other data services from different compatible networks.

THE IIA PROTOTYPE

This section describes our experiences of implementing the above approach and experimenting with the IIA prototype. The following description focuses on the implementation of the relevant components and services of IIA and does not include all implemented services. The described prototype has been implemented and is being used in ten clinical research centres.

The architecture of the current prototype has followed, at its core, the general implementation of grid-based applications for the distributed middleware. Although, grid-based services assume more static binding behaviour, which often and lack semantic support, they provide an ideal distributed infrastructure. Thus the decision is to use a grid infrastructure but modify or add components to employ semantically rich problem models combined with domain ontologies, supported by knowledge services.

The problem models, EQAM, combined with the terminology and knowledge services are the backbone of this approach to enable the semantic interoperability in the current prototype. They enabled semantic-awareness through the architecture to individual data sources. However, the richness of the semantic-awareness in the architecture depends, to a great extend, on the richness of the terminologies and knowledge services. While there always will potentially be limitations of the richness of terminologies and their mappings, the key is to enable observing and recognising it in the respective data services. There needs to exist a feedback mechanism to recognise and quantify semantic shortcomings where they exist. Given the legacy nature of electronic health records, it would be difficult to assume completeness in the knowledge services that include all terminologies. However, the key is that this approach enables extensibility, allowing the addition of terminologies while maintaining the integrity of the results of problem model instances, which is critical in the clinical domain.

We found only very minimal changes needed to the domain and data governance ontologies across services deployed at the different clinical centres. While the prototype was implemented only in three different clinical centres, they represented a reasonable sample of the primary care domain in the UK. However, it can be a time consuming task to create domain ontologies for a given domain, this was noted for the first prototype given the lack of knowledge of the interdisciplinary collaboration and evaluation of potential contributing standards. However, this can be improved once these steps are overcome especially for other domains. The mapping between the domain ontology and data sources is a straightforward mechanism and easily configurable.

The data governance ontology was expressed in terms of roles and privileges of access. Roles and Privileges are expressed in relation to the domain ontology concepts opposed to the individual instances of data elements. This enabled dynamically enacting roles in accordance with service data governance policies and allowed extensibility not only in defining new roles but also variations in same roles across services with no physical co-relation to or dependency on individual instances or changes of mappings.

The meta-registry was implemented using a modified version of the jUDDI version 3.0. It was extended to allow storing semantic meta-data about individual data services beyond the simple service registration data that supports. The meta-data included, in addition to WSDL-type information, descriptions of the content, used codings, available clinical data types in relation to the domain ontology, data changes and service support information. It also included annotations of individual domain ontology mappings and data governance constraints. These are used by the IIA to enable dynamic discovery of and binding to individual data services. Although, it may appear that the current prototype relies on the assumption that meta-data is kept up-to-date for successful dynamic binding, our experiments have shown little change tendency in the core semantic elements that may affect the system. In fact, in one case, it was a substantial change in the underlying EHR system itself for which the data service needed to be re-configured, including the mapping ontologies. However, to be exhaustive more experiments are needed to examine the extent of change on its semantic-awareness extensibility.

CONCLUSION

This chapter presented the interoperability challenges in eHealth systems and argued that they face similar challenges to those in service-oriented architecture except with focus on data-intensive needs. We assert that using semantic interoperability standards is not sufficiently scalable approach for complex data-intensive closed domains such as eHealth, and that a domain-based semantic driven approach is a more suitable adaptive solution.

The chapter outlined an approach to dynamic semantic interoperability based on extensible semantically enriched problem models and domain ontologies. It described briefly the relevant implementation of the approach as part of the IIA prototype and presented some initial results reflecting on its advantages, potential requirements and limitations.

ACKNOWLEDGMENT

This work has been funded in part by the NIHR. We would like to thanks all members of the ePCRN project for their input and valuable contributions to the ePCRN development of this paper.

REFERENCES

Akkiraju, R., Farrell, J., & Miller, J. (2005). *Web Service Semantics-WSDL-S*. Technical Note, Version 1.0, April, 2005. Available at: http://lsdis.cs.uga.edu/library/download/WSDL-S-V1.html

Ankolekar, A., Burstein, M., Hobbs, J. R., Lassila, O., Martin, D., McDermott, D., ... Sycara, K. (2002, June), *DAML-S: Web service description for the semantic web*. International Semantic Web Conference, Italia. doi:10.1007/3-540-48005-6_27

Bache, R., Miles, S, & Taweel, A. (2013). An adaptable architecture for patient cohort identification from diverse data sources. *J Am Med Inform Assoc, 20*(e2).

Cruz, I. F., & Xiao, H. (2009). Ontology Driven Data Integration in Heterogeneous Networks. *Complex Systems in Knowledge-based Environments: Theory, Models, and Applications, 168*, 75–98.

El-Khatib, H. T., Williams, M. H., MacKinnon, L. M., & Marwick, D. H. (2002). Using a Distributed Approach to Retrieve and Integrate Information from Heterogeneous Distributed Databases. *The Computer Journal*, *45*(4), 381–394. doi:10.1093/comjnl/45.4.381

Ethier, J. F., Dameron, O., Curcin, V., McGilchrist, M., Verheij, R. A., Arvanitis, T. A., & Burgun, A. et al. (2013). A unified structural/terminological interoperability framework based on LexEVS: Application to TRANSFoRm. *Journal of the American Medical Informatics Association*, *20*(5), 986–994. doi:10.1136/amiajnl-2012-001312 PMID:23571850

Farooq, A., & Shah, A. (2010). Similarity Identification and Measurement between Ontologies. *Journal of American Science*, *6*(4), 67–85.

García, J. M., Junghans, M., Agarwal, S., & Ruiz-Cortés, A. (2013). Integrating semantic Web services ranking mechanisms using a common preference model. *Knowledge-Based Systems*, *49*, 22–36. doi:10.1016/j.knosys.2013.04.007

Garde, S., Knaup, P., Hovenga, E., & Heard, S. (2007, December). Towards Semantic Interoperability for Electronic Health Records: Domain Knowledge Governance for *open*EHR Archetypes. *International Journal of Medical Informatics*, *76*(Supplement 3), S334–S341. doi:10.1016/j.ijmedinf.2007.02.004 PMID:17392019

Issarny, V., & Bennaceur, A. (2013). Composing Distributed Systems: Overcoming the Interoperability Challenge. *Lecture Notes in Computer Science*, *7866*, 168–196. doi:10.1007/978-3-642-40615-7_6

Jakobovits, R. (1997). Integrating Autonomous Heterogeneous Information Sources. *Principles for Digital Library Development Communications of the ACM*, *44*(5), 49–54.

Kandpal, A., Goudar, R. H., Chauhan, R., Garg, S., & Joshi, K. (2014). Effective Ontology Alignment: An Approach for Resolving the Ontology Heterogeneity Problem for Semantic Information Retrieval. *Advances in Intelligent Systems and Computing*, *243*, 1077–1087. doi:10.1007/978-81-322-1665-0_110

Lee, W., Lee, M., Choi, Y., Choi, D., Cho, M., Song, S., . . . Yoon, H. (2013). ETL-based interoperable data management system. In Multimedia Tools and Applications. Springer.

Lin, J., Zou, J., & Yao, G. (2013). Application Discovery of Semantic Web Service Based on Qos Ontology. *Information Technology Journal*, *12*(20), 5501–5504. doi:10.3923/itj.2013.5501.5504

Liu, C. H., Chen, S. L., & Huang, T. Y. (2013). Data flow analysis and testing for OWL-S semantic web service compositions. *International Journal on Computer Science and Engineering*, *8*(4), 349–360. doi:10.1504/IJCSE.2013.057299

Martin, D., Burstein, M., & Hobbs, J. R. (2004). *Website.* Available at http://www.w3.org/Submission/OWL-S/

Martin, D., Burstein, M., McDermott, D., McIlraith, S., Paolucci, M., Sycara, K, McGuinness, D., Sirin, E. & Srinivasan, N. (2007), Bringing Semantics to Web Services with OWL-S. *Journal of World Wide Web, 10*(3).

Martin, L., Anguita, A., & Graf, N. (2011). ACGT: Advancing clinico-genomic trials on cancer—four years of experience. *Studies in Health Technology and Informatics*, *169*, 734–738. PMID:21893844

Musen, M. A. (1998). Domain ontologies in software engineering: Use of Protégé with the EON architecture. *Methods of Information in Medicine*, (37): 540–550. PMID:9865052

Naml, T., Aluc, G., & Dogac, A. (2009). An Interoperability Test Framework for HL7-Based Systems. *IEEE Transactions on Information Technology in Biomedicine*, *13*(3), 389–399. doi:10.1109/TITB.2009.2016086 PMID:19304492

NCI. (2014). Available at https://wiki.nci.nih.gov/display/LexEVS/LexEVS+6.0

Orguna, B., & Vub, J. (2006). HL7 ontology and mobile agents for interoperability in heterogeneous medical information systems. *Computers in Biology and Medicine*, *36*(7–8), 817–836. doi:10.1016/j.compbiomed.2005.04.010 PMID:16139263

Sheth, A. P. (1998). Changing Focus on Interoperability in Information Systems: From System, Syntax, Structure to Semantics. In M. F. Goodchild, M. J. Egenhofer, R. Fegeas, & C. A. Kottman (Eds.), *Interoperating Geographic Information Systems*. Kluwer.

Shvaiko, P., & Euzenat, J. (2013). Ontology Matching: State of the Art and Future Challenges. *IEEE Transactions on Knowledge and Data Engineering*, *25*(1), 158–176. doi:10.1109/TKDE.2011.253

Stead W., Miller R., Musen M. & Hersh, W. (2000), Integration and Beyond: Linking Information from Disparate Sources and into Workflow. *AMIA*, (7), 135-145.

Taweel, A., Rector, A., et al. (2006). Grid-based Collaborative Secure Distributed Biomedical Research System. *The Universal Computer Science Journal, 12*(1), 80-98.

Taweel, A., Rector, A., Kalra, D., Rogers, J., et al. (2004). Joining up Healthcare with Clinical and Post-Genomic Research. In *Proceedings of Health Computing 2004*.

Visser, P. R. S., Jones, D. M., Bench-Capon, T. J. M., & Shave, M. J. R. (1997, March). *An analysis of ontology mismatches; heterogeneity versus interoperability*. AAAI 1997 Spring Symposium on Ontology Engineering, Stanford, CA.

Wache, H., Wache, T., Vögele, U., Visser, H., Stuckenschmidt, G., Schuster, N. H., & Hübner, S. (2001), Ontology-based Integration of Information - A Survey of Existing Approaches. In *Proceedings of IJCAI-01 Workshop: Ontologies and Information Sharing*.

Wu, M., Wang, Z., Zhang, A., & Yang, H. (2009). Ontology-driven Heterogeneous Geographic Data Set Integration. In *Proceedings of the 2009 WRI Global Congress on Intelligent Systems*. doi:10.1109/GCIS.2009.347

Chapter 9
SOA Governance in Healthcare:
Beyond Early Ideas to a Structured Framework

Konstantinos Koumaditis
University of Piraeus, Greece, & Aarhus University, Denmark

Marinos Themistocleous
University of Piraeus, Greece & University of Coimbra, Portugal

ABSTRACT

This chapter depicts the gradual development of a conceptual SOA Governance Framework tailored for healthcare organisations. The proposed framework presented herein is based on the authors' previous research and includes nine SOA Governance elements that need to be considered during the SOA process. The identification and conceptualisation of the elements were grounded in the normative literature and further developed to include healthcare specific aspects. This comes as a method to overcome the limitations identified in normative literature and enhance the elements' conceptualisation. Besides, the authors propose a unique design combining nine elements of SOA Governance with SOA Critical Success Factors (CSFs) and Healthcare Information Systems (HIS) challenges. This proposal aims to pinpoint attributes and guidelines for each element, required to successfully govern SOA and tackle longstanding HIS challenges. The framework is intended to be used as a decision supporting tool for SOA Governance in a healthcare setting.

DOI: 10.4018/978-1-4666-9870-3.ch009

INTRODUCTION

Economic conditions demand that Healthcare Information Technologies (HIS) deliver ever more business value. Today, HIS play a more and more important role in the provision of healthcare. The scope and complexity of HIS projects has increased, requiring excellent project management to fully realize the benefits of such an investment. Unfortunately, healthcare projects are associated with considerable failure rates or having significant cost or budget overruns (Kaplan & Harris-Salamone, 2009). Both research and anecdotal evidence suggests that many HIS projects struggle to meet functionality and quality targets. Research has identified multiple reasons for these challenges in HIS projects, such as: project escalation, poor risk management, failure to manage user expectations, poor software development or project management processes, or inability to learn from past mistakes and successes (Dwivedi et al., 2013; Lunt et al., 2011). Yet, integrated technologies that have been employed by healthcare organisations, to tackle these challenges, have not shown great levels of adoption due to their barriers, like: (a) high costs, (b) resistance to change, (c) organisational issues, (d) high complexity, (e) large scale of change, (f) time consuming implementation and (g) politics.

Consequently, the necessity for integrated HIS in a safer, interoperable and more manageable environment motivated organizations to consider the adoption of paradigms, such as SOA. SOA can be beneficial for a healthcare organisation as it provides interoperability and integration of the legacy HIS, attributes need in modern healthcare organisations.

Nevertheless, despite SOA benefits Heffner (2009) indicates that, 41% of SOA users in the Global 2000 firms believe that: (a) SOA has delivered less benefit than expected, (b) 17% claim they face problems and (c) will not expand SOA use. This reveals that even though SOA is considered a valuable architectural paradigm its application, efficiency and performance are affected by various factors. These statistics indicate that almost half the companies that implement SOA have not figured out how to benefit from their projects. This is attributed to unclear or weak governance planning (Stephens, 2008). In a recent research on the global status of IT governance standards and models (like COBIT, ITIL/ISO20000 etc.) the findings reveal a tendency to adopt such frameworks, but also a lack of a clear "winner" amongst them. For example, amongst 834 business executives, from 21 countries and 10 industries reveal that ISO20000 or ITIL is referred in 28% of them, while COBIT in 12% (ITGI., 2011). Yet, out of the 839 respondents only 10% have been healthcare executives, thus the percentages drop lower regarding their focus on IT governance in healthcare.

In an attempt to study this issue, we focused on SOA CSFs in healthcare, like: (a) alignment of SOA, organization, human and legal aspects, (b) clear goals set from the beginning of the endeavour, (c) complexity introduced to the system, (d) cost, funding and sponsoring the SOA project, (e) SOA culture that can create support and communication between the stakeholders, (f) experience, skills and training of the employees, (g) governance plan to provide compliance and check services concerning capability, security and strategic business alignment, (h) long-term planning to include reusable services that fit future business, (i) adequate measurement of the compliance and performance, (j) maturity identification and progress of the organization in aspects as IT, organization etc., (k) identification of the right candidate projects/pilots, (l) security risks (data confidentiality, access control), (m) detailed roadmap, (n) adequate standards (e.g. XML, WSDl, REST, HL7 etc.), (o) a team with understanding and experience in change management and clear vision of SOA, and (p) testing of the services and impact (Koumaditis, Themistocleous, Mantzana, & Souliotis, 2012).

The outcome of the review, demonstrates that the most frequently reported CSF in the cases reviewed is SOA Governance. In a nutshell, they report that SOA implementations require governance mechanisms to excel, otherwise the architecture will end up complex, uncontrolled, brittle and eventually discarded (Marks, 2008). A failure in a healthcare organisation's IT infrastructure is not an option as the literature is full of cases where healthcare IT failures cost patients' lives (Fitzgerald & Russo, 2005; Johnson, 2011; Kaplan & Harris-Salamone, 2009). This motivates us to study SOA Governance in healthcare.

SOA Governance is a research area with many issues (e.g. scope, model, associations) uncharted. In an attempt to fill this literature void, in a previous publication we introduced a set of SOA Governance issues that we were asked to revisit and provide a more structured and detailed approach in this publication (Koumaditis, Themistocleous, & Morabito, 2013). In doing so, resulting in the development of a framework that can be used to support decision-making on SOA Governance issues.

The remaining of the chapter is structured as follows Section 2 presents the HIS need for integration, Section 3 the SOA Governance literature review, Section 4 the SOA Governance Framework in healthcare, Section 5 the research methodology, Section 6 the discussion and Section 7 conclusions and future research agenda.

HEALTHCARE INFORMATION SYSTEMS: NEED FOR INTEGRATION

Healthcare delivery is a complex practice which uses different devices and machines for performing tests, monitoring patients and completing tasks, spread across many organisations, surgery rooms, patients' wards, and medical labs. All these devices need specific vendor based interfaces to communicate with computers. These interfaces are implemented based on specific protocols and much often there is a lack of integration amongst them or an increased cost to integrate them (Rhoads, Cooper, Fuchs, Schluter, & Zambuto, 2010).

Independent initiatives like: (a) Integrating the Healthcare Enterprise (IHE) and (b) Meaningful Use provide standards (e.g. HL7, DICOM, etc.) and guidelines (e.g. EHR) to enhance the interoperability and information sharing among healthcare organisations (HealthIT, 2014; IHE, 2012). An enabler of these standards is the SOA paradigm. An example of this is the recognized Healthcare Services Specification Program (HSSP) program, which is a collaborative effort between standards groups HL7 and OMG to address interoperability challenges within the healthcare sector, operating on SOA (HSSP, 2013). Additionally, HSSP's working groups emphasise on the need of an effective SOA Governance model, which they portray as a critical dimension to SOA implementations, as it becomes the guidance, the oversight, the enforcement, and ultimately the compliance mechanism needed for SOA (HL7/OMG, 2010).

Additionally, HIS integration has been associated with various aspects, amongst others: strategic, social, and/or organisational (Finnegan & Hamid, 2009). In this regard, there is a common tendency to address HIS integration by an overall approach, seen as integrated patient centered care (Leventhal, Taliaferro, Wong, Hughes, & Mun, 2012). Integrated patient centered care reflects on integrated HIS (with elements as e-health services) requiring coordination across professionals, facilities, support systems that is continuous over time and between patient visits (Singer et al., 2011). This approach is observed on national healthcare strategies that encourage patient involvement in their healthcare treatment. Moreover, in the USA and Europe, online personal health records that allow patients to manage their health data have emerged (Black et al., 2011).

For example in Finland, this integration trend can be observed in a legislation that allows citizens to access and interact with their own Electronic Healthcare Records (EHRs), ePrescriptions and audit-logs via the Internet (Ruotsalainen, Iivari, & Doupi, 2008). Following similar legislative opportunities worldwide, patients increase their involvement with HIS. This is a growing involvement, seen in parallel with mechanisms for the collection of information (obtained by mobile and other sources) in order to develop an enhanced, complete and integrated view of citizens health status. The latter is reflected in Electronic Health Records (EHRs) and Personal Health Records (PHRs), which are being enriched and exploited by different actors and stakeholders (i.e. health and care professionals, citizens, nutrition experts, hospitals, etc) in the health ecosystem. Three general PHR models have been proposed (Detmer, Bloomrosen, Raymond, & Tang, 2008): a) the stand-alone model, b) Electronic Health Record (EHR) system, and c) the integrated one, which is an interoperable system providing linkage with a variety of patient information sources such as EHRs, home diagnostics, insurance claims etc. The main types of health information supported by PHRs are problem lists, procedures, major illnesses, provider lists, allergy data, home-monitored data, family history, social history and lifestyle, immunizations, medications and laboratory tests (Halamka, Mandl, & Tang, 2008; Tang, Ash, Bates, Overhage, & Sands, 2006). Widely known PHR platforms in terms of centralized web-based portals include Dossia (www.dossia.org) and Microsoft Health Vault (www.healthvault.com/) platforms. Many systems presented in literature offer integration with already established PHRs platforms (Reti, Feldman, & Safran, 2009; Zhou, Yang, Álamo, Wong, & Chang, 2010). Early experiences from the adoption of PHR-based systems have been found to be positive, showing that such systems can be feasible, secure, and well accepted by patients (Jennett & Watanabe, 2006). Nonetheless, today's EHRs and PHRs are far from being what the citizens consider as of value to their health, since for the public view, health means more than being disease-free.

Following this trend for patients' empowerment, academics, practitioners and patients advocate in favor of the patient centered healthcare systems. Still the aforementioned advocates have not yet reached a concise definition of Patient-Centered e-Health (PCEH) that is shared across the research disciplines that focus on health and Information Technology (IT) (Wilson & Strong, 2014). The lack of consensus can be attributed, amongst other, (a) on the number of challenges that are involved in transitioning healthcare delivery to a more patient-centered system and (b) the lack of proof-of-concept through well-documented and effective PCEH projects.

Many of these applications are based on SOA as HIS can be easily delivered to both desktop and mobile computer devices using for instance Java and Visual Studio development environments. Mobile technologies and especially smart phones support patients and professionals to interact with integrated EHR and other e-health applications. This is an emerging area of e-health, given the term m-health (Chatterjee, Chakraborty, Sarker, Sarker, & Lau, 2009). Sarasohn-Kan (2010) report that a major mobile application vendor provides 5,805 health, medical and fitness applications with 73% of them used by patients and 27% by healthcare professionals (Sarasohn-Kahn, 2010). The aforementioned approaches empower the patients and allows them to take their own measurements, and provide verbal and written inputs (Clemensen, Rasmussen, Denning, & Craggs, 2011).

Clearly, except the introduction of standards (e.g. HL7) all these endevours require adequate healthcare specific SOA Governance to be developed and run in a manageable way. SOA can facilitate the plan to redesign HIS towards patient-centred systems in parallel to end-to-end integration (Bhandari & Snowdon, 2011; Leventhal et al., 2012; Papakonstantinou, Malamateniou, & Vassilacopoulos, 2010). Moreover, Business Process Management (BPM) techniques and tools bridges SOA and aligns business processes (based on patient needs) to end-to-end integration (Koufi, Malamateniou, Papakonstantinou, & Vassilacopoulos, 2010; Strnadl, 2007). Thus, SOA can transform heterogeneous and incompatible systems in a patient-centred environment of cooperating services based on healthcare business processes and services (Bhandari & Snowdon, 2011). SOA can be directly associated with patient centred design, as sub-categories of SOA like User-Centred SOA (UCSOA) can facilitate the redesign of HIS towards a patient centred design including support for the end user (e.g. patient) (Chang, He, Tsai, Xiao, & Chen, 2006; Lizcano, Soriano, Reyes, & Hierro, 2009). Furthermore, SOA can assist in the m-health endeavors by providing interoperable services, support diverse processing efficiently, enable cross-platform communication and adapt dynamically to meet changing needs (Firat, Moser, & Melliar-Smith, 2008; Themistocleous, Azab, Kamal, Ali, & Morabito, 2012). In addition to this, SOA interoperability can be seen as a way to minimise medical errors, by providing data exchange accurately, effectively, securely and consistently (Mantzana, Koumaditis, & Themistocleous, 2011).

The value of SOA can be realised from a management point of view, when SOA incorporates a well-developed SOA Governance framework (Biske, 2008). This way, SOA Governance ensures an organisation is (a) pursuing an appropriate SOA strategy aligned with business goals, and (b) is executing that strategy in accordance with guidelines and constraints defined by a body of SOA principles and policies (Marks, 2008). By focusing on SOA Governance healthcare organisations can better address issues like complexity, security, standards, education/training and even provide the backbone for more capabilities like cloud computing. In the following section the authors address SOA Governance.

SOA GOVERNANCE LITERATURE REVIEW

Literature indicates that literature reviews especially when addressing a new area of research (e.g. SOA Governance) is required to be rigorous and comprehensibly described (Levy & Ellis, 2006). Only then can readers assess the exhaustiveness of the review and other scholars in the field can more confidently (re)use the results in their own research (vom Brocke et al., 2009). Following this view we proceeded to a rigorous review of the normative literature (Koumaditis & Themistocleous, 2013) which resulted in the creation of a SOA Governance concept map, as seen in Figure 1. Due to limited space, the authors will not proceed to analyse the concept map for this publication, but in the following paragraph briefly discuss its use.

Figure 1. SOA Governance Concept Map

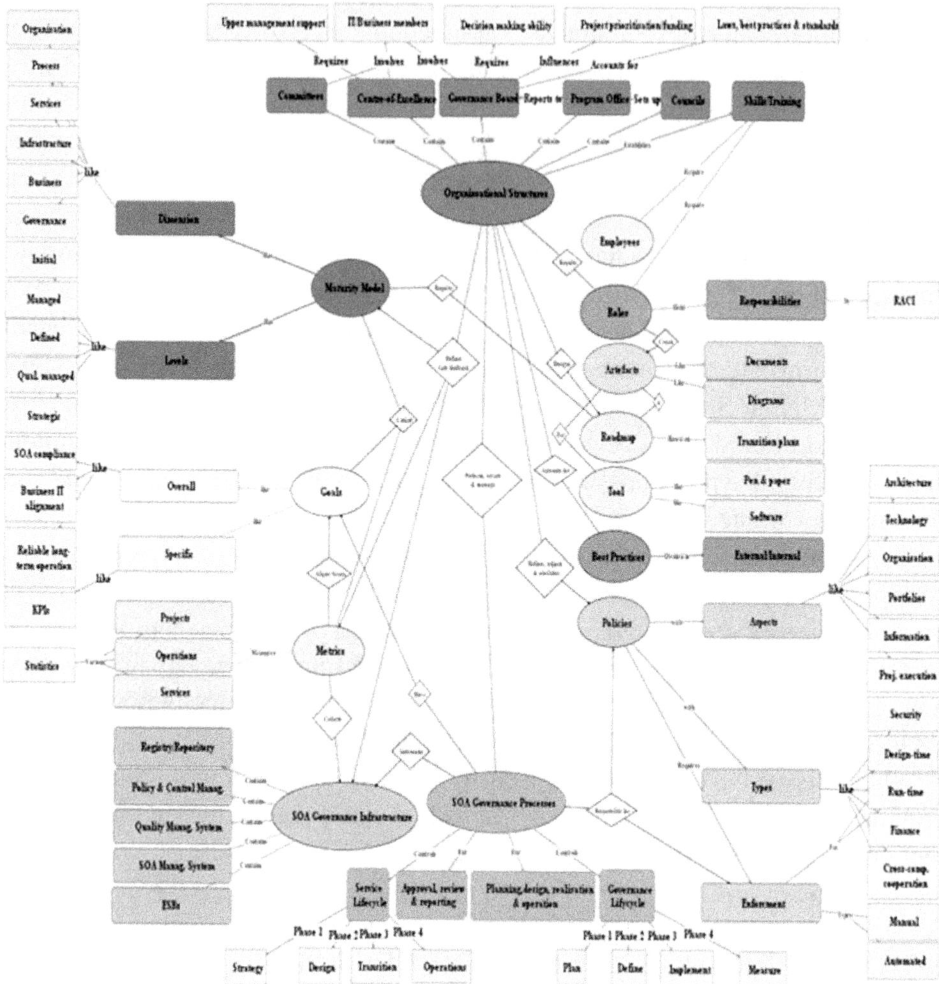

The SOA Governance concept map provides not only a graphical representation of the main concepts, but aids in the discussion of the similarities (common elements), differences (scale, detail and analysis) and limitations (confusion, overlapping, and lack of testing and healthcare aspects).

Moreover, the similarities contribute in the construction of the SOA Governance Framework as they provide the common elements and understanding to create the proposition. On the other hand, the differences and limitations as overlapping and confusion, allowed the authors to discard elements as 'employees', 'artefacts', 'tool' and 'goals'. The decision for exclusion was based on an individual basis. For example, the employees concept overlaps with the organisational structure concept as they both refer to the same notion, while the latter was more frequently observed in the literature and portrayed in more comprehensive conceptualization, thus the first was discarded. The remaining nine common SOA Governance concepts, structure the main elements of the SOA Governance Framework. These elements are:

- **Organisational Structure:** Includes a range of high level structures (e.g. Centre-of-Excellence, boards, offices) and committees/councils dedicated to SOA Governance,
- **Roles:** Concept is identified as newly created or already applied roles with SOA related responsibilities,
- **Maturity Model:** Is an assessment mechanism who provides a comparison between current and future states of SOA aspects (like IT, process, organization),
- **Roadmap:** Concept is portrayed as a transition plan that provides guidance through the SOA endeavor,
- **SOA Governance Infrastructure:** Manages governance information, automates processes, enforces policies and collects metrics,
- **Policies:** Comprise rules for deploying and managing SOA with the aid of enforcement mechanisms (manual or automated)
- **Metrics:** Provides visibility of essential parameters of the SOA initiative,
- **Best Practices***:* To collect experiences and supports the successful implementation of SOA,
- **SOA Governance Processes:** Deal with the management and execution of SOA based on the service lifecycle.

Yet, the authors identified limitations in the normative literature as limited scope and analysis of the concepts (e.g. above mentioned nine elements). To this, the authors propose the following additions:

- The *Organisational Structure* needs to be designed as to compensate for the weaknesses of the current organisational IT structures and incorporate a defined engagement approach with the rest of the organization,
- A list of *Roles* needs to be incorporated in this element exemplifying the corresponding responsibilities,
- Design guidelines to aid in the conceptualization of a *Roadmap* are added to this element,
- The Goal/Questions/Metric method (see (Basili et al., 2010) is utilized as a guideline for *Metrics* element,
- As part of the *Best Practices* element a categorization is included,

- *SOA Governance Processes* are portrayed in four phases: plan, design, implement, measure, and additional attributes are provided for each.

Another limitation identified by the authors is that the nine concepts are tailored for a non-specific sector, whereas the authors emphasise on the need to include healthcare specific aspects as a failure in an IT project directly impacts and endangers patients' quality of care and well-being (Fitzgerald & Russo, 2005; Johnson, 2011; Kaplan & Harris-Salamone, 2009). Thus, the authors propose the use of the SOA CSFs as additions to the nine common issues. This unique grouping is presented in the following section of this chapter.

SOA GOVERNANCE FRAMEWORK FOR HEALTHCARE

Following the literature review findings of the previous section, the authors proposed the main nine elements that a SOA Governance Framework may consist, namely: (a) Organisational Structures, (b) Roles, (c) Roadmap, (d) Best Practices, (e) Policies, (f) SOA Governance Processes, (g) SOA Governance Infrastructure, (h) Metrics, and (i) Maturity Model. This is identified as the first component of our proposition. The second component are specific additions that were introduced as guidelines to enhance them, like: (a) SOA Governance structure guidelines, (b) example list of SOA roles and responsibilities, (c) SOA roadmap design guidelines, (d) method to construct metrics, (e) best practices categorisation guidelines, and (f) SOA Governance phases and their attributes (examples of the latter). In this section and as a third component, the authors propose specific additions (based on SOA CSFs in healthcare) to the nine elements so as to tackle their lack of healthcare specific conceptualisation. The aforementioned synthesis can be graphically observed in Figure 2.

Figure 2. SOA Governance Framework Synthesis

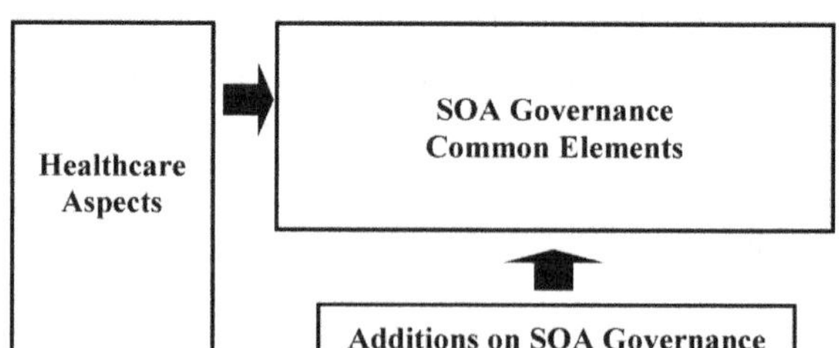

In more detail, the process of addressing the SOA CSFs is presented in the following paragraphs.

- **Alignment:** Beimborn et al., (2009) suggest that well established SOA Governance structures positively influence the structural dimension of IT/ business alignment. The authors agree with the aforementioned view and believe that organisational structures can address this CSF with attributes as dedicated committees and/or individuals who hold alignment related roles and responsibilities (e.g. strategy manager). These individuals can then set specific goals like SOA compliance (e.g. alignment with legal, internal regulations) and business/IT alignment (these goals are also supported by Niemann (2010)), implement SOA Governance processes, design policies that influence the alignment and using appropriate metrics measure and control the level of complexity.
- **Clear Goals:** This is a broadly defined CSF that can be implied for all the elements of the proposed SOA Governance Framework. For example, SOA Governance processes and metrics have specific goals that are set by organisational structures and individuals holding roles in these structures. It is our understanding that the clear definition of these goals is placed on the clarity of the concept they address and the skills of the individuals defining them. Thus, we propose to include in the organisational structure element the guidelines: (a) responsible to set clear goals for all elements and (b) involve individuals with skills that can set clear goals so as to address this CSF.
- **Complexity:** We argue that identifying sources that increase the overall complexity in a system can be placed as a responsibility in individual roles. For example, the SOA architect holds the responsibility for designing and implementing the logical/physical architecture and thus can foresee and manage in some extent the complexity introduced by the implementation. Additionally, individuals with these kinds of responsibilities (e.g. complexity related) can collectively under an organisational structure (e.g. committee, interest groups) or more informally (e.g. intranets, wikis) address potential complexity issues. Yet, as complexity was also identified as a HIS challenge we emphasise the need for this CSF to be adequately addressed. Literature suggestions recommend the utilisation of SOA metric systems that can measure design-time and run-time services and predict unwanted levels of complexity (Hirzalla, Cleland-Huang, & Arsanjani, 2009). We agree with this suggestion and propose that the metrics element (metrics that measure system complexity) need to be utilised so as to provide better governance of the complexity factor.

- **Cost:** Cost and more precisely funding was included in the organisational structure element that can control in certain extent the funding of SOA projects. However, it is our belief that for this CSF to be better dealt the creation of committees in charge of cost planning and control that can also identify service/project sponsors within or outside the organisation, is required. Additionally, funding can be added as an area in the SOA maturity model, so as the healthcare organisation can compare the progress of business processes, technology and other areas with financial data and better govern this factor.
- **Culture:** We argue that the organisational structure can cultivate a SOA friendly culture and gain the trust and cooperation with the rest of the healthcare organisation. This may involve specific governance processes that promote SOA and its beneficial parameters (e.g. educational and communication planning). Thus, we propose the aforementioned additions in the corresponding elements.
- **Experience and Training:** This CSF including the requirements of experienced personnel and additional training is in great extent covered by the SOA organisational structures' and SOA Governance processes' elements.
- **Governance:** It is our understanding that the proposed SOA Governance elements (Part A and B) and healthcare aspect added in this section (Part C) can address all the requirements for governance (as an CSF) in a healthcare organisation.
- **Long-Term Planning:** We argue that the CSF identified as long-term planning can be represented by the SOA maturity model as a more elaborate approach. For example, one of the application areas that a SOA maturity model examines is the services, these are described starting from an initial and reaching to a final maturity level, expressed in a similar progressive way as in a long-term plan. Thus, we identify this approach to be a useful tool for SOA Governance and propose its utilisation to address this CSF.
- **Measurement:** It can be stated that this CSF can be addressed by the metrics element, as they hold similar conceptualisation, with emphasis on the role of the SOA Governance infrastructure in the collection of metrics and diffusion of feedback about them.
- **Maturity Identification:** The authors accept that this CSF can be represented by the SOA maturity model element.
- **Project Identification:** It can be argued that this factor is addressed as part of the SOA organisational structure and also it is the authors' belief that specific roles, like strategy manager, SOA architect and SOA designer, are responsible for the project identification.

- **Resources:** This CSF is described as a multifaceted one with parameters as financial (budget), technical (software/hardware), and staff (experts, implementation team, consultants) aspects. The financial parameter can be addressed similarly the cost CSF (e.g. from organisational structures and SOA maturity model elements). As far as the technical aspect we believe that is covered by the SOA Governance infrastructure element conceptualisation, since both refer to adequate resources as software and hardware systems. Additionally, the introduction of the roles element can resemble the staffing aspect of this CSF.
- **Risk:** It can be stated that this CSF is addressed by the proposed roles of security manager and tester regarding the security and error risk, and from the organisational structure element regarding the funding and sponsoring risk (in the form of dedicated committees or groups). Yet, it is our understanding that data security and patients' confidentiality are clearly a significant challenge to healthcare and beyond the organisational structures and roles, specific testing, standards, policies and best practices are needed. These will be discussed in the following paragraphs.
- **Roadmap:** It can be stated that this CSF can be addressed by the roadmap element,
- **Roles:** We argue that this CSF can be addressed by the roles element.
- **Standards:** SOA is based on established global standards (e.g. XML, UDDI, SOAP, WSDL, BPEL and REST). In healthcare the standards related to information coding and sharing (e.g. SNOMED, HL7) or protocols (e.g. DICOM) that enhance the interoperability and improve the way HIS share information are usually developed from national central standardisation bodies or independent organisations like IHE (IHE, 2012). This combination between SOA and healthcare standards is an important factor for SOA implementations, regarding aspects of security, interoperability and QoS. Thus, it is our belief that such standards need to be incorporated as best practices and utilised accordingly. In charge of such best practices can be organisational structures (e.g. committees, interest groups) that can identify the standards, evaluate them and recommend them as best practices and thus minimise the risk in issues like: security, access control and medical errors. Additionally, this activity can be included as a SOA Governance process (e.g. standardisation process).
- **Team:** We argue that this CSF can be addressed by the SOA Governance organisational structures element.
- **Testing:** This CSF was identified requiring tools and methods to test the integration approaches and services before the actual service implementation. The authors extents this CSF's importance to testing in both design-

and run-time SOA and believes that specific roles like tester, infrastructure and SOA architect, service developer, process and security manager with the aid of SOA Governance infrastructure can control the criticality of this factor. These roles include a wide spectrum of responsibilities related to testing like error localization for service developer, and/or maintenance for process manager and of course testing for the tester role. Yet, it is our understanding that since testing was identified as a HIS challenge, additional emphasis is required to address this factor. Thus, proposes governance processes that address this factor to be included in the SOA Governance processes element, which with the aid of SOA Governance infrastructure can provide testing capabilities. Furthermore, these processes can be placed in the best practices element and form guidelines that minimize errors.

Up till now, most of the SOA Governance elements were introduced in parts, as common elements in Part A, additions to these elements in Part B and healthcare aspects of the elements in Part C. Following is the synthesis of the nine SOA Governance elements, as the proposed SOA Governance Framework, as depicted in Figure 3.

Figure 3. Proposed SOA Governance Framework

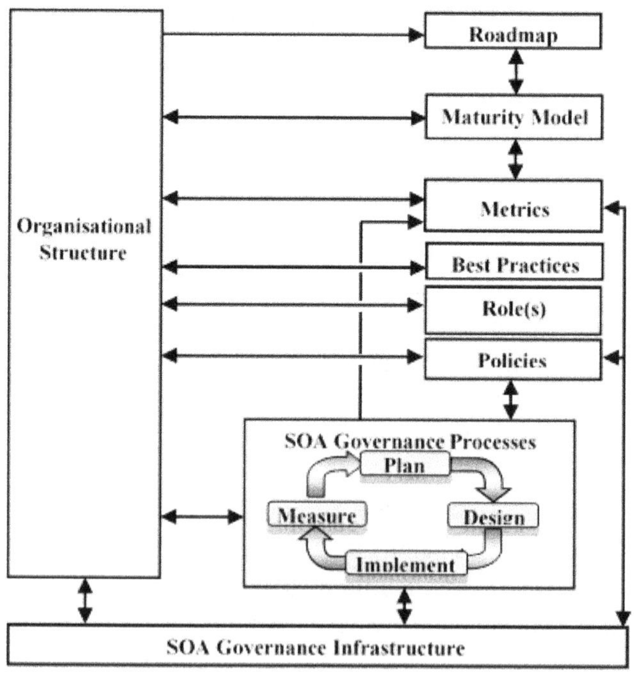

The proposed framework in Figure 3 makes a novel contribution at two levels. Firstly, at a conceptual level, it identifies and proposes nine elements that should be considered during the SOA Governance process. The identification of the nine elements is based on the theoretical works conducted by others in this area (see (Koumaditis & Themistocleous, 2013)). As a result, the conceptualisation of the elements is grounded in the normative literature. In addition to this, the framework incorporates additions that are gathered from additional literature resources beyond the ones that composed the elements. This comes as a method to overcome the limitations identified in normative literature and enhance the elements' conceptualisation. Moreover, the authors propose a unique formulation combining the identified common elements of SOA Governance (seen in Part A and B), the SOA CSFs and HIS challenges. This proposal aims to pinpoint attributes and guidelines for each element, required to successfully govern a SOA and tackle longstanding HIS challenges. Secondly, at a practical level, the proposed framework contributes towards a better understanding of the research area (SOA Governance in healthcare).

RESEARCH METHODOLOGY

To test the SOA governance framework an interpretive qualitative research approach is proposed, with the aid of a case study. The decision to utilize such a research strategy was based on the need to study the SOA governance issues surrounding SOA implementations and on the unique nature of healthcare itself.

In more detail, healthcare can be characterized by unique issues, such as: (a) the interactive nature of practitioner/patient relationships, (b) patients' subjective experiences of illness, (c) their own personal understanding of human suffering and (d) stakeholders behavior and interpersonal interactions (A. Miles, 2009). The aforementioned characteristics of healthcare drive effective clinical process to rely not to a single but rather several different kinds of knowledge (e.g. medical, anthropological and instrumental). Consequently, giving the required depth of understanding that can be applied to a given problem situation. The same principle, as in clinical practice, is useful to be applied to the research methodology so as to research a healthcare setting (Fossey, Harvey, McDermott, & Davidson, 2002). Additionally, as to understand the interplay between stakeholders (clinical and non-clinical) and IS, emphasis is required on the meanings, concepts, definitions, characteristics, descriptions and associations rather than numbers and statistics. Thus, as a more suitable candidate the interpretive qualitative research approach is followed in this research, as it can relate closely to the healthcare aspect of the research. Additionally, qualitative research methods are being used increasingly in evaluations of computer systems and IT both within and outside healthcare (Kaplan & Maxwell, 2005). Furthermore, the use to consider a case study strategy is supported, as it is a widely used research mechanism for examining IS frameworks and supports the investigation of: (a) little-known phenomena (SOA governance in healthcare) and (b) complex processes (SOA implementation) in their natural setting (Bairi & Manohar, 2011).

Therefore, the authors propose a qualitative research with three stages: (a) research design, (b) data collection and (c) data analysis, as seen in Figure 4.

DISCUSSION

Healthcare is a unique sector not only due to its relevance to human life, but also due to the big amount of: (a) complexity, (b) legacy systems, (c) data and (d) resources utilized each year. Yet, the development of SOA Governance in healthcare and its impact to healthcare organizations remains unexposed to research. Such research will undoubtedly provide a more compelling basis for the utilization of SOA and a more controlled environment for HIS integration.

This chapter deals with this important research area and addressed HIS integration challenges. These challenges certainly will be very real over the next few years as governance and management of IT projects, as we continue to embrace SOA projects across widely distributed HIS. To this end and with the help of a rigorous literature review the authors developed and proposed a SOA Governance Framework

Figure 4: Research Methodology Design

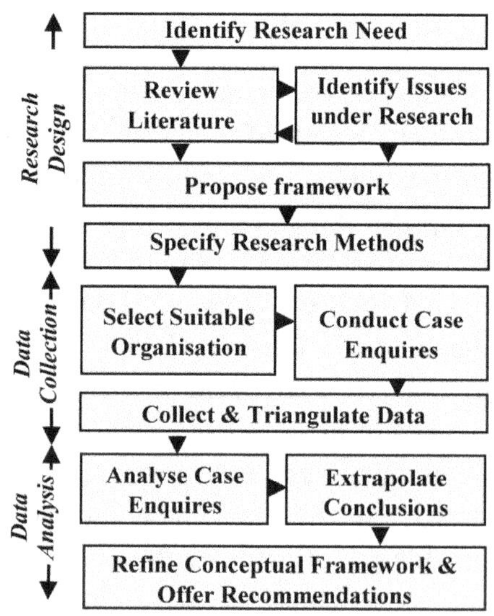

that can address these challenges. An overview of the proposed SOA Governance Framework was presented in Figure 3. Without a doubt, further research is required to enhance our understanding and impact of such proposition in a healthcare organization. To do this, we already brought forward a qualitative research methodology plan (e.g. Figure 4). Yet, further research actions are needed. These are discussed in the following section.

FUTURE RESEARCH DIRECTIONS

The authors have planned to test the SOA Governance Framework with key SOA players in healthcare such as: (a) public and private hospitals and (b) healthcare organizations (e.g. insurance funds). It is our view that the data gathered from the empirical arena will strengthen, refine and highlight our proposition.

Following the aforementioned actions, we also propose to transform the proposed SOA Governance elements' structure and the framework itself (e.g. refined form) into a large-scale survey questionnaire, instant of using interpretive epistemology. Clearly, this approach would not have been possible previously, since the framework did not exist. Miles and Huberman (1994) discuss such a research design starting with a qualitative approach that provides an initial exploratory phase, whose outcomes may be used to create quantitative instruments (e.g. surveys) to collect new data. It is our understanding that such large-scale survey may offer the opportunity to establish generic significance to the issues related to the proposed SOA Governance Framework. In surveying a representative sample of organisations the elements' characteristics related to the proposed framework can be better verified and understood.

REFERENCES

Bairi, J., & Manohar, M. (2011). Critical success factors in gaining user customer satisfaction in outsourced IT services. *Journal of Enterprise Information Management, 24*(6), 475–493. doi:10.1108/17410391111166530

Basili, V., Lindvall, M., Regardie, M., Seaman, C., Heidrich, J., Münch, J., & Trendowicz, A. et al. (2010). Linking Software Development and Business Strategy Through Measurement. *Computer, 43*(4), 57–65. doi:10.1109/MC.2010.108

Beimborn, D., Joachim, N., Schlosser, F., & Streicher, B. (2009). *The Role of IT/Business Alignment for Achieving SOA Business Value - Proposing a Research Model.* Paper presented at the 15th Americas Conference on Information Systems, San Francisco, CA.

Bhandari, G., & Snowdon, A. (2011). Design of a patient-centric, service-oriented health care navigation system for a local health integration network. *Behaviour & Information Technology*, 1–11. doi:10.1080/0144929x.2011.563798

Biske, T. (2008). *SOA Governance*. Birmingham, UK: Packt Publishing Ltd.

Black, A. D., Car, J., Pagliari, C., Anandan, C., Cresswell, K., Bokun, T., & Sheikh, A. et al. (2011). The Impact of eHealth on the Quality and Safety of Health Care: A Systematic Overview. *PLoS Medicine*, *8*(1), e1000387. PMID:21267058

Chang, M., He, J., Tsai, W., Xiao, B., & Chen, Y. (2006). *UCSOA: User-Centric Service-Oriented Architecture*. Paper presented at the IEEE International Conference on e-Business Engineering, Shanghai, China.

Chatterjee, S., Chakraborty, S., Sarker, S., Sarker, S., & Lau, F. Y. (2009). Examining the success factors for mobile work in healthcare: A deductive study. *Decision Support Systems*, *46*(3), 620–633. doi:10.1016/j.dss.2008.11.003

Clemensen, J., Rasmussen, J., Denning, A., & Craggs, M. (2011). *Patient Empowerment and New Citizen Roles through Telehealth Technologies - The Early Stage*. Paper presented at the Third International Conference on eHealth, Telemedicine, and Social Medicine, Gosier, France.

Detmer, D., Bloomrosen, M., Raymond, B., & Tang, P. (2008). Integrated personal health records: Transformative tools for consumer-centric care. *BMC Medical Informatics and Decision Making*, *8*(1), 45. doi:10.1186/1472-6947-8-45 PMID:18837999

Dwivedi, Y., Ravichandran, K., Williams, M., Miller, S., Lal, B., Antony, G., & Kartik, M. (2013). IS/IT Project Failures: A Review of the Extant Literature for Deriving a Taxonomy of Failure Factors. In Y. Dwivedi, H. Henriksen, D. Wastell, & R. De' (Eds.), *Grand Successes and Failures in IT. Public and Private Sectors* (Vol. 402, pp. 73–88). Springer Berlin Heidelberg. doi:10.1007/978-3-642-38862-0_5

Finnegan, D., & Hamid, K. (2009). Information systems (IS) integration approaches in healthcare: a critical review. In W. Currie & D. Finnegan (Eds.), Integrating Healthcare With Information and Communications Technology. London: Radcliffe Publishing.

Firat, K., Moser, L., & Melliar-Smith, M. (2008). Building a Distributed E-Healthcare System Using SOA. *IT Professional*, *10*(2).

Fitzgerald, G., & Russo, N. (2005). The turnaround of the London ambulance service computer-aided despatch system (LASCAD). *European Journal of Information Systems*, *14*(3), 244–257. doi:10.1057/palgrave.ejis.3000541

Fossey, E., Harvey, C., McDermott, F., & Davidson, L. (2002). Understanding and evaluating qualitative research. *The Australian and New Zealand Journal of Psychiatry*, *36*(6), 717–732. doi:10.1046/j.1440-1614.2002.01100.x PMID:12406114

HL7/OMG. (2010). The Practical Guide for SOA in Health Care. *Healthcare Services Specification Project.* Retrieved 01.10.10, 1.0, from http://hssp.wikispaces.com/file/view/2008-12-29+SOA%2BHealthcare%2BPractical%2BGuide%2Bv1.0.pdf

Halamka, J., Mandl, K., & Tang, P. (2008). Early Experiences with Personal Health Records. *Journal of the American Medical Informatics Association*, *15*(1), 1–7. doi:10.1197/jamia.M2562 PMID:17947615

Health, I. T. (2014). Meaningful Use Definition & Objectives. *EHR Incentives & Certification.* Retrieved 04.05., 2014, from http://www.healthit.gov/providers-professionals/meaningful-use-definition-objectives

Heffner, R. (2009). *Forrester Report: Survey Results Show SOA Governance Improves SOA Benefit Realization.* Academic Press.

Hirzalla, M., Cleland-Huang, J., & Arsanjani, A. (2009). A Metrics Suite for Evaluating Flexibility and Complexity in Service Oriented Architectures. In G. Feuerlicht & W. Lamersdorf (Eds.), Service-Oriented Computing – ICSOC 2008 Workshops. Springer Berlin Heidelberg.

HSSP. (2013). *Healthcare Services Specification Program.* Retrieved 19.01.2013, from http://hssp.wikispaces.com/

IHE. (2012). *Integrating the Healthcare Enterprise.* Retrieved 01.03.2011, 2011., from http://www.ihe.net/

ITGI. (2011). Global Status Report on the Governance of Enterprise I.T. (GEIT). In Global Status Research. Rolling Meadows, IL: IT Governance Institute.

Jennett, P., & Watanabe, M. (2006). Healthcare and Telemedicine: Ongoing and Evolving Challenges. *Disease Management & Health Outcomes*, *14*(1).

Johnson, C. W. (2011). Identifying common problems in the acquisition and deployment of large-scale, safety–critical, software projects in the US and UK healthcare systems. *Safety Science*, *49*(5), 735–745.

Kaplan, B., & Harris-Salamone, K. D. (2009). Health IT success and failure: Recommendations from literature and an AMIA workshop. *Journal of the American Medical Informatics Association: JAMIA*, *16*(3), 291–299. doi:10.1197/jamia.M2997 PMID:19261935

Kaplan, B., & Maxwell, J. (2005). Qualitative Research Methods for Evaluating Computer Information Systems: Evaluating the Organizational Impact of Healthcare Information Systems. Springer New York.

Koufi, V., Malamateniou, F., Papakonstantinou, D., & Vassilacopoulos, G. (2010). In G. A. Papadopoulos, W. Wojtkowski, G. Wojtkowski, S. Wrycza, & J. Zupancic (Eds.), *Using ESB and BPEL for Evolving Healthcare Systems Towards Pervasive, Grid-Enabled SOA Information Systems Development* (pp. 167–175). Springer, US.

Koumaditis, K., & Themistocleous, M. (2013). *SOA Governance from a Healthcare Perspective.* Paper presented at the IADIS International Conference e-Health 2013, Prague, Czech Republic.

Koumaditis, K., Themistocleous, M., Mantzana, V., & Souliotis, K. (2012). *A Proposition of Critical Sucess Factors Influencing SOA Implementation in Healthcare.* Paper presented at the European Conference on Information Systems, Barcelona, Spain.

Koumaditis, K., Themistocleous, M., & Morabito, V. (2013). New Trends in Healthcare Information Systems (HIS) Integration. In I. M. Miranda & M. M. Cruz-Cunha (Eds.), Handbook of Research on ICTs for Healthcare and Social Services: Developments and Applications (Vol. 1). IGI Global.

Leventhal, T., Taliaferro, P., Wong, K., Hughes, C., & Mun, S. (2012). The Patient-Centered Medical Home and Health Information Technology. *Telemedicine Journal and e-Health, 18*(2), 145–149. doi:10.1089/tmj.2011.0130 PMID:22304440

Levy, Y., & Ellis, T. J. (2006). A Systems Approach to Conduct an Effective Literature Review in Support of Information Systems Research. *Informing Science Journal, 9*(9), 181–212.

Lizcano, D., Soriano, J., Reyes, M., & Hierro, J. (2009). A user-centric approach for developing and deploying service front-ends in the future internet of services. *Int. J. Web Grid Serv., 5*(2), 155–191. doi:10.1504/IJWGS.2009.027572

Lunt, N., Smith, R., Exworthy, M., Green, S., Horsfal, D., & Mannion, R. (2011). Medical Tourism: Treatments, markets and health system implications: A scoping review. In OECD (Ed.), *International Trade in Health Services* (Vol. 1, p. 55). Paris, France: Directorate for Employment,Labour and Social Affairs.

Mantzana, V., Koumaditis, K., & Themistocleous, M. (2011). *Healthcare IS Interoperability: Challenges and Solutions.* Paper presented at the HEALTHINF 2011: International Conference on Health Informatics, Rome, Italy.

Marks, E. (2008). *Service-Oriented Architecture (SOA) Governance for the Services Driven Enterprise.* Wiley.

Miles, A. (2009). Complexity in medicine and healthcare: People and systems, theory and practice. *Journal of Evaluation in Clinical Practice*, *15*(3), 409–410. doi:10.1111/j.1365-2753.2009.01204.x PMID:19522904

Miles, M., & Huberman, A. (1994). *Qualitative Data Analysis: An Expanded Sourcebook* (2nd ed.). Thousand Oaks, CA: Sage.

Niemann, M., Miede, A., Wolfgang, J., Repp, N., & Steinmetz, R. (2010). Structuring SOA Governance. *International Journal of IT/Business Alignment and Governance*, *1*(1), 58–75.

Papakonstantinou, D., Malamateniou, F., & Vassilacopoulos, G. (2010). A SOA approach to the implementation of an electronic medical record. *International Journal of Applied Systemic Studies*, *3*(3), 343–352. doi:10.1504/IJASS.2010.034626

Reti, S. R., Feldman, H. J., & Safran, C. (2009). Governance for Personal Health Records. *Journal of the American Medical Informatics Association*, *16*(1), 14–17. doi:10.1197/jamia.M2854 PMID:18952939

Rhoads, J., Cooper, T., Fuchs, K., Schluter, P., & Zambuto, R. P. (2010). Medical device interoperability and the Integrating the Healthcare Enterprise (IHE) initiative. *Biomedical Instrumentation & Technology,* 21-27.

Ruotsalainen, P., Iivari, A., & Doupi, P. (2008). Finland's strategy and implementation of citizens' access to health information. *Studies in Health Technology and Informatics*, *137*, 379–385. PMID:18560100

Sarasohn-Kahn, J. (2010). *How smartphones are changing health care for consumers and providers*. California HealthCare Foundation. Retrieved from http://www.chcf.org/

Singer, S., Burgers, J., Friedberg, M., Rosenthal, M., Leape, L., & Schneider, E. (2011). Defining and measuring integrated patient care: Promoting the next frontier in health care delivery. *Medical Care Research and Review*, *68*(1), 112–127. doi:10.1177/1077558710371485 PMID:20555018

Stephens, E. (2008). *Managing IT investment - The role of EA and SOA with governance*. Paper presented at the SOA in Healthcare realizing quality-of-care, Chicago, IL.

Strnadl, C. (2007). Bridging Architectural Boundaries Design and Implementation of a Semantic BPM and SOA Governance Tool Service-Oriented Computing – ICSOC 2007 (Vol. 4749, pp. 518-529). Springer Berlin / Heidelberg.

Tang, P., Ash, J., Bates, D., Overhage, J., & Sands, D. (2006). Personal Health Records: Definitions, Benefits, and Strategies for Overcoming Barriers to Adoption. *Journal of the American Medical Informatics Association*, *13*(2), 121–126. doi:10.1197/jamia.M2025 PMID:16357345

Themistocleous, M., Azab, N., Kamal, M., Ali, M., & Morabito, V. (2012). Location-Based Services for Public Policy Making: The Direct and Indirect Way to e-Participation. *Information Systems Management*, *29*(4), 269–283. doi:10.1080/10580530.2012.716743

vom Brocke, J., Simons, A., Niehaves, B., Riemer, K., Plattfaut, R., & Cleven, A. (2009). *Reconstructing the Giant: On the Importance of Rigour in Documenting the Literature Search Process.* Paper presented at the ECIS 2009, Verona, Italy.

Wilson, V., & Strong, D. (2014). Editors' Introduction to the Special Section on Patient-centered e-Health: Research Opportunities and Challenges. *Communications of the Association for Information Systems*, *34*(15).

Zhou, F., Yang, H., Álamo, J., Wong, J., & Chang, C. (2010). Mobile Personal Health Care System for Patients with Diabetes. In Y. Lee, Z. Z. Bien, M. Mokhtari, J. Kim, M. Park, J. Kim, H. Lee, & I. Khalil (Eds.), Aging Friendly Technology for Health and Independence. Springer Berlin Heidelberg.

KEY TERMS AND DEFINITIONS

HIS Integration: The alignment of HIS in an interoperable environment.

HIS Interoperability: The ability of HIS to work together and exchange information.

HIS: Information systems designed to facilitate healthcare services.

PCEH: Patient Centered e-health.

SOA Governance: Important mechanisms that ensure the reliable long-term operation of an SOA.

SOA: An architectural paradigm to build ecosystems of services.

Chapter 10
Healthy 3.0:
Healthcare Digital Dimensions

Maria Teresa Borges Tiago
University of Azores, Portugal

Francisco Emanuel Batista Amaral
University of Azores, Portugal

Flávio Tiago
UAC, Portugal

Sandra Silva
Unidade de Saúde de Ilha de S. Miguel Azores, Portugal

ABSTRACT

Over the past few years, healthcare practice has evolved to include new forms of information and communication technologies, and healthcare providers have begun to leverage IT solutions and the internet to reach consumers in transformative ways. There is a common thought both in business and academia that the technology adoption process is a key component of success and allows firms to achieve and sustain competitive advantages. Therefore, this research attempts to reinforce the assessment of ICT impacts on healthcare, analyzing it from two different perspectives: 1) firm performance, which is measured as a combination of induced and intangible benefits beyond the traditional financial benefits; and 2) healthcare providers' acceptance and adoption of ICT tools. To assess the first perspective, a structural equation model was applied to a large database sample covering firms from 17 European countries. The results reinforce the importance of induced and structural benefits in firms' overall performance. The second perspective was analyzed only for the Portuguese healthcare providers sample. These results can be a starting point for rethinking the healthcare models emphasizing the perspectives of Healthy 2.0 and considering that patients' technological pattern evolution will lead to Healthy 3.0 in the short term. Nevertheless, some questions remain unanswered regarding the impacts of the ICT acceptance process on overall benefits; therefore, future research will focus on this domain.

DOI: 10.4018/978-1-4666-9870-3.ch010

INTRODUCTION

It is no longer enough to consider the impact and role of information and communication technologies (ICTs) at firm and industry levels. Much has been written about these matters (Inklaar, O'Mahony, & Timmer, 2005; Jennings, Clifford, Fox, O'Connell, & Gardner, 2015; Pilat, 2004; M. B. Tiago & Tiago, 2013; Van Ark, Inklaar, & McGuckin, 2003), but the vast technological changes that occurred require that the scope of these researches be broadened.

Traditionally, and taking into account the results found in previous studies, the impact of ICT can be perceived as detailed in: 1) the contribution of ICT investment to capital intensity; 2) the contribution of the technological adoption model to a firm's performance; 3) the spillovers of rapid innovation by the use of ICT; 4) the competitive and dynamic effects of ICT on a firm's turbulence in terms of entry, exit, and the mobility of market shares of incumbents; and 5) the empowerment of strategic dimensions through the use of ICT tools (Fracolli et al., 2014). Nowadays, there needs to be the added consideration of the role and impact of ICT in the communication flows of the firms, regardless of internal or external context. In these contexts, the web developments influenced the flows of information creation and sharing. Additionally, the initial Web evolved into Web 2.0, reflecting a gradual growth in terms of popularity and resources and the emergence of new tools that meet users' need for interactivity with information (Tekli et al., 2013).

ICT-related sectors are often characterized as high-tech and knowledge-intensive industries, since they rely deeply on the use of ICT tools to leverage an internal innovation process When approaching other service sectors, the impacts of ICT adoption are perceived as lower (I. Chang, 2007). There has been much discussion of the role that recent advances in ICTs could play in improving health service systems in developing countries, as well as other services industries with traditionally lower levels of technology connected to healthcare (Hadgkiss & Renzaho, 2014).

Drawing on the existing literature, this chapter attempts to analyze: 1) the impacts of ICT in healthcare services firms' performance; 2) the adoption and acceptance of ICT patterns of physicians and nurses; and, 3) to unveil some of the trends in the healthcare sector driven from ICT use in European countries. Therefore, a conceptual model was developed for understanding and investigating the different contributions achieved by the adoption of ICT in this sector.

The data used in this research came from the 2006 e-business watch survey, covering 834 health services firms in 17 countries (Belgium, Bulgaria, Czech Republic, Denmark, Finland, Greece, Spain, France, Hungary, Ireland, Italy, Latvia, The Netherlands, Norway, Poland, Sweden, and the UK). The survey was enlarged with data gathered in Portugal regarding physicians' and nurses' use of technology-based systems.

In general, our findings support the conceptual framework presented and the results obtained can be used as a support tool in ICT decision makers' processes, since it clearly states the overall benefits of ICT successful implementation as well as presents the global performance impacts achieved with an integrated IS framework. Some useful preliminary insights are produced, however, leaving a considerable number of issues for future research, including the possibility of extending the research to include new tools and perspectives.

This chapter is organized in the following manner. The next section summarizes the literature related to the adoption of ICT tools by healthcare firms. The third section of the chapter formalizes the major points presented in the conceptual model and translates them into hypotheses. In the fourth section, the methodology is applied and the results are presented. The fifth section offers concluding remarks about the some of the major issues, controversies, and problems, as well as suggests solutions and future research paths.

BACKGROUND

In the mid-1980s, information and communication technologies have achieved a dominant role, leading to several changes in the internal organizational environment, regardless of the sector. In today's competitive global context, such technologies act as an imperative in two ways: 1) reducing the uncertainties related to production and services processes (Henderson et al., 2012), as well as supporting administrative tasks (Dewett & Jones, 2001; Sheng, Chang, Teo, & Lin, 2013) and subsequent achievement of sustainable competitive advantage (McKee, Varadarajan, & Pride, 1989); and 2) narrowing the distance between providers and customers, allowing a continuum of information flow that enhances overall service quality (Darkins, Foster, Anderson, Goldschmidt, & Selvin, 2013; Egea, González, & Menéndez, 2015; Kumar, Novak, & Tomkins, 2010; McGowan et al., 2012).

These changes impel rethinking firms' strategies concerning the digital domain: as IT investments that need to be performed to enhance performance; and, as a daily tool between service providers and clients that needs to be spread out and regulated.

A review of the existing literature related to information and communication technologies and IS impacts on organizational performance may enable a more effective implementation of these tools and how organizations can take advantage of their application (Bayo-Moriones, Billón, & Lera-López, 2013; Eder & Igbaria, 2001). According to the results of several research studies, such as the papers of Papastathopoulos, et al. (2007) and Peansupap and Walker (2005), there are two main reasons that tend to influence greatly the way firms handle the acceptance and implementation of ICTs: the level of investment involved and failure rates or past experiences of failure associated with the implementation of ICT applications.

More, the debate regarding the use of ICT seeks to determine which firms' characteristics enhance the adoption of ICT and enhance their impact on organizational performance (Dewett & Jones, 2001; Liao, 2003). In this sense, the literature suggests as adoption enablers' firms' characteristics, strategy commitment and external environment. This concept has stimulated the study of the elements and drivers of adoption of ICT/IS use in recent years (Bayo-Moriones et al., 2013; Bayo-Moriones & Lera-López, 2007; Liao, 2003; Liu & Liu, 2008; Papastathopoulou et al., 2007; Schillewaert, Ahearne, Frambach, & Moenaert, 2005; Wild & Griggs, 2008; Yi & Hwang, 2003 ; Zhu & Kraemer, 2002; Zhu, Kraemer, & Dedrick, 2004).

Information technology has become a common asset in health services industry in the past four decades and has gained widespread usage (Rahimi & Vimarlund, 2007). Thus, it's hard to picture health care services with absence of information and communication technology tools (I. Chang, 2007; M.-Y. Chang, Pang, Tarn, Liu, & Yen, 2015; Hung, Hung, Tsai, & Jiang, 2010). Nevertheless, the evaluation of the outcomes, the benefits and inhibitors associated with IT-based systems in medical informatics is still a challenge.

Nowadays, it is clear that ICT offers tremendous opportunities to improve daily-base activities in healthcare sector. One of the main reasons for the growing importance of IT in this sector relies on the fact that IT is consider to be an enabler to handle the enormous amount of information related to patients. The identified determinants, which would influence the future implementation of electronic healthcare systems, can be classified into six major categories: (1) Technology, (2) Acceptance, (3) Organization, (4) Financing; (5) Adoption; and, (6) Policy and Legislation (see Figure 1).

The use of *technology* in health services can be observed in regular operations such as electronic patient records access, decision support systems which helps clinical actions, among others (Ammenwerth, Gräber, Herrmann, Bürkle, & König, 2003; Buntin, Burke, Hoaglin, & Blumenthal, 2011; Egea et al., 2015). The following table presents some of these applications and the research made around them (see table 1).

After summarizing all these works that analyze the use of digital tools on healthcare, it seems very cliché to define the concept of healthcare, but the panoply of definitions and uses found in literature impels us to do so. Therefore, in this work "Health care" is considered as the broad concept, which encompasses diagnosis and treatment of patients, education of staff, patients and the general public, and administrative activities (Fischer & Soyez, 2015).

From the results of multiple studies, it can be seen that information technologies such as electronic patient records, electronic health records, e-prescribing, decision

Figure 1. ICT adoption dimensions in healthcare sector

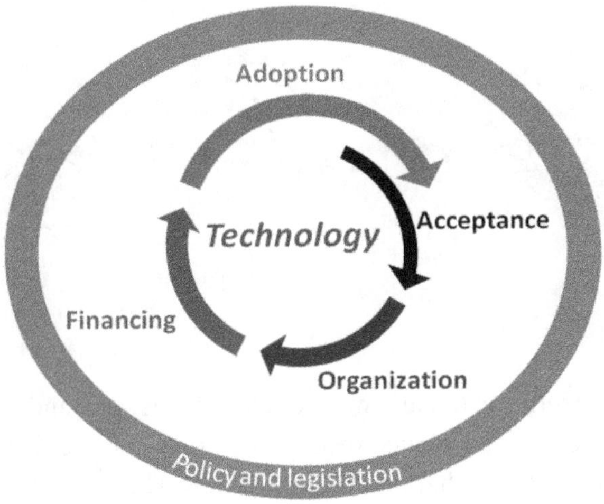

Table 1. Examples of research performed on technology tools adopt in healthcare services

Authors (Year)	ICT Tool Analyzed
Laerum et al (2003); Stengel et al (2004)	Computer-based documentation
Wang (2003); Adams et al (2003); Hier et al (2004); Likourezos et al (2004)	Electronic medical record
Hippisley-Cox, et al. (2003); Mäkelä et al (2005)	Electronic patient record
Ammewerth et al (2003)	Computer-based nursing process
Baum et al (2004)	Helpdesk in HIS
Laerum et al (2004)	Hospital information system
Scott et al (2005)	Electronic health record
Persaud et al (2005); Steventon et al. (2012); Darkins et al. (2013); Henderson et al. (2012)	Telehealth
Noble et al (2005)	Telemedicine
Ahmad, Hudak, Bercovitz, Hollenberg, & Levinson (2006)	Electronic consultation
Buntin, Burke, Hoaglin, & Blumenthal (2011); Rahimi and Vimarlund (2007)	Health information system
Lau (2011)	Web 2.0 Tools
McGowan et al (2012); Fischer and Soyez (2015)	Social media applications
Costa Fabricio F Costa (2013)	PatientsLikeMe social network
Egea et al. (2015)	Adoption of Internet technologies by physicians

Figure 2. IT and Medical evolution
Source: Adapted from Fabricio F. Costa (2013)

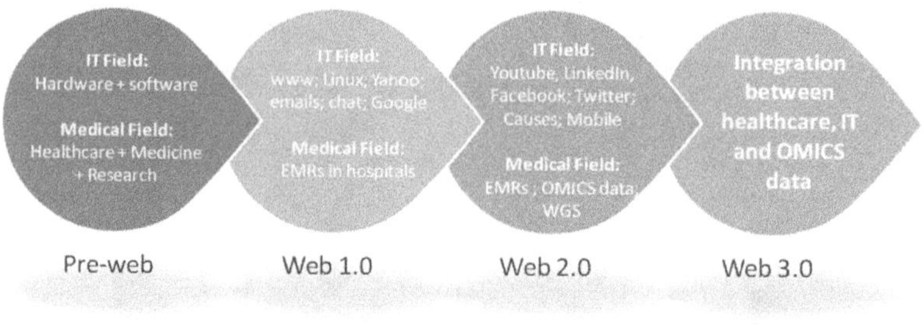

support systems, electronic management of chronic disease, and bar coding of drugs and biological products can reduce health care costs and medical errors (Ammenwerth, Schnell-Inderst, Machan, & Siebert, 2008; Bates et al., 1998), as well as improve the communication between all stakeholders (Lau, 2011; McGowan et al., 2012). However, implementation of these information technologies has lagged in most European nations as well as the United States, leaving a question unanswered: *if the adoption of ICT has so many positive contributions, why it's use still so reduce and controversial?*

The quest for revealing this answer leads us to the second dimension – *acceptance* – and to its four different domains: social and ethical barriers; interoperability of systems; technology organizational environment and end-users acceptance.

ICT adoption and especially internet use is rapidly changing the landscape of health information (Ahmad et al., 2006; Sharma, Kilian, & Leung, 2014). Nevertheless, the potential arise from this electronic elements is far bigger then what is been explore. The full capacity use is still constrained by social and ethical barriers.

The work of Fabricio F. Costa (2013) added to this field by incorporating the technology as a catalyst and enhancer of healthcare over time (see Figure 2).

Since web 2.0, big data start to be used and in these processes the primary stakeholders in the decision of, and the impact of, are the patients, the researchers, and the other healthcare providers. Additionally, it can be considered in the participations of payers and other regulators. With web 3.0, genetic, genomic and other "OMICS" information tends to be integrated to help services providers to deliver a person-driven healthcare.

Thus, as mention by Jensen et al. (2009) and reinforce by Fabricio F. Costa (2013) and Brothers and Rothstein (2015), clients' questions regarding data privacy and security led to smaller rates of implementation of electronic health systems. By one hand, the legal frames in different countries constrain the use and electronic diffusion of patients' records. By other hand the patient and the physician have ethical and personal concerns regarding the adoption of these tools, especially when these enable the access by third parts (Brothers & Rothstein, 2015).

Lucas (2008) examining the adoption of ICT in developing countries uncover some of the potential problems related to the technology environment of each business unit. To this author in the short term is quite easy to have goods results driven from the adoption of ICT. Nevertheless, this initial small-scale success aren't guarantee of sustainable large-scale benefits or even long term success. The main reasons for this septic framework are related to robustness of sophisticated electronic equipment; the availability of technical staff to operate, maintain and support the equipment adopt; the complexity of hardware and software failures; the adequate training programs; the proper funding to finance routine operating expenses, maintenance costs and the frequent needs for upgrades; and the end-users commitment and knowledge regarding the system benefits and applications.

The second dimension is related to interoperability of the information systems, since healthcare providers use information systems with several different types of data and user interfaces (Macedo & Isaías, 2009) and standardized output is need. Until recently, IT products available for healthcare providers were mostly designed for large organizations and were costly. And, as Brannigan (1985) suggested, the major problem with IT acquisition is not the initial decision process, but the complete final analyses of adequacy of the system to the health care providers needs. Technical verification and validation are important keys during system development, but their validation after implementation is critical.

The fast and growing adoption, combine with the need to evaluate the outcome of the investment, include the "technology assessment" as a crucial element of health policy (Fischer & Soyez, 2015). Thus, back in 1990, in a conference held in Montpellier, Flagle et al. (1991) stated out the importance of (1) ''develop a dialogue between the fields of medical informatics and Health Technology Assessment''; and (2) ''to issuing recommendations about the methodological requirements for evaluating Health Information Systems''.

As research in other fields suggests, the adoption and acceptance of ICT tools requires a set of human, organizational and technological conditions. Since the seventies, research on information systems has contribute to a better understanding of the advantages related to the use of IS and the facilitators factors of an ICT acceptance process (Hadgkiss & Renzaho, 2014; Pilat, 2004). The work of Davies (1989) brought some light to his matter, introducing a new framework of analysis – Technological Acceptance Model and since then several studies have been conducted analyzing the adoption of technologies by end users (T. C. Davis et al., 1993). On his model, Davis examines the mediating role of perceived ease of use and perceived usefulness in their relation between systems characteristics (external variables) and the probability of system use (an indicator of system success). An update version of his research -TAM2- has presented several years later and the overall results explain almost 40% of systems use. In both works the emphasis has been set on end users performance. This model has been test in healthcare sector (M.-Y. Chang et al., 2015; Hu, Chau, Sheng, & Tam, 1999; Raitoharju, 2005) and the results pointed to the fact that individual impacts are often neglected when evaluating ICT initiatives as well as the IT stress as a factor of IT acceptance.

Another approach is to analyze the customization of the systems to healthcare providers' main characteristics. Considering the strong push for clinical leadership in the development and procurement of information technology in health care, it's surprising the lack of clinical input acknowledge by IT system' developers (Heathfield, Pitty, & Hanka, 1998).

The lack of participation and commitment to the system implementation and outcome continuous to be consider the major factor in the failure of information technology in health services (Lucas, 2008). More recent work has built on the practice perspective recognizing the importance of contextual environment in ICT adoption. Existing work practices may shape and be shaped by the introduction of new ICTs (Egea et al., 2015; Hadgkiss & Renzaho, 2014).

Back in the earliest nineties, Tornatzky and Fleischer (1990) present a framework which assess technological and organizational environment through three key dimensions - the organizational context, technological context and the surrounding context. Since then, the TOE model has been widely used, since it helps to understand the technological path of the firm.

Papastathopoulou (2007) and Peansupap and Walker (2005), present two other strong reasons that tend to influence greatly the way firms handle the acceptance and implementation of ICTs: the level of investment involved and failure rates or past experiences of failure associated with the implementation of ICT applications. These ideas introduce us in to the fourth dimension: *financing*.

Despise the reports revealing that electronic medical records provide financial benefits by helping to reduce costs and improve revenues, few formal cost-benefit analyses have been performance (Jennings et al., 2015). Wang et al (2003) analyzed the results obtain by organizations during a 5 year period driven from the adoption of ICT. According to these authors the healthcare firm had two majors costs associated with this implementation: systems cost, which are related to system implementation, support and maintenance; and induce cost, which are related to the process of converting paper-base operations in digital operations. These two domains had an overall cost of almost $50.000, which was lower than the benefits achieved of $86.400. The benefits obtained in the process were found to be especially savings in drug expenditure, reduction of cost in radiology and decreasing of billing expenditure costs. Similar conclusions were found in the work of Ruland and Ravn (2003), Hillestad et al. (2005) and Lapointe and Rivard (2006). However, traditional financial and accounting methods of evaluation are not totally suitable in this case, because there are some intangible, indirect and even strategic benefits related to IT implementation that need to be considered (Grembergen & Amelinckx, 2002).

Looking at the healthcare sector, back in the 70s, among others authors, Ware, Davies and Stewart (1977) suggested the increasing importance of customer/patient satisfaction with medical and healthcare services. Almost four decades after those statements, patients' satisfaction remains a critical aspect; however, as services literature notes, the need for employees' satisfaction is a driver for customers' satisfaction, since the healthcare service outcome is dependent on their performance (Anderson, Fornell, & Rust, 1997). Several studies conducted to measure patients' overall satisfaction confirm the importance of physicians and nurses in this process (Jennings et al., 2015).

The fifth dimension comprises the *adoption* of different healthcare information technologies to improve the quality of healthcare services. In this sense, improving the quality of care and customer satisfaction are key factors that need to be considered and that can push healthcare providers to adopt more ICT tools (Hung et al., 2010). These tools can improve services quality, since it changes the model of health services delivery (Jennings et al., 2015). Some examples of such services include educating patients about their diseases, online follow-ups, monitoring of symptoms, and clarifying doubts about diseases. To support these new services, adoption healthcare providers can exploit different IT applications.

Innovative companies found that Web 2.0 collaborative applications could be introduced in their current or new implementations of intranets, bringing them advantages in internal communication with employees. Given the characteristics of blogs, RSS and wikis, they are the most used Web 2.0 tools to facilitate communication, collaboration and sharing of internal information.

Several studies have examined the Web 2.0 intranets tools (Lai & Turban, 2008; Richter, Stocker, Müller, & Avram, 2013) and the outcomes of their use:

- **Wikis:** Collaboration, audit, internal training, knowledge management;
- **Blogs:** in-house training, communication, sharing, definition of social responsibility, knowledge management;
- **RSS:** News, information and knowledge management.

At a macro level, these information flows can promote inward sharing, outward sharing, inbound sharing and outbound sharing (Drapeau & Wells, 2009; Murphy, 2010). Looking at the inward sharing in healthcare organizations, the mere fact that providers belong to small groups who work together within the organization improves their subjective wellbeing, and allows them to share knowledge easily between colleagues to gain expert status, to collect feedback and to improve overall job satisfaction (Murphy, 2010).

The outbound level and the outward sharing have gained relevance in the past decade with the explosive growth of the Internet, which stimulated social behaviour exchanges and consequently modified human daily activities, habits and interactions. Online communities explore the ubiquity of the web and bring people together from all over the globe, allowing them to share knowledge and promote a collective dialog (Budden, Anthony, Budden, & Jones, 2011; Kumar et al., 2010).

In this context, healthcare institutions were forced to adopt a user-centric model that doesn't focus on diseases, but on the user as an involved member of the decision-making process, with capabilities to choose between different health options and preventive health behaviors. As a result, the "P4 Medicine" model seeks to change the medicine perspective from reactive to proactive, aiming to maximize individual health rather than just treat the causes of disease. The P4 in this model stands for: predictive, preventive, personalized, and participatory (Fabricio F Costa, 2013).

On the second and fourth P, the use of social networks leverages the doctor/patient interaction, allowing the sharing of information among patients as the network (Fabricio F Costa, 2013). A good example is the PatientsLikeMe social network.

The potential of social networks and other Web 2.0 tools to establish new health services cannot be ignored. These services are known as Healthy 2.0, which reflects the use of social media by health professionals and patients in order to customize treatments and promote health education (Sharma et al., 2014).

Several studies analyzed the adoption of social networking to mediate the communication flows between organizations and patients, and unveiled the most common applications: health information and dissemination campaigns, and tele-assistance and monitoring. But these studies also revealed that social networks are been used by patients as a community in order to share and search information and experiences with peers, to keep and search medication information, and to use an interactive medication database (Fabricio F Costa, 2013; Dhillon, Wünsche, & Lutteroth, 2013; Sharma et al., 2014).

More, this approach leads to the use of OMICS and other big data driven-content, but also requires a human-IT approach that enhances the adoption and use of technology by all stakeholders (Fischer & Soyez, 2015).

So, the question that remains unanswered is: if technology enables healthcare providers' to deliver a high quality service, why some many are reluctant to engage in a more digital service? This question finds a partial answer in the legal domain, since some of the inhibitors found in the literature are related with legal risk and privacy concerns (Classen et al., 2011).

The last dimension cover refers to *policy and legislation* and finish what can be consider as the cycle of adoption of ICT in healthcare (see, Figure 1). In this domain there are no general rules and guides, since it's deeply associated with national health systems policy and they differ from one country to another. Nevertheless, there are some common points that need to be considered: patients' privacy rights and their legal protection (Jensen et al., 2009); security standards which allow a common language between players (Gritzalis, 1997); and, clinicians activity rules and structure (Buntin et al., 2011).

The Council of European Professional Informatics Societies, back in 2005, produce a report considering the Standardization for ICT Security and one of the sections was devoted to analyze the ICT security standards for healthcare applications. The authors advocate that Health informatics standards were essential to achieve the goals of e-Health in Europe, supporting interoperability between systems and patient information exchange between health organizations and protecting patients and clinicians' privacy rights. Pirnejad et al. (2007) suggested that the first steps in establishing an international application with adequate data protection safeguards rely in building an Inter-organizational communication network (IOCN) in healthcare with appropriated strategies safeguarding security measures. For instance, in the European case the directive "CEN EN14484 (2003) International transfer of Personal health data" covered data protection and established specific terms of exchange data with third countries.

Although healthcare researchers and information system investigators have studied ICT adoption to some extent, there are still few conceptual bases available to assess the global information and communication technology contribution to overall healthcare business success. There is also limited data regarding the combined acceptance and adoptions of these ICT tools by physicians, nurses and patients. When analyzing these assessments with a business-value approach, weaknesses assume a major role. Therefore, the next section attempts to minimize these gaps.

CONCEPTUAL FRAMEWORK AND HIPOTHESES

In the last three decades information technology in health care has existed and has gained widespread usage (Ammenwerth et al., 2004). Nevertheless, there are also hazards related with information technology in health care driven from the challenges and innovations adoption process and measurement.

For more than a decade it is widely believed that broad adoption of electronic medical record (EMR) systems will lead to major health care savings, reduce medical errors, and improve health care services (Marques, Oliveira, Dias, & Martins, 2011). However, the measurement of ICT impacts covers the assessment of the quality, value and their applications in the health care environment, the improvement of health information applications and the enabling of an evidence-based health informatics practice.

Thus, as it happens in other industries, the cost-benefits evaluation of IT implementation cannot be performed only base in traditional financial and accounting methods. Literature review revealed some intangible, indirect and even strategic benefits related to IT implementation that need to be considered, most of them common in IT domain (Grembergen & Amelinckx, 2002). Thus, there is undoubtedly a need to develop a better comprehension of ICT healthcare adoption impacts on global results.

The application of IT literature in this subject may shed some light on the measurement of the success of these initiatives (Romano Jr & Fjermestad, 2001). Yoon et al. (1995) suggested a framework based on five levels: business profitability, improved decision performance, level of system usage, perceived benefits and user satisfaction. The work of Eder and Igbaria (2001) analyses the impact of ICT on business performance and stressed that there are some indirect effects which need to be consider. More recently, Bayo-Moriones and Lera-López (Bayo-Moriones et al., 2013; 2007) suggested that the positive impacts identified are not limited to increased productivity and reduced costs, influencing intermediate performance measures such as process efficiency, quality of services, organizational improvements, knowledge flows and customer satisfaction.

These last elements (quality of services, knowledge flows and customer satisfaction) can be improved by technology, but as mentioned previously, are dependent on end-user acceptance and adoption (I. Chang, 2007; Holden & Karsh, 2010; Jennings et al., 2015). From previous works, three sets of players need to be considered when adopting an HIS: patients (Hall & Dornan, 1988; Norum, Grev, Moen, Balteskard, & Holthe, 2003; Scalone et al., 2008); nurses (Abbott & Coenen, 2008; Verdegem & Verhoest, 2009) and physicians (Egea et al., 2015; Hunt, Haynes, Hanna, & Smith, 1998; Van Der Meijden, Tange, Troost, & Hasman, 2003; Verdegem & Verhoest, 2009).

In order to improve the success of information technology implementations, different models grounded in behavioral science or using theories that identify conditions and determinants of success are used (M.-Y. Chang et al., 2015; Hadgkiss & Renzaho, 2014; Heathfield et al., 1998; Holden & Karsh, 2010; Hunt et al., 1998; Mathieson, 1991; Norum et al., 2003). Nevertheless, as IT literature has evolved, these models have been tested separately and in a more-or-less restricted set of IT implementation procedures. In the healthcare setting, user behavior is influenced not only by the end-user personal framework, but also by a multifactor structure at the group, organizational and patient level. In this context, the defining of suitable multi-level intervention has been overlooked and this is the gap that the current research attempts to fulfill.

Figure 3. Conceptual Model

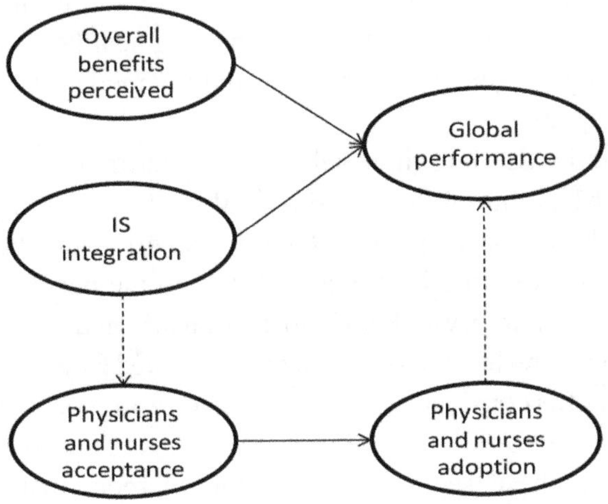

For this purpose, a significantly modified version of the original TAM was used, integrating the concepts presented by King & He (2006), and considering the relationships among the three main TAM variables—perceived ease of use, perceived usefulness and behavioral intention to use—and considering the three sets of players.

The research model, as shown in Figure 3, illustrates an examination of the productivity flows considering not only the operational process but also intangibles domains, which affects healthcare systems adoption and results. This framework also identifies metrics that can be used to measure the intangibles benefits. Each perspective is evaluated according to the appropriate metrics.

The primary research question to consider is this: What are the benefits engages in performance, considering it as global productivity increasing, trough the implementation of ICT? And what is the impact of operational process (integrated IS) on global productivity performance? Besides measuring the convergence of a technological approach with a business value approach, our aim is to discover the direct nature of the impact of intangible benefits in healthcare firms' outcome.

The model is validated by using a structure equation model to test the hypotheses. The measurement model is done by using Confirmatory Factor Analysis (CFA). We will see later that the observable variables (indicators) we selected are measures of latent variables (factors). We assume that IT process and benefits driven from organization acceptance of IT have a direct effect on successful IS application. Therefore, we assume that the healthcare productivity performance gains are explained not only by the standard use of information systems, but also by the perceptions of organizational, technical and productivity gains.

Two sets of postulates were put together: first, considering as a theoretical base for the development of these postulates the literature on information systems and healthcare fields that evaluates the factors impacting healthcare performance; and, second, considering as a theoretical background the models related to technology adoption and acceptance.

The first is subdivided into three subsets and measures the impact of the three different kinds of benefits; following the results found by other researchers and bringing to HIS the measurement of intangible benefits already consider in other IT domains. The induce benefits are consider as all the benefits arise in terms of security, efficiency, reliability and staff satisfaction driven from the adoption of ICT. The financial benefits reflect the financial gains resulted from ICT implementation. The structural benefits consider the gains obtained from process modifications and operational cost reductions.

The second hypothesis seeks to confirm the inference that there is a positive impact of overall benefits on global healthcare productivity and consequently on healthcare firms' performance. The third hypothesis sought to identify a positive impact of the interoperability and integration of IS on global productivity performance, as an agent driving the optimize adoption and use of ICTs.

Another set of three questions was defined for each different set of players, based on the conceptual model present by King & He (2006). Therefore, the fourth hypothesis considers that the perceived ease of use of the implemented system impacts positively the acceptance of global HIS. The fifth proposition considers that healthcare providers' perception of the ICT usefulness impacts positively the acceptance of HIS. The last hypothesis advocates that behavioral intention, driven from personal past experiences and expectations, impacts positively HIS acceptance.

DATA TREATMENT AND RESULTS

To validate the first set of assumptions, data was collected from a sample of 834 European healthcare firms in a total of 17 countries (Belgium, Bulgaria, Czech Republic, Denmark, Finland, Greece, Spain, France, Hungary, Ireland, Italy, Latvia, The Netherlands, Norway, Poland, Sweden and UK) and covering seven dimensions of analysis: (1) ICT infrastructure and e-business software systems; (2) automated data exchange; (3) e-standards and interoperability issues; (4) Innovation activity of the company; (5) ICT skills requirements and ICT costs; (6) ICT impacts, drivers and inhibitors; and (7) background information about the company.

Initially we used a set of descriptive statistics that allowed for a greater sensitivity to the data (Sekaran, 2006). Such descriptive statistics also acted as guide for the multivariate statistics later on performed (Hair, Anderson, Tatham, & Black, 1998). Some notes about the sample used.

Distribution of firm size, measured by the number of employees, shows that almost half of the firms are micro- and small-size firms (around 50.7%). Around 99% of the firms in the sample have access to Internet and from those 28.7% use a wireless access. The importance of having ICT department at firm structure was measure and 49% of the sample currently employs ICT practitioners. The importance give to the lack of ICT department was measure by their impact on global ICT strategy and management (37.5% considers it a great deal), in ICT network architecture (56.4% considers it a huge concern), in ICT security (52.1% consider important) and maintenance (35.4% consider it important).

When asked about the IT solutions adopted by their firms, the highest percentage of respondents refers the use of pharmacy management system, as we can observe in the following figure 4.

The model was estimated by the Maximum Likelihood method in the AMOS package. The model goodness of fit may be considered acceptable according to the values of some goodness-of-fit index, although the chi-square test statistic ($\chi 2$ = 626,4; df =321; p-value = 0,000) is significant, implying a bad fit. However, as is well known, this test has serious limitations — namely its dependence on the sample size and on the number of indicators. In general, for large sample sizes the chi-square statistic is significant, and in the present case the sample size is quite large (n = 834) (Hair et al., 1998). For that reason, it is usual to evaluate the goodness of the fit by a set of index, also presented in Figure 4.

After global model fit has been assessed, the numerical results were evaluated in order to test their support of the research question. The numerical results can be obtained directly from the path coefficients of the structural model presented in Figure 5. We refer to standardised coefficients that account for scale effects and serve as indicators of the relative importance of the variables.

The measures for global model fit included in Figure 5 suggest that our model fits the underlying data well (Hair et al., 1998) and all the paths were statistically significant.

Our findings generally support the conceptual framework previously presented. The three dimensions used to compose the overall benefits achieved trough ICT adoption are all significant and validate trough the confirmatory factor analysis performed. Induce benefits, financial benefits and structural benefits explained 76 percent, 72 percent and 79 percent respectively regarding the variance in the overall benefits construct. As a result, hypothesis H1 is not rejected. A reference needs to be made regarding the relative similar value achieved in terms of financial benefits, reinforcing the perspective token in this research.

Figure 4. Percentage of adoption of different HIS

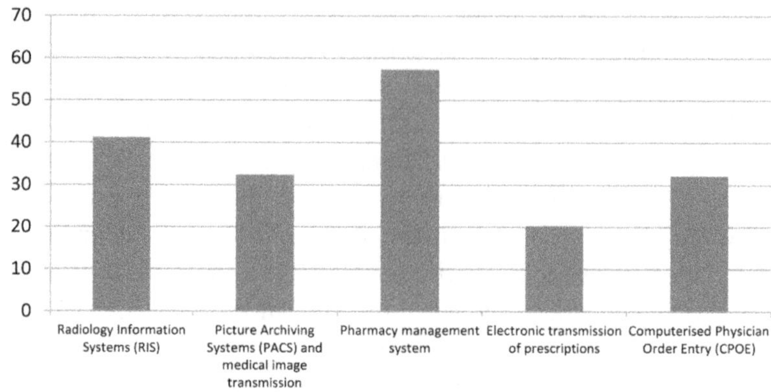

The results also allow concluding that the overall benefits contribute with 59 percent to global performance, so hypothesis H2 is not rejected.

The indirect effects existent in the model were also assessed. From those arises the strong relationship between interoperability of HIS and reduction of cost.

On the other hand, the results show that the construct "integrated IS", which is related to the interoperability between HIS present in the firm, contributes with 81 percent to global performance, implying that our hypothesis H3 is confirmed.

Figure 5. Structural equation model and estimation results (model 1)

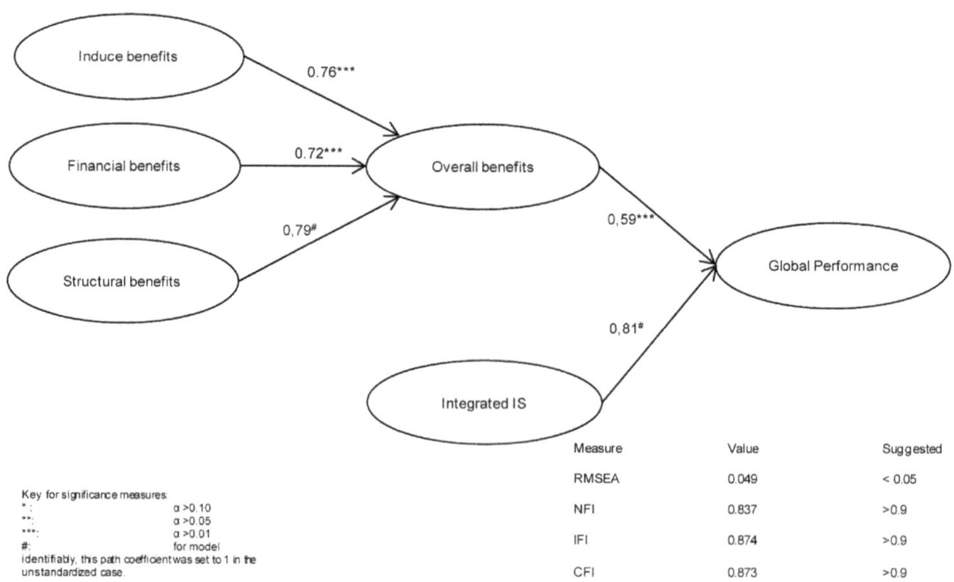

A last note needs to be made relative to the value achieved in this path, which is greater than the relationship found between overall benefits and global productivity.

To validate the second subset of assumptions, data was collected from a sample of Portuguese physicians and nurses, covering four dimensions of analysis: 1) perceptions regarding the ease of use of current systems, 2) perceptions regarding impact of use, 3) behavioural intention to use ICT tools, and 4) past experience and demographics. Taking into consideration that the TAM will produce different results if the users being questioned have a) used the technology being tested previously and b) had a choice in whether to use the technology, the questionnaire will target healthcare providers with experience in the use of HIS.

Again, we used a set of descriptive statistics that allowed for a greater sensitivity to the data. As shown below, the sample has a higher representation of nurses, and in both profiles, the average age is quite low. This reflects the higher propensity of the millennial generation to use ICT tools, since the sample only gathered the data of individuals who actually used technology (see Figure 6).

All physicians use a computer at the hospital or clinic where they operate, other than the EMR, but only 23% report using it in private clinic. Looking closely at the perceived ease of use of electronic patient records, female physicians present a more positive perception of this tool: 50% consider EPR very easy to use. Since there seems to exist a significant difference between female and male physicians (Gefen & Straub, 1997; Lu, Yu, Liu, & Yao, 2003; Venkatesh & Morris, 2000), the analysis was performed based on perceived gender differences. All nurses refer to using a computer for their daily records and show evidence of having a longer experience in doing so (average time of usage: 5 years). Regarding the physician-patient rela-

Figure 6. Demographic profile of healthcare providers' using ICT tools

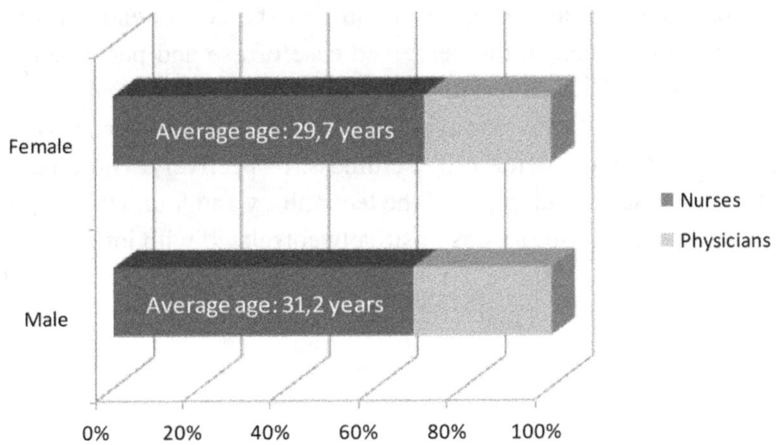

Figure 7. Structural equation model and estimation results (model 2)

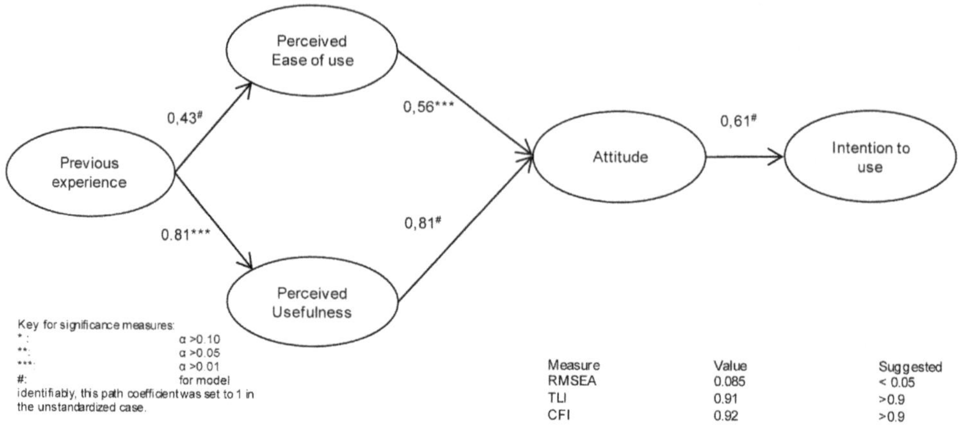

tionship, physicians are not convinced that the use of EMR improves the quality of medical care received by patients (44.7%), but 65.8% believe that it helps them perform better. Looking at nurses' answers, 56% believe that EMR does not improve the quality of medical care received by patients.

A second structural model was estimated by the Maximum Likelihood method in the AMOS package. After global model fit was assessed, the numerical results were evaluated in order to test their support of the research question. The numerical results can be obtained directly from the path coefficients of the structural model presented in Figure 7. We refer to standardised coefficients that account for scale effects and serve as indicators of the relative importance of the variables.

When performing multi-group analysis, the sample size of the groups being compared should be roughly equal. Since, in our sample, the number of nurses was larger, it wasn't possible to perform a multi-group analysis.

Once more, our findings, in general, support the conceptual framework. The dimensions used to compose the perceived ease of use and perceived usefulness are all significant and validate with the confirmatory factor analysis performed. Previous experience with the use of IT systems explained 43 and 81 percent of perceived ease of use and perceived usefulness, respectively. These results unveil some difficulties with the adoption of the technology and found that support of the attitude toward using ICT tools was positively correlated with intention behaviour. A note needs to be made relative to the value achieved in perceived usefulness and attitude towards use, which is greater than the relationship found between perceived ease of use and attitude.

DISCUSSION AND CONCLUSION

The digital era bring with it enormous challenges that healthcare firms can embrace, especially if we consider the facilities associated with the gathering of information about customers, suppliers, markets, and supply — and the easy processing of information regarding processes, and services, which can also be easily spread to the clients and other publics.

Even though academic researchers and practitioners alike praise information and communication technologies adoption (M.-Y. Chang et al., 2015; Hadgkiss & Renzaho, 2014; Marques et al., 2011), perhaps the most significant gap in the literature is the lack of large-scale empirical evidence showing that ICT makes a difference to the overall performance of the firm and determining which factors are critical to leverage overall performance.

The goal of the current study was twofold: 1) to identify the nature of the relationship between overall performance and these benefits, as well as the relationship with interoperability of HIS; and 2) to determine if the individual's acceptance of a technology is determined by its perceived usefulness and perceived ease of use. For this purpose, a set of propositions were developed: the first relies on exploring the nature of the benefits that can be achieved during the implementation and use of ICT tools; the second is based on the relationship between these benefits and healthcare performance; the third relies on the fact that most healthcare firms use more than one HIS, and for that reason, interoperability between all the systems can be crucial to global performance; the fourth and fifth predict that ease of use and usefulness will influence an individual's attitudes toward, intention to use, and acceptance of the technology. Therefore, our aim is to develop a new interpretation that offers fresh insights and understanding.

Given the nature of relationship between variables that is consider, the use of structural equation model is suitable. Based on the results of our two models, we can draw the following conclusions:

- Bayo-Moriones and Lera-López (2007) reported that the positive impacts occurred in an organization were not limited to increased productivity and reduced costs, but also influencing intermediate performance measures. The present work reinforces these ideas in the healthcare sector, presenting induces benefits achieved from ICT adoption.
- When comparing our results with the ones found by Egea et al. (2015), who also study European healthcare providers relationship with technologies, a positive trend seems to appear. This might be a sign that Europeans are more willing to adopt technologies which is fairly positive if considering the down-

turn economic context and that those TI-solutions are quite effective in lower-resource settings.

- Our results confirmed some prior research regarding the relationship between interoperability of HIS and global performance (Macedo & Isaías, 2009; M. B. Tiago & Tiago, 2013), since we found a strong relationship between these constructs. In addition, indirect effects were also found, especially between interoperability of HIS and reduction of cost, which is an important dimension of global performance.
- Even though prior research on HIS field does not consider the intangible benefits of an adoption of ICT, we can empirically show that induce benefits influences the composition of total benefits. It means that this tendency, already observed in other IS domains, needs to be considered when evaluating the outcome of ICT investments.
- We validate the construct of global healthcare performance integrating measurement metrics besides the financial and accounting, following the path introduce by the work of Grembergen and Amelinckx (2002) and already tested in other domains (Maria Teresa Borges Tiago, Couto, Tiago, & Vieira, 2007; M.T.B. Tiago, Couto, Tiago, & Vieira, 2008).
- Our results also point to the existence of relevant benefits driven from structural processes which suffer improvements from the adoption of ICT, in line with Eder and Igbaria (2001), that had suggested the impact of some indirect effects on firms performance due to the use of ICT.
- The most surprising fact is, however, related to the relative contribution of financial benefits to total benefits. Since this is the most common dimension of analysis adopted by firms, we were expecting to find here the biggest contribution of all three dimensions. But, regardless your expectation, the impact found was strong but the smallest of all three.
- When looking at the results of the second sample, gender and age differences were found in terms of ICT adoption and benefit perceptions, which was already suggested in previous works (Gefen & Straub, 1997; Lu et al., 2003; Venkatesh & Morris, 2000).
- In the work of McGowan, et al (2012) focusing on social media usage by physicians, the authors stated that the frequency of usage is influenced primarily by positive attitudes toward the technology, perceiving that the technology is easy to use, and perceiving the technology to be useful to achieve better performance outcomes. Similar results were found in our sample.
- Our results also point to a lower relationship between perceived ease of use and attitude. These results might reflect the minimal training and customization of the IT systems used in the healthcare facilities in the sample.

- Our results didn't allow us to conclude if there was statistical evidence that physicians' and nurses have different behavior intentions regarding ICT. However, looking at the data we can infer that regarding to ICT acceptance and adoption the outcomes are not significantly different, which is quite unique when compare with the results from other studies regarding cost and quality of service provided by nurses and physicians (Jennings et al., 2015).

We caution readers to consider that the induce benefits and structural dimensions of HIS await future research and that the conclusions presented are related to the present samples used. For these reasons they cannot be generalized.

Issues, Controversies, Problems

It is often stated that healthcare is lagging in the rear of others sectors of our society when it comes to the adoption and use of ICT. If we look carefully at healthcare organizations strategic choices in terms of investment in this area, we still notice that the investments are consider as pilot projects and are disperse and with reduce or none IS architecture. This limited investment in ICT has been a rational choice since the measurement of the gains is still scarce. Besides, compensation mechanisms, public recognition and pressure, and consumer demand have not created a strong enough incentive for healthcare organizations to accept the financial costs and face up to the non-financial obstacles to ICT implementation.

However, the fast growth of web-based platforms that facilitate online social behavior has significantly modified the nature of human activities, habitats, and interactions (T. Tiago & Veríssimo, 2014). And service providers that neglect ICT investments are clearly loosing focus on consumer, regardless of the industry.

One of the major challenges concerning the ICT adoption is end users' acceptance. But who are these end users? Until a few years, the healthcare sector was focused on internal stakeholders. With the evolution of both medical and IT fields, the focus shift and started to integrate external stakeholders too.

From an internal perspective, if it is a common domain to recognize related to ICT adoption the reduction of medical errors, delays and misdiagnosis. But, it's also common to find references to the reduction of human relation or contact between physicians, patients and nurses. Thus, if for some this is a benefic consequence of ICT, for others, it is a lack of conformity that is damaging the outcome of the service. In short, if healthcare providers were rewarded for safety and quality results, they would be more likely to invest in ICT and promote an IT culture inside healthcare services stakeholders.

From a patient perspective, there is a wide range of benefits that can be achieved from the use of ICT, such as efficiency, convenience, richer and participate information, and social network application. As previously mentioned the Healthy 2.0 model answers to some of the challenges that the healthcare sector faces (Fabricio F. Costa, 2013). Again, this model relies on the end-user's acceptance and adoption, meaning that healthcare providers need to be motivated to adopt a digitally active posture.

Considering that for patients and relatives, through information communication technologies have a number of benefits including efficiency, convenience, richer and participative information, and accessibility, is relatively common to find these participants on social networks and in search motors looking for answers. With semantic web, big data and new OMICS technologies have been targeted, since it can enable a more efficient, low-cost and large-scale generation and analysis of biomedical data and personalize IT-driven healthcare service.

Especially considering that in the near future information sharing among the various health-specific social networks, and with the generic social networks (Facebook, Twitter), using Web 3.0 technology will improve the patient/provider relationship in all 4P's, paving the way for the development of new IT tools, such as Healthy 3.0.

However, the adoption of a Healthy 3.0 scenario requires that healthcare providers consider that the information and the digital sharing are trustworthy and valid. Additionally, it requires that they are ready to adopt these technologies and ultimately embrace them as a format for providing new services and lifelong learning.

In the meantime, governments and national service entities try to develop mechanisms through policy and legislation to minimize the effects of these inhibitors' and promote ICT standardization and capable pathways within the national service frameworks.

In essence, the ICT adoption process reveals six dimensions that need to be consider in order achieving success and points out to the importance of three major players in the process: physicians, patients or clients and nurses. If all these stakeholders are awareness of the benefits of ICT to the entire organization, the acceptance of ICT will be easier and the financial and productivity gains are greater. Thus, we can consider that the success of these initiatives relies on developing an ICT environment inside and outside the healthcare firm.

Solutions and Recommendations

Our comments are given with Portugal as main background for the healthcare sector together with a global understanding of the healthcare systems in other European countries and the USA. So, looking at the model present in this study several considerations can be made.

The first suggestion we make is related with acknowledge by all stakeholders the total benefits and not only the financial benefits of ICT implementation. In order to overall acknowledge of induce and structure benefits, a communication strategy

Figure 8. Healthy 3.0: healthcare digital dimensions

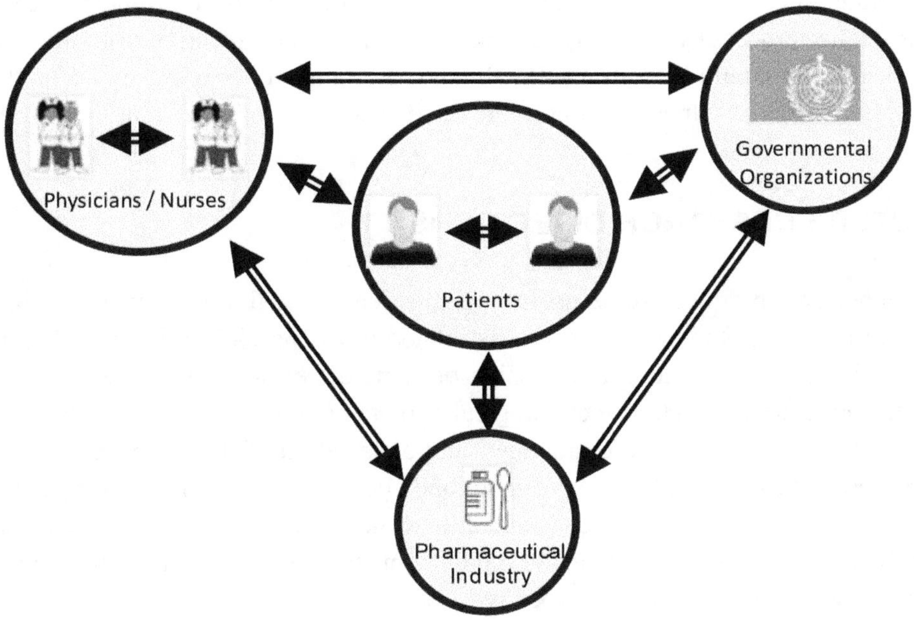

needs to be set considering the three different major players: clients, physicians and nurses and their contact points with ICT. For instance, the communication with the last two publics can be executed trough training and public recognition of the outcomes. The success of this process relies on multiple actors' structure, as shown in Figure 8.

Therefore, our suggestions included reinforcing harmonization activities between the existing entities of a national health system (NHS), starting with the clear identification of the players and their specific needs, followed by the development of specific ITS base on the identified needs. Afterwards, a certification procedure for e-health standards and adoptions should be promote, considering that such a process would allow interoperability of systems and the increasing of end-user orientation.

Since the orientation should be focus on the end-user several actions should take place. Regarding health services clients, the emphasis needs to be on demystifying the concerns related to privacy and security. In this process, communication plays a crucial role and needs to reflect the organizations' commitment in leverage digital technologies to provide better, ubiquitous and less expensive services to customers.

The other two types of end-users should sense the support of their board, which is clear when auscultation during ITS development and implementation occurs; training and customization of ICT tools is provide; and global and personal efforts are recognize and compensate.

With the adoption of this matrix the intangible benefits can be identify and enlarge and interoperability of systems is assured. Nonetheless, to promote an easier acceptance process by inside players, the start timing and executive commitment is critical. This should be combined with the use of a team of expert innovators that will have as goals educate and promote the development of an IT culture.

FUTURE RESEARCH DIRECTIONS

This research produces some useful insights, leaving still a number of issues for future research. One of these issues is related to the possibility of extending the study in order to consider an inclusion of some dimensions of the technological acceptance model, such as technological personal readiness. Similarly, this study could be expanded covering the views and expectation of the three main players consider in this work: physicians, nurses and clients. The analysis of their perspective on this matter can reinforce some of the conclusions achieved, challenge some of the outcomes of this work and certainly contribute to a deeper understanding of healthcare IS evolution and prospective.

Another path to follow regards the new ways of healthcare delivery, the new public and their solicitations. This will require additional IS functionalities, been an interesting field for future research.

CONCLUSION

The results generated some interesting findings. First, the data support our conceptualization for the global benefits construct. Within global benefits elements, all have a positive impact on the maximization of firms ICT-driven benefits and consequently global performance. Secondly, the findings allow us to conclude that induce benefits have a positive indirect impact on global productivity. Thus, financial and intangible benefits appear to greater than what was usual accounted, paying back the initial investments made by the healthcare firms. Nonetheless, the size of the effect for this relationship was smaller than would be expected.

According to these results, the concept of integrated systems as an important dimension of overall results equation is reinforced. So, managers should consider the use of HIS competencies to improve everyday services process. Namely, taking advantage of the benefits such as reducing structural and operational costs, increasing employees' motivation and satisfaction, improving services quality as pointed out by others researches.

More, healthcare providers should be motivated to adopt ICT tools as an important opportunity to engage customers and perform a high-quality service.

REFERENCES

Abbott, P. A., & Coenen, A. (2008). Globalization and advances in information and communication technologies: The impact on nursing and health. *Nursing Outlook, 56*(5), 238-246. e232.

Ahmad, F., Hudak, P. L., Bercovitz, K., Hollenberg, E., & Levinson, W. (2006). Are Physicians Ready for Patients With Internet-Based Health Information? *Journal of Medical Internet Research, 8*(3), e22. doi:10.2196/jmir.8.3.e22 PMID:17032638

Ammenwerth, E., Brender, J., Nykanen, P., Prokosch, H. U., Rigby, M., & Talmon, J. (2004). Visions and strategies to improve evaluation of health information systems: Reflections and lessons based on the HIS-EVAL workshop in Innsbruck. *International Journal of Medical Informatics, 73*(6), 479–491. doi:10.1016/j.ijmedinf.2004.04.004 PMID:15171977

Ammenwerth, E., Gräber, S., Herrmann, G., Bürkle, T., & König, J. (2003). Evaluation of health information systems--problems and challenges. *International Journal of Medical Informatics, 71*(2-3), 125–135. doi:10.1016/S1386-5056(03)00131-X PMID:14519405

Ammenwerth, E., Schnell-Inderst, P., Machan, C., & Siebert, U. (2008). The effect of electronic prescribing on medication errors and adverse drug events: A systematic review. *Journal of the American Medical Informatics Association, 15*(5), 585–600. doi:10.1197/jamia.M2667 PMID:18579832

Anderson, E. W., Fornell, C., & Rust, R. T. (1997). Customer satisfaction, productivity, and profitability: Differences between goods and services. *Marketing Science, 16*(2), 129–145. doi:10.1287/mksc.16.2.129

Bates, D. W., Leape, L. L., Cullen, D. J., Laird, N., Petersen, L. A., & Teich, J. M. et al. (1998). Effect of Computerized Physician Order Entry and a Team Intervention on Prevention of Serious Medication Errors. *Journal of the American Medical Association, 280*(15), 1311–1316. doi:10.1001/jama.280.15.1311 PMID:9794308

Bayo-Moriones, A., Billón, M., & Lera-López, F. (2013). Perceived performance effects of ICT in manufacturing SMEs. *Industrial Management & Data Systems, 113*(1), 117–135. doi:10.1108/02635571311289700

Bayo-Moriones, A., & Lera-López, F. (2007). A firm-level analysis of determinants of ICT adoption in Spain. *Technovation*, *27*(6-7), 352–366. doi:10.1016/j.technovation.2007.01.003

Brannigan, V. (1985). Acceptance Testing-The Critical Problem in Software Acquisition. *IEEE Transactions on Bio-Medical Engineering*, *BME-32*(4), 295–299. doi:10.1109/TBME.1985.325451 PMID:3838735

Brothers, K. B., & Rothstein, M. A. (2015). Ethical, legal and social implications of incorporating personalized medicine into healthcare. *Personalized Medicine*, *12*(1), 43–51. doi:10.2217/pme.14.65 PMID:25601880

Budden, C. B., Anthony, J. F., Budden, M. C., & Jones, M. A. (2011). Managing the evolution of a revolution: Marketing implications of internet media usage among college students. *College Teaching Methods & Styles Journal (CTMS), 3*(3).

Buntin, M. B., Burke, M. F., Hoaglin, M. C., & Blumenthal, D. (2011). The benefits of health information technology: A review of the recent literature shows predominantly positive results. *Health Affairs*, *30*(3), 464–471. doi:10.1377/hlthaff.2011.0178 PMID:21383365

Chang, I., Hwang, H.-G., Hung, M.-C., Lin, M.-H., & Yen, D. C. (2007). Factors affecting the adoption of electronic signature: Executives' perspective of hospital information department. *Decision Support Systems*, *44*(1), 350–359. doi:10.1016/j.dss.2007.04.006

Chang, M.-Y., Pang, C., Tarn, J. M., Liu, T.-S., & Yen, D. C. (2015). Exploring user acceptance of an e-hospital service: An empirical study in Taiwan. *Computer Standards & Interfaces*, *38*, 35–43. doi:10.1016/j.csi.2014.08.004

Classen, D. C., Resar, R., Griffin, F., Federico, F., Frankel, T., & Kimmel, N. et al. (2011). 'Global trigger tool'shows that adverse events in hospitals may be ten times greater than previously measured. *Health Affairs*, *30*(4), 581–589. doi:10.1377/hlthaff.2011.0190 PMID:21471476

Costa, F. F. (2013). Social networks, web-based tools and diseases: Implications for biomedical research. *Drug Discovery Today*, *18*(5), 272–281. doi:10.1016/j.drudis.2012.10.006 PMID:23103282

Darkins, A., Foster, L., Anderson, C., Goldschmidt, L., & Selvin, G. (2013). The design, implementation, and operational management of a comprehensive quality management program to support national telehealth networks. *Telemedicine Journal and e-Health*, *19*(7), 557–564. doi:10.1089/tmj.2012.0263 PMID:23705961

Davis, F. D., Bagozzi, R. P., & Warshaw, P. R. (1989). User acceptance of computer technology: A comparison of two theoretical models. *Management Science*, *35*(8), 982–1003. doi:10.1287/mnsc.35.8.982

Davis, T. C., Jackson, R. H., George, R. B., Long, S. W., Talley, D., & Murphy, P. W. et al. (1993). Reading ability in patients in substance misuse treatment centers. *Substance Use & Misuse*, *28*(6), 571–582. doi:10.3109/10826089309039648 PMID:8098019

Dewett, T., & Jones, G. R. (2001). The role of information technology in the organization: A review, model, and assessment. *Journal of Management*, *27*(3), 313–346. doi:10.1177/014920630102700306

Dhillon, J. S., Wünsche, B. C., & Lutteroth, C. (2013). *An online social-networking enabled telehealth system for seniors: a case study*. Paper presented at the Fourteenth Australasian User Interface Conference.

Drapeau, M., & Wells, I. (2009). *Social software and national security: An initial net assessment*. DTIC Document.

Eder, L. B., & Igbaria, M. (2001). Determinants of intranet diffusion and infusion. *Omega*, *29*(3), 233–242. doi:10.1016/S0305-0483(00)00044-X

Egea, J. M. O., González, M. V. R., & Menéndez, M. R. (2015). *E-Health Services Adoption by European General Practitioners Assessing the Different Roles of Marketing Theory and Practice in the Jaws of Economic Uncertainty*. Springer.

Fischer, S., & Soyez, K. (2015). *Trick or Treat: Assessing Health 2.0 and Its Prospects for Patients, Providers and Society Challenges and Opportunities in Health Care Management*. Springer.

Flagle, C., Grémy, F., & Perry, S. (1991). *Assessment of Medical Informatics Technology*. Paper presented at the Joint Working Conference.

Fracolli, L. A., Gomes, M. F. P., Nabão, F. R. Z., Santos, M. S., Cappellini, V. K., & Almeida, A. C. C. (2014). Primary health care assessment tools: A literature review and metasynthesis. *Ciencia & Saude Coletiva*, *19*(12), 4851–4860. doi:10.1590/1413-812320141912.00572014 PMID:25388193

Gefen, D., & Straub, D. W. (1997). Gender differences in the perception and use of e-mail: An extension to the technology acceptance model. *Management Information Systems Quarterly*, *21*(4), 389–400. doi:10.2307/249720

Grembergen, W., & Amelinckx, I. (2002). *Measuring and Managing E-business Projects through the Balanced Scorecard*. Paper presented at the 35th Hawaii International Conference on System Science, Hawaii, HI. doi:10.1109/HICSS.2002.994395

Gritzalis, D. (1997). A baseline security policy for distributed healthcare information systems. *Computers & Security*, *16*(8), 709–719. doi:10.1016/S0167-4048(97)00009-6

Hadgkiss, E. J., & Renzaho, A. M. (2014). The physical health status, service utilisation and barriers to accessing care for asylum seekers residing in the community: A systematic review of the literature. *Australian Health Review*, *38*(2), 142–159. PMID:24679338

Hair, J., Anderson, R., Tatham, R., & Black, W. (Eds.). (1998). *Multivariate Data Analysis*. Prentice Hall.

Hall, J. A., & Dornan, M. C. (1988). Meta-analysis of satisfaction with medical care: Description of research domain and analysis of overall satisfaction levels. *Social Science & Medicine*, *27*(6), 637–644. doi:10.1016/0277-9536(88)90012-3 PMID:3067359

Heathfield, H., Pitty, D., & Hanka, R. (1998). Evaluating information technology in health care: Barriers and challenges. *BMJ (Clinical Research Ed.)*, *316*(7149), 1959–1961. doi:10.1136/bmj.316.7149.1959 PMID:9641938

Henderson, C., Knapp, M., Fernández, J.-L., Beecham, J., Hirani, S., Beynon, M., . . ., Doll, H. (2012). Cost-effectiveness of telehealth in people with social care needs: the Whole Systems Demonstrator cluster randomised trial. *International Journal of Integrated Care, 12*(Suppl1).

Hillestad, R., Bigelow, J., Bower, A., Girosi, F., Meili, R., Scoville, R., & Taylor, R. (2005). Can electronic medical record systems transform health care? Potential health benefits, savings, and costs. *Health Affairs*, *24*(5), 1103–1117. doi:10.1377/hlthaff.24.5.1103 PMID:16162551

Hippisley-Cox, J., Pringle, M., Cater, R., Wynn, A., Hammersley, V., & Coupland, C. et al. (2003). The electronic patient record in primary care-regression or progression? A cross sectional study. *British Medical Journal*, *326*(7407).

Holden, R. J., & Karsh, B. T. (2010). The technology acceptance model: Its past and its future in health care. *Journal of Biomedical Informatics*, *43*(1), 159–172. doi:10.1016/j.jbi.2009.07.002 PMID:19615467

Hu, P. J., Chau, P. Y. K., Sheng, O. R. L., & Tam, K. Y. (1999). Examining the technology acceptance model using physician acceptance of telemedicine technology. *Journal of Management Information Systems*, *16*(2), 91–112. doi:10.1080/07421222.1999.11518247

Hung, S.-Y., Hung, W.-H., Tsai, C.-A., & Jiang, S.-C. (2010). Critical factors of hospital adoption on CRM system: Organizational and information system perspectives. *Decision Support Systems*, *48*(4), 592–603. doi:10.1016/j.dss.2009.11.009

Hunt, D. L., Haynes, R. B., Hanna, S. E., & Smith, K. (1998). Effects of computer-based clinical decision support systems on physician performance and patient outcomes. *Journal of the American Medical Association*, *280*(15), 1339. doi:10.1001/jama.280.15.1339 PMID:9794315

Inklaar, R., O'Mahony, M., & Timmer, M. (2005). ICT and Europe's productivity performance. industry level growth account comparisons with the United States. *Review of Income and Wealth*, *51*(4), 505–536. doi:10.1111/j.1475-4991.2005.00166.x

Jennings, N., Clifford, S., Fox, A. R., O'Connell, J., & Gardner, G. (2015). The impact of nurse practitioner services on cost, quality of care, satisfaction and waiting times in the emergency department: A systematic review. *International Journal of Nursing Studies*, *52*(1), 421–435. doi:10.1016/j.ijnurstu.2014.07.006 PMID:25443302

Jensen, J., Tøndel, I. A., Jaatun, M. G., Meland, P. H., & Andresen, H. (2009). *Reusable Security Requirements for Healthcare Applications*. Academic Press.

King, W. R., & He, J. (2006). A meta-analysis of the technology acceptance model. *Information & Management*, *43*(6), 740–755. doi:10.1016/j.im.2006.05.003

Kumar, R., Novak, J., & Tomkins, A. (2010). Structure and evolution of online social networks. *Link Mining: Models, Algorithms, and Applications*, 337-357.

Lai, L. S., & Turban, E. (2008). Groups formation and operations in the Web 2.0 environment and social networks. *Group Decision and Negotiation*, *17*(5), 387–402. doi:10.1007/s10726-008-9113-2

Lapointe, L., & Rivard, S. (2006). Getting physicians to accept new information technology: Insights from case studies. *Canadian Medical Association Journal*, *174*(11), 1573–1578. doi:10.1503/cmaj.050281 PMID:16717265

Lau, A. S. (2011). Hospital-based nurses' perceptions of the adoption of Web 2.0 tools for knowledge sharing, learning, social interaction and the production of collective intelligence. *Journal of Medical Internet Research*, *13*(4), e92. doi:10.2196/jmir.1398 PMID:22079851

Lee, M. A., & Yom, Y. H. (2007). A comparative study of patients' and nurses' perceptions of the quality of nursing services, satisfaction and intent to revisit the hospital: A questionnaire survey. *International Journal of Nursing Studies*, *44*(4), 545–555. doi:10.1016/j.ijnurstu.2006.03.006 PMID:16687147

Liao, S. H. (2003). Knowledge management technologies and applications - literature review from 1995 to 2002. *Expert Systems with Applications*, *25*(2), 155–164. doi:10.1016/S0957-4174(03)00043-5

Liu, M.-S., & Liu, N.-C. (2008). Sources of knowledge acquisition and patterns of knowledge-sharing behaviors--An empirical study of Taiwanese high-tech firms. *International Journal of Information Management*, *28*(5), 423–432. doi:10.1016/j.ijinfomgt.2008.01.005

Lu, J., Yu, C. S., Liu, C., & Yao, J. E. (2003). Technology acceptance model for wireless Internet. *Internet Research*, *13*(3), 206–222. doi:10.1108/10662240310478222

Lucas, H. (2008). Information and communications technology for future health systems in developing countries. *Social Science & Medicine*, *66*(10), 2122–2132. doi:10.1016/j.socscimed.2008.01.033 PMID:18343005

Macedo, M., & Isaías, P. (2009). Patient Standardization Identification as a Healthcare Issue. *Human Interface and the Management of Information. Information and Interaction*, 566-575.

Marques, A., Oliveira, T., Dias, S. S., & Martins, M. F. O. (2011). Medical Records System Adoption in European Hospitals. *The Electronic Journal Information Systems Evaluation*, *14*(1), 89–99.

Mathieson, K. (1991). Predicting user intentions: Comparing the technology acceptance model with the theory of planned behavior. *Information Systems Research*, *2*(3), 173–191. doi:10.1287/isre.2.3.173

McGowan, B. S., Wasko, M., Vartabedian, B. S., Miller, R. S., Freiherr, D. D., & Abdolrasulnia, M. (2012). Understanding the factors that influence the adoption and meaningful use of social media by physicians to share medical information. *Journal of Medical Internet Research*, *14*(5), e117. doi:10.2196/jmir.2138 PMID:23006336

McKee, D. O., Varadarajan, P. R., & Pride, W. M. (1989). Strategic Adaptability and Firm Performance: A Market-Contingent Perspective. *Journal of Marketing*, *53*(3), 21–35. doi:10.2307/1251340

Murphy, G. D. (2010). *Using Web 2.0 tools to facilitate knowledge transfer in complex organisational environments: a primer*. Academic Press.

Norum, J., Grev, A., Moen, M. A., Balteskard, L., & Holthe, K. (2003). Information and communication technology (ICT) in oncology. Patients' and relatives' experiences and suggestions. *Supportive Care in Cancer*, *11*(5), 286–293. PMID:12690539

Papastathopoulou, P., Avlonitis, G. J., & Panagopoulos, N. G. (2007). Intraorganizational information and communication technology diffusion: Implications for industrial sellers and buyers. *Industrial Marketing Management*, *36*(3), 322–336. doi:10.1016/j.indmarman.2005.10.002

Peansupap, V., & Walker, D. (2005). Factors enabling information and communication technology diffusion and actual implementation in construction organisations. *Electronic Journal of Information Technology in Construction*, *10*, 193–218.

Pilat, D. (2004). The ICT productivity paradox: Insights from micro data. *OECD Economic Studies*, *38*(1), 37–65.

Pirnejad, H., Bal, R., Stoop, A. P., & Berg, M. (2007). Inter-organisational communication networks in healthcare: Centralised versus decentralised approaches. *International Journal of Integrated Care*, *7*(2). PMID:17627296

Rahimi, B., & Vimarlund, V. (2007). Methods to evaluate health information systems in healthcare settings: A literature review. *Journal of Medical Systems*, *31*(5), 397–432. doi:10.1007/s10916-007-9082-z PMID:17918694

Raitoharju, R. (2005). *When Acceptance is not Enough-Taking TAM-Model into Healthcare*. Academic Press.

Richter, A., Stocker, A., Müller, S., & Avram, G. (2013). Knowledge management goals revisited: A cross-sectional analysis of social software adoption in corporate environments. *Vine*, *43*(2), 132–148. doi:10.1108/03055721311329927

Romano, N. C. Jr, & Fjermestad, J. (2001). Electronic commerce customer relationship management: An assessment of research. *International Journal of Electronic Commerce*, *6*(2), 61–113.

Ruland, C. M., & Ravn, I. H. (2003). Usefulness and effects on costs and staff management of a nursing resource management information system. *Journal of Nursing Management*, *11*(3), 208–215. doi:10.1046/j.1365-2834.2003.00381.x PMID:12694368

Scalone, L., Mantovani, L. G., Krol, M., Rofail, D., Ravera, S., & Grazia Bisconte, M. et al. (2008). Costs, quality of life, treatment satisfaction and compliance in patients with -thalassemia major undergoing iron chelation therapy: The ITHACA study. *Current Medical Research and Opinion*, *24*(7), 1905–1917. PMID:18507891

Schillewaert, N., Ahearne, M. J., Frambach, R. T., & Moenaert, R. K. (2005). The adoption of information technology in the sales force. *Industrial Marketing Management, 34*(4), 323–336. doi:10.1016/j.indmarman.2004.09.013

Sekaran, U. (2006). *Research methods for business*. Wiley India Pvt. Ltd.

Sharma, S., Kilian, R., & Leung, F.-H. (2014). Health 2.0—Lessons Learned Social Networking With Patients for Health Promotion. *Journal of Primary Care & Community Health*.

Sheng, M., Chang, S.-Y., Teo, T. S., & Lin, Y.-F. (2013). Knowledge Barriers, Knowledge Transfer, and Innovation Competitive Advantage in Healthcare Settings. *Management Decision, 51*(3), 1–1. doi:10.1108/00251741311309607

Steventon, A., Bardsley, M., Billings, J., Dixon, J., Doll, H., Hirani, S., . . . Henderson, C. (2012). Effect of telehealth on use of secondary care and mortality: findings from the Whole System Demonstrator cluster randomised trial. *BMJ: British Medical Journal, 344*.

Tekli, J., Rjeily, A. A., Chbeir, R., Tekli, G., Houngue, P., Yetongnon, K., et al. (2013). *Semantic to intelligent web era: building blocks, applications, and current trends*. Paper presented at the Fifth International Conference on Management of Emergent Digital EcoSystems.

Tiago, M. B., & Tiago, F. (2013). *Roadmaps for Future ICT Use in the Health Sector Handbook of Research on ICTs and Management Systems for Improving Efficiency in Healthcare and Social Care*. IGI Global. doi:10.4018/978-1-4666-3990-4.ch035

Tiago, M. T. B., Couto, J. P., Tiago, F., & Vieira, A. C. (2007). Knowledge management:An overview of European reality. *Management Research News, 30*(2), 100–114. doi:10.1108/01409170710722946

Tiago, M. T. B., Couto, J. P. A., Tiago, F. G., & Vieira, J. A. C. (2008). The missing link between virtual CRM and e-business performance1. *International Journal of Business and Management, 2*(1).

Tiago, T., & Veríssimo, J. (2014). Digital marketing and social media: Why bother? *Business Horizons, 57*(6), 703–708. doi:10.1016/j.bushor.2014.07.002

Tornatzky, L. G., & Fleischer, M. (1990). *The processes of technological innovation*. Lexington Books.

Van Ark, B., Inklaar, R., & McGuckin, R. H. (2003). ICT and productivity in Europe and the United States Where do the differences come from? *CESifo Economic Studies, 49*(3), 295–318. doi:10.1093/cesifo/49.3.295

Van Der Meijden, M., Tange, H., Troost, J., & Hasman, A. (2003). Determinants of success of inpatient clinical information systems: A literature review. *Journal of the American Medical Informatics Association*, *10*(3), 235–243. doi:10.1197/jamia.M1094 PMID:12626373

Venkatesh, V., & Morris, M. G. (2000). Why don't men ever stop to ask for directions? Gender, social influence, and their role in technology acceptance and usage behavior. *Management Information Systems Quarterly*, *24*(1), 115–139. doi:10.2307/3250981

Verdegem, P., & Verhoest, P. (2009). Profiling the non-user: Rethinking policy initiatives stimulating ICT acceptance. *Telecommunications Policy*, *33*(10-11), 642–652. doi:10.1016/j.telpol.2009.08.009

Wang, S. J., Middleton, B., Prosser, L. A., Bardon, C. G., Spurr, C. D., & Carchidi, P. J. et al. (2003). A cost-benefit analysis of electronic medical records in primary care. *The American Journal of Medicine*, *114*(5), 397–403. doi:10.1016/S0002-9343(03)00057-3 PMID:12714130

Ware, J. E., Davies, A. R., & Stewart, A. L. (1977). *The measurement and meaning of patient satisfaction: a review of the literature*. Rand Corporation.

Wild, R., & Griggs, K. (2008). A model of information technology opportunities for facilitating the practice of knowledge management. *Vine*, *38*(4), 490–506. doi:10.1108/03055720810917732

Yi, M. Y., & Hwang, Y. (2003). Predictingthe use of web-based information systems: Self-efficacy, enjoyment, learning goal orientation, and the technology acceptance model. Int. *J. Human-Computer Studies*, *59*(4), 431–449. doi:10.1016/S1071-5819(03)00114-9

Yoon, Y., Guimaraes, T., & O'Neal, Q. (1995). Exploring the factors associated with expert systems success. *Management Information Systems Quarterly*, *19*(1), 83–106. doi:10.2307/249712

Zhu, K., & Kraemer, K. (2002). E-commerce Metrics for Net-enhanced Organizations: Assessing the Value of e-commerce to Firm Performance in the Manufacturing Sector. *Information Systems Research*, *13*(3), 275–295. doi:10.1287/isre.13.3.275.82

Zhu, K., Kraemer, K., & Dedrick, J. (2004). Information Technology payoff in e-business environments: Na international perspective of value creation of e-business in the financial service industry. *Journal of Management Information Systems*, *21*(1), 17–54.

ADDITIONAL READING

Andersen, S. T., & Jansen, A. (2011). Innovation in ICT-Based Health Care Provision. [IJHISI]. *International Journal of Healthcare Information Systems and Informatics*, *6*(2), 14–27. doi:10.4018/jhisi.2011040102

Anderson, J., & Aydin, C. (2005). Overview: Theoretical perspectives and methodologies for the evaluation of healthcare information systems. *Evaluating the Organizational Impact of Healthcare Information Systems*, 5-29.

Anderson, L. M., Scrimshaw, S. C., Fullilove, M. T., Fielding, J. E., & Normand, J. (2003). Culturally competent healthcare systems* 1: A systematic review. *American Journal of Preventive Medicine*, *24*(3), 68–79. doi:10.1016/S0749-3797(02)00657-8 PMID:12668199

Andreassen, H. K. (2010). What does an e-mail address add?-Doing health and technology at home. *Social Science & Medicine*. PMID:21208702

Antheunis, M. L., Tates, K., & Nieboer, T. E. (2013). Patients' and health professionals' use of social media in health care: Motives, barriers and expectations. *Patient Education and Counseling*, *92*(3), 426–431. doi:10.1016/j.pec.2013.06.020 PMID:23899831

Bakker, A. R. (2002). Health care and ICT, partnership is a must. *International Journal of Medical Informatics*, *66*(1-3), 51–57. doi:10.1016/S1386-5056(02)00036-9 PMID:12453558

Black, E., Light, J., Black, N. P., & Thompson, L. (2013). Online Social Network Use by Health Care Providers in a High Traffic Patient Care Environment. *Journal of Medical Internet Research*, *15*(5), e94. doi:10.2196/jmir.2421 PMID:23685530

Chaudhry, B., Wang, J., Wu, S., Maglione, M., Mojica, W., & Roth, E. et al. (2006). Systematic review: Impact of health information technology on quality, efficiency, and costs of medical care. *Annals of Internal Medicine*, *144*(10), 742. doi:10.7326/0003-4819-144-10-200605160-00125 PMID:16702590

Cheong, L. H., Armour, C. L., & Bosnic-Anticevich, S. Z. (2013). Primary health care teams and the patient perspective: A social network analysis. *Research in Social & Administrative Pharmacy*, *9*(6), 741–757. doi:10.1016/j.sapharm.2012.12.003 PMID:23395532

Doarn, C. R., Yellowlees, P., Jeffries, D. A., Lordan, D., Davis, S., & Hammack, G. et al. (2008). Societal drivers in the applications of telehealth. *Telemedicine Journal and e-Health*, *14*(9), 998–1002. doi:10.1089/tmj.2008.0111 PMID:19035816

Doherty, R. B. (2010). The certitudes and uncertainties of health care reform. *Annals of Internal Medicine, 152*(10), 679. doi:10.7326/0003-4819-153-1-201007060-00235 PMID:20378676

Garg, A. X., Adhikari, N. K. J., McDonald, H., Rosas-Arellano, M. P., Devereaux, P., & Beyene, J. et al. (2005). Effects of computerized clinical decision support systems on practitioner performance and patient outcomes. *Journal of the American Medical Association, 293*(10), 1223. doi:10.1001/jama.293.10.1223 PMID:15755945

Grajales, F. J. III, Sheps, S., Ho, K., Novak-Lauscher, H., & Eysenbach, G. (2014). Social Media: A Review and Tutorial of Applications in Medicine and Health Care. *Journal of Medical Internet Research, 16*(2). PMID:24518354

Hamid, A., & Sarmad, A. (2011). Multi-Dimensional Criteria for the Evaluation of E-Health Services.

Hansen, D. P., Gurney, P., Morgan, G., & Barraclough, B. (2011). The Australian e-Health Research Centre: Enabling the health care information and communication technology revolution. *The Medical Journal of Australia, 194*(4), S5–S7. PMID:21401490

Hippisley-Cox, J., & Pringle, M. (2004). Prevalence, care, and outcomes for patients with diet-controlled diabetes in general practice: Cross sectional survey. *Lancet, 364*(9432), 423–428. doi:10.1016/S0140-6736(04)16765-2 PMID:15288740

Kawamoto, K., Houlihan, C. A., Balas, E. A., & Lobach, D. F. (2005). Improving clinical practice using clinical decision support systems: A systematic review of trials to identify features critical to success. *BMJ (Clinical Research Ed.), 330*(7494), 765. doi:10.1136/bmj.38398.500764.8F PMID:15767266

Mars, M., & Scott, R. E. (2010). Global e-health policy: A work in progress. *Health Affairs, 29*(2), 237–243. doi:10.1377/hlthaff.2009.0945 PMID:20348067

Moffatt, J., Eley, D., & Eley, J. M. D. (2011). Barriers to the up-take of telemedicine in Australia–a view from providers. *Rural and Remote Health, 11*(1581). PMID:21385004

Nickelson, D. W. (1998). Telehealth and the evolving health care system: Strategic opportunities for professional psychology. *Professional Psychology, Research and Practice, 29*(6), 527–535. doi:10.1037/0735-7028.29.6.527

Orszag, P. R., & Emanuel, E. J. (2010). Health care reform and cost control. *The New England Journal of Medicine, 363*(7), 601–603. doi:10.1056/NEJMp1006571 PMID:20554975

Parish, M. B., & Yellowlees, P. (2014). The Rise of Person-Centered Healthcare and the Influence of Health Informatics and Social Network Applications on Mental Health Care. In *Mental Health Informatics* (pp. 17–39). Springer Berlin Heidelberg. doi:10.1007/978-3-642-38550-6_2

Park, E., Baek, S., Ohm, J., & Chang, H. J. (2014). Determinants of player acceptance of mobile social network games: An application of extended technology acceptance model. *Telematics and Informatics*, *31*(1), 3–15. doi:10.1016/j.tele.2013.07.001

Sánchez, J. L., Savin, S., & Vasileva, V. (2005). *Key success factors in implementing electronic medical records in University Hospital of Rennes. L'Ecole Nationale de la Santé Publique* (pp. 1–59). Rennes, Rennes, France: National School of Public Health.

While, A., & Dewsbury, G. (2011). Nursing and information and communication technology (ICT): A discussion of trends and future directions. *International Journal of Nursing Studies*, *48*(10), 1302–1310. doi:10.1016/j.ijnurstu.2011.02.020 PMID:21474135

KEY TERMS AND DEFINITIONS

Healthy 3.0: Adoption of Web 3.0 technology-based tools to improve the patient/provider relationship.

HIS Measurement: Methods to evaluate outputs and outcomes of the use of IT-based systems in medical informatics.

ICT Acceptance: Individual and firms 'attitudes regarding technology and their intention to use.

ICT Induce Benefits: Intangible benefits achieved by the adoption and use of ICT in healthcare.

ICT Performance: ICT can give significant boost productivity gains of a firm, which can be measure through financial and non-financial metrics.

ICT ROI: Financial accountable benefits driven from the value gains and cost reduction.

ICT Support: Technical and training support in daily basis and board commitment to ICT use, measure by recognition of efforts and compensation.

Conclusion

From a management perspective, these new challenges have forced Healthcare Stakeholders (HS) to look at different healthcare management concepts that could alleviate the problem of information explosion. The following are some of the new paradigms and concepts that have caught the attention of HS.

EVIDENCE-BASED MEDICINE (EBM)

EBM is defined as the conscientious, explicit and judicious use of current best evidence in making decisions about the care of individual patients (Cowling, Newman, & Leigh, 1999). A typical EBM process starts with an identification of knowledge gaps in current healthcare treatment processes, followed by a search for the best evidence. This is then succeeded by a process to aid in the selection of appropriate electronic data and information sources and IT applications that focus on clinical competencies in context of the evidence generated.

The next step is to carry out a critical appraisal of the best evidence identified by carrying out checks for accuracy and diagnostic validity of the procedures and treatments identified by the best evidence generated. The costs and benefits of alternative procedures (i.e. the current best evidence procedure/treatment being recommended) are then considered. The last step is its application to patient healthcare which calls for integration of the identified evidence with the General Practitioners' (GP) clinical expertise so as to provide best treatment and care (Cowling, Newman, & Leigh, 1999).

MODEL OF INTEGRATED PATIENT PATHWAYS (MIPP/IPP)

It has been argued that the model of integrated patient pathways (MIPP/IPP) is a more comprehensive concept for HIs (Schmid & Conen, 2000). As the acronym suggests, IPPs aim to enable better support for HIs by focusing on the creation of clinical guidelines for commonly accepted diagnostic and therapeutic procedures at a defined level of quality. This would lead to cost efficient treatment. It could be argued that IPP calls for in-house development of standardised clinical treatment procedures for some pre-defined diagnoses and treatments.

IPP aims to ensure that patients receive the right treatment which is based upon best practice guidelines that have sufficient evidence to warrant the label of "best practice" and which have been proven to be clinically adequate (Schmid & Conen, 2000). They argue that when a hospital tries to implement IPP, it will automatically go through a circular chain process that calls for identifying sources of best practice, converting them to organisation-wide implementation practices and then, based upon their performance, converting them to benchmarks.

CLINICAL GOVERNANCE (CG)

Clinical governance (CG) was first introduced in the UK in a National Health Service (NHS) white paper (Firth-Cozens, 1999) and calls for an integrated approach to quality, team development, clinical audit skills, risk management skills, and information systems. A typical CG process can be delineated into a sequential process that calls for (a) the means to disseminate knowledge about relevant evidence from research, (b) best treatments rather than focusing just on recognition of poor treatments, (c) better appreciation of what IT-led solutions can do for clinical governance and (d) knowing what data and information is available so as to provide baselines for best care and treatments.

The NHS has witnessed the incorporation and development of many approaches that support and promote effective health care, but in practice, none of them have been successful (Melvin, et.al, 1999). The problem may lie in the lack of proper systems to support the measurement of clinical organisational effectiveness in a healthcare delivery context (Zairi & Whymark, 1999).

One of the biggest challenges in having concise summaries of the most effective clinical practices is establishing what is meant by "quality in healthcare" (Sewell, 1997). Measurement standards in clinical practice will change from each context. This is attributed to the linkage between measurement standards and values and the expectations of the individual HS which, in turn, originate from the shared values, expectations to which all the HS subscribe (Sewell, 1997).

In the UK, the NHS has started to support the concept of clinical governance by identifying individual best effective clinical practices. This process provides concise summaries of the most effective clinical practices in all key clinical areas. Summaries that are successfully substantiated are then disseminated throughout the NHS (Melvin, et.al, 1999). It has noted that the USA, Canada, Australia and New Zealand have adopted a formal accreditation system for the healthcare sector based upon the ISO 9000 approach (Sewell, 1997).

COMMUNITY HEALTH INFORMATION NETWORKS (CHIN)

The rationale behind the CHIN concept is to allow users to collect data which could be used to formulate best practice protocols for effective treatment at a low-cost, i.e., clinical best evidence practices for both healthcare diagnosis and delivery (Kennedy, 1995). It was anticipated that the advent of CHINs, in conjunction with Internet technologies, would empower HS to provide healthcare to patients in real time whilst being in geographically-distinct locations (Kennedy, 1995; Morrissey, 2000).

The advent of CHIN was accompanied by a wave of new technologies that focused on establishing electronic connectivity amongst different HS, creating the visage of a virtual e-healthcare system (Mercer, 2001; Pryga & Dyer, 1992). This allowed CHINs to transmit healthcare information across departmental and organisational boundaries. As CHINs developed further, it became clear that the existing technological infrastructure was inadequate in empowering appropriate healthcare stakeholders with contextually accurate information at the precise time in the right format (Mercer, 2001).

The failure of existing healthcare management concepts to tackle the information overload in healthcare has strengthened the case for incorporating the KM paradigm in healthcare (Mercer, 2001 and Health Canada, Online). The need for integration of KM in healthcare has been supported by Jurisica et al. (2001) who note that systematic knowledge management (i.e. support for acquisition, representation, organisation, usage, and evolution of knowledge in its many forms) can alleviate problems caused due to the information explosion in the biomedical domain.

It has been argued that future healthcare stakeholders would need to combine management skills with clinical knowledge (Stefl, 1997). The way forward for HIs is to "integrate clinical knowledge bases at the point of care…thereby rendering it more accessible" which would call for streamlining clinical knowledge into the workflow of healthcare processes (Blumenfeld, 1997, pp. 44). KM can assist in this context, as it is a multi-disciplinary paradigm, which uses technology to support the acquisition, generation, codification and transfer of knowledge in the context of specific organisational process (see section 2.3).

The very nature of healthcare processes calls for physicians to use both KM strategies [(1) codification strategy and (2) personalisation strategy] (Wyatt, 2001). The codification strategy could be very effective for repetitive healthcare processes for routine medical conditions (e.g. influenza) whilst the personalisation strategy could be more suitable for variations of routine medical conditions and non-routine medical conditions (e.g. Meningitis).

In the UK, the National Health Service (NHS) emphasis has concentrated on KM strategies supporting codification to standardise treatment of routine cases. The aim of the NHS is to create "a standard approach…for dissemination based on best NHS practice…to raise performance to that of the best units (Wyatt, 2001, pp. 6).

KM: HEALTHCARE SUCCESS STORIES

The biggest success story of KM in Healthcare is the discovery of Viagra. Pfizer were testing a new angina drug and the results were not promising. However, a few researchers noticed that the angina drug improved male sexual potency. They asked around and found that the best-suited management team to exploit this was in the USA. The findings were then sent from the UK to the US and history was made. What is unique about this was that the UK based researchers had no idea of the importance of their work, but due to an effective KM infrastructure, they were able to locate the best experts to look at their work. If this KM infrastructure was not there, the findings angina drug could so easily have landed on the desk of the wrong person who could have simply filed them away not realizing their significance (Tyler, 1999).

In another study, a group of physicians observed that they needed new or clinically important information only once or twice a week, and could meet these needs by consulting a textbook or journal. The same groups of same physicians were then questioned while seeing patients and in less then half a day, up to 16 requirements for new, clinically important data were identified. When a test was carried out to confirm if they could confirm what the information needs would actually be met by looking at textbooks or asking colleagues, it was found that only 30 per cent of these information needs could be met by looking at textbooks or asking colleagues. The study concluded that for the same group about eight clinical decisions a day might have been altered if the necessary information had been available (Rowland and Harris, 1998).

The process of creating new drugs has been conventionally divided into two main phases: (1) Discovery and (2) Clinical development. In clinical development, one of the main challenges is to gather sufficient evidence that validates the use of the drug, both from safety and efficacy issues. The logistics and costs of clinical development trials as seen below can be overwhelming.

A clinical development trial for a recently approved drug by the US based Federal Drug Administration's (FDA) Cardiovascular and Renal Drugs Advisory Committee involved 11000 patients in 27 countries and 700 treatment centers (Koretz & Lee, 1998). On average, pharmaceutical companies spend about US $350 million over a period of 8 to 12 years to bring an archetypal new drug to the consumers and the average submission reports on 60 clinical trials and the report typically runs into thousands of pages (Koretz & Lee, 1998).

Conclusion

Hoffmann-LaRoche – a leading pharmaceutical organisation was facing a similar challenge. Hoffmann-LaRoche was investigating new ways of reducing the time taken to launch a new product on the market and commenced a KM program. The results were astonishing. Before the introduction of the KM programme, an average drug used to cost $250 million and used to take five to eight years to develop. Now, the savings of the KM programme are estimated at $90 million. Even more remarkable was the result achieved in getting US FDA approval for the distribution of pharmaceutical products. After the introduction of the KM programme, the time taken for US FDA approval fell from three years to nine months (Seeman, Online).

The major contention of this book is that KM can assist the healthcare industry. Future healthcare systems would see increased interest in knowledge recycling of the collaborative learning process acquired from previous healthcare industry practices. The healthcare sector has been exclusively focussed on IT to meet challenges as described in this section. This research reiterates that this challenge cannot be met by an IT led solution alone.

Organisational aspects, such as KM initiatives, should be incorporated within the technological revolution that is speeding across healthcare industry. There needs to be a balance between organisational and technological aspects of the healthcare process i.e. one cannot exist without the other.

It is important that clinicians take a holistic view of their organisation. This requires clinicians to have an understanding of IT in a healthcare context and a shared vision of the organisation. KM can help the healthcare sector to make tacit knowledge explicit and re-purposed via new IT innovations. This book concludes with the assessment that the KM concept is an important and appropriate vehicle to guide medical informatics and the healthcare sector into the new millennium.

REFERENCES

Blumenfeld, B. (1997). Integrating knowledge bases at the point of care. *Health Management Technology*, *18*, 44–46. PMID:10169797

Cowling, A., Newman, K., & Leigh, S. (1999). Developing a competency framework to support training in evidence-based healthcare. *International Journal of Health Care Quality Assurance*, *12*(4), 149–159. doi:10.1108/09526869910272509

Firth-Cozens, J. (1999). Clinical governance development needs in health service staff. *Clinical Performance and Quality Health Care*, *7*(4), 155–160. doi:10.1108/14664109910315569 PMID:10947388

Health Canada. (1998). *Vision and strategy for knowledge management and IM/IT for Health Canada.* Available from http://www.hc-sc.gc.ca/iacb-dgiac/km-gs/english/vsmenu_e.htm

Jurisica, I., Wolfley, J. R., Rogers, P., Bianca, M. A., Glasgow, J. I., Weeks, D. R., & Luft, J. R. et al. (2001). Intelligent decision support for protein crystal growth. *IBM Systems Journal, 40*(2), 394–409. doi:10.1147/sj.402.0394

Kennedy, M. (1995). Integration fever. *Computerworld, 29*(14), 81–83.

Koretz, S., & Lee, G. (1998). Knowledge management and drug development. *Journal of Knowledge Management, 2*(2), 53–58. doi:10.1108/13673279810249387

Melvin, K., Wright, J., Harrison, S. R., Robinson, M., Connelly, J., & Williams, D. R. (1999). Effective practice in the NHS and the contribution from public health: A qualitative study. *British Journal of Clinical Governance, 4*(3), 88–97. doi:10.1108/14664109910309638

Mercer, K. (2001). Examining the impact of health information networks on health system integration in Canada. *Leadership in Health Services, 14*(3), 1–30. doi:10.1108/13660750110399928

Morrissey, J. (2000, May 29). The eVolution of a CHIN. *Modern Healthcare,* ▪▪▪, 42–43. PMID:11067123

Pryga, E., & Dyer, C. (1992). The AHA's national health reform strategy: An overview. *Trustee, 45*(5), 10. PMID:10117814

Rowland, H., & Harris, L. (1998). Doctor know. *People Management, 4*(5), 50–52. PMID:9798566

Schmid, K., & Conen, D. (2000). Integrated patient pathways: "MIPP" - A tool for quality improvement and cost management in health care: Pilot study on the pathway "Acute Myocardial Infarction". *International Journal of Health Care Quality Assurance, 13*(2), 87–92. doi:10.1108/09526860010319541

Seeman, P. (1997). *Managing knowledge at Hoffman-LaRoche.* Available from: http://www.businessinnovation.ey.com/mko/pdf/HOFFCASE.PDF

Sewell, N. (1997). Continuous quality improvement in acute health care: Creating a holistic and integrated approach. *International Journal of Health Care Quality Assurance, 10*(1), 20–26. doi:10.1108/09526869710159598 PMID:10166023

Stefl, M. E. (1997). The commentaries: A summary. *Frontiers of Health Services Management, 13*, 26–27.

Tyler, G. (1999). Well, what d'ya know? *Management Services*, *43*(6), 28–32.

Wyatt, J. C. (2000). 7 Intranets. *Journal of the Royal Society of Medicine*, *93*(10), 530–534. PMID:11064692

Zairi, M., Whymark, J., & Cooke, M. (1999). Best practice organisational effectiveness in NHS Trusts Allington NHS Trust case study. *Journal of Management in Medicine*, *13*(5), 298–307. doi:10.1108/02689239910274134 PMID:10787499

Compilation of References

Abbott, P. A., & Coenen, A. (2008). Globalization and advances in information and communication technologies: The impact on nursing and health. *Nursing Outlook, 56*(5), 238-246. e232.

Abelein, U., & Paech, B. (2013). Understanding the Influence of User Participation & Involvement on System Success–a Systematic Mapping Study. *Empirical Software Engineering*, 1–54.

Abelein, U., & Paech, B. (2014). State of Practice of User-Developer Communication in Large-Scale IT Projects. In *Requirements Engineering: Foundation for Software Quality* (pp. 95–111). Springer International Publishing. doi:10.1007/978-3-319-05843-6_8

Abu-Hasaballah, K., James, A., & Aseltine, R. H. Jr. (2007). Lessons and pitfalls of interactive voice response in medical research. *Contemporary Clinical Trials, 28*(5), 593–602. doi:10.1016/j.cct.2007.02.007 PMID:17400520

Adewale, O. S. (2004). An Internet-based telemedicine system in Nigeria. *International Journal of Information Management, 24*(3), 221–234. doi:10.1016/j.ijinfomgt.2003.12.014

Adler-Milstein, J., & Bates, D. W. (2010). Paperless healthcare: Progress and challenges of an IT-enabled healthcare system. *Business Horizons, 53*(2), 119–130. doi:10.1016/j.bushor.2009.10.004

Aggelidis, V. P., & Chatzoglou, P. D. (2012). Hospital information systems: Measuring end user computing satisfaction (EUCS). *Journal of Biomedical Informatics, 45*(3), 566–579. doi:10.1016/j.jbi.2012.02.009 PMID:22426283

Ahmad, F., Hudak, P. L., Bercovitz, K., Hollenberg, E., & Levinson, W. (2006). Are Physicians Ready for Patients With Internet-Based Health Information? *Journal of Medical Internet Research, 8*(3), e22. doi:10.2196/jmir.8.3.e22 PMID:17032638

AIHW. (2007). *National Indicators for Monitoring Diabetes: Report of the Diabetes Indicators Review Subcommittee of the National Diabetes Data Working Group: AIHW cat. no. CVD 38.* Canberra: AIHW.

AIHW. (2008). *Diabetes: Australian Facts 2008.* Canberra: Australian Institute of Health and Welfare.

Akkiraju, R., Farrell, J., & Miller, J. (2005). *Web Service Semantics-WSDL-S*. Technical Note, Version 1.0, April, 2005. Available at: http://lsdis.cs.uga.edu/library/download/WSDL-S-V1.html

Alaghehband, F. K., Rivard, S., Wu, S., & Goyette, S. (2011). An Assessment of the Use of Transaction Cost Theory in Information Technology Outsourcing. *The Journal of Strategic Information Systems*, *20*(2), 125–138. doi:10.1016/j.jsis.2011.04.003

Aldrich, D., & Masera, P. (1999). *Mastering the Digital Market Place*. New York, NY: John Wiley & Sons.

Alemagno, S. A., Cochran, D., Feucht, T. E., Stephens, R. C., Butts, J. M., & Wolfe, S. A. (1996). Assessing substance abuse treatment needs among the homeless: A telephone-based interactive voice response system. *American Journal of Public Health*, *86*(11), 1626–1628. doi:10.2105/AJPH.86.11.1626 PMID:8916533

Alemi, F., Stephens, R. C., Javalghi, R. G., Dyches, H., Butts, J., & Ghadiri, A. (1996). A randomized trial of a telecommunications network for pregnant women who use cocaine. *Medical Care*, *34*(suppl 10), OS10–OS20. doi:10.1097/00005650-199610003-00002 PMID:8843933

Alizadeh, R., Panahi, F., Saghafinia, M., Alizadeh, K., Barakati, N., & Khaje-Daloee, M. (2012). Impact of Trauma Dispatch Algorithm Software on the Rate of Missions of Emergency Medical Services. *Trauma Monthly*, *17*(3), 319–322. doi:10.5812/traumamon.6341 PMID:24350116

Allen-Davis, J. T., Beck, A., Parker, R., Ellis, J. L., & Polley, D. (2002). Assessment of vulvovaginal complaints: Accuracy of telephone triage and in-office diagnosis. *Obstetrics and Gynecology*, *99*(1), 18–22. doi:10.1016/S0029-7844(01)01670-2 PMID:11777504

Allen, S. I. (1969). The telephone as a computer input-output terminal for medical information. *Journal of the American Medical Association*, *208*(4), 673–679. doi:10.1001/jama.1969.03160040081012 PMID:5818568

Alpay, L. L., Henkemans, O. B., Otten, W., Rövekamp, T. A., & Dumay, A. C. (2010). E-health applications and services for patient empowerment: Directions for best practices in The Netherlands. *Telemedicine Journal and e-Health*, *16*(7), 787–791. doi:10.1089/tmj.2009.0156 PMID:20815745

Alpay, L., Verhoef, J., Xie, B., Te'eni, D., & Zwetsloot-Schonk, J. (2009). Current challenge in consumer health informatics: Bridging the gap between access to information and information understanding. *Biomedical Informatics Insights*, *2*(1), 1. PMID:20419038

American Telemedicine Association. (n.d.). *What is Telemedicine & Telehealth*. Retrieved from; http://www.americantelemed.org/files/public/abouttelemedicine/What_Is_Telemedicine.pdf

Ammenwerth, E., Brender, J., Nykanen, P., Prokosch, H. U., Rigby, M., & Talmon, J. (2004). HIS-EVAL workshop participants. Visions & strategies to improve evaluation of health information systems: Reflections & lessons based on the HIS-EVAL workshop in Innsbruck. *International Journal of Medical Informatics*, *73*(6), 479–491. doi:10.1016/j.ijmedinf.2004.04.004 PMID:15171977

Ammenwerth, E., Gräber, S., Herrmann, G., Bürkle, T., & König, J. (2003). Evaluation of health information systems--problems and challenges. *International Journal of Medical Informatics*, *71*(2-3), 125–135. doi:10.1016/S1386-5056(03)00131-X PMID:14519405

Ammenwerth, E., Schnell-Inderst, P., Machan, C., & Siebert, U. (2008). The effect of electronic prescribing on medication errors and adverse drug events: A systematic review. *Journal of the American Medical Informatics Association*, *15*(5), 585–600. doi:10.1197/jamia.M2667 PMID:18579832

Anderson, E. W., Fornell, C., & Rust, R. T. (1997). Customer satisfaction, productivity, and profitability: Differences between goods and services. *Marketing Science*, *16*(2), 129–145. doi:10.1287/mksc.16.2.129

Anderson, J. G. (2007). Social, ethical and legal barriers to e-health. *International Journal of Medical Informatics*, *76*(5), 480–483. doi:10.1016/j.ijmedinf.2006.09.016 PMID:17064955

Anderson, M. M., Boly, L. D., & Deck, R. W. (1996). Remote clinic/patient monitoring for multicenter trials. *Controlled Clinical Trials*, *17*(5), 407–414. doi:10.1016/S0197-2456(96)00021-9 PMID:8932973

Ankolekar, A., Burstein, M., Hobbs, J. R., Lassila, O., Martin, D., McDermott, D., … Sycara, K. (2002, June), *DAML-S: Web service description for the semantic web.* International Semantic Web Conference, Italia. doi:10.1007/3-540-48005-6_27

Anton, J. (2000). The past, present and future of customer access centers. *International Journal of Service Industry Management*, *11*(2), 120–130. doi:10.1108/09564230010323534

Aoki, K., & Bray, E. H. (2006). Learning styles of distance learners in Japan: Cultural considerations.*Proceedings of the 11th Annual Conference of the European Learning Styles Information Network.*

Arnaert, A., & Macfarlane, F. (2011). Telehealth Nursing in Canada: Opportunities for Nurses to Shape the Future. In Telenursing (pp. 29-45). Springer London.

Arnstein, S. R. (2007). A ladder of citizen participation. *Journal of the American Institute of Planners*, *35*(4), 216–224. doi:10.1080/01944366908977225

Aron, R., Clemons, E. K., & Reddi, S. (2005). Just right outsourcing: Understanding and managing risk. *Journal of Management Information Systems*, *22*(2), 37–55.

Arsand, E., Tufano, J., Ralston, J., & Hjortdahl, P. (2008). Designing mobile dietary management support technologies for people with diabetes. *Journal of Telemedicine and Telecare*, *14*(7), 329–332. doi:10.1258/jtt.2008.007001 PMID:18852310

Artalejo, J. R., Economou, A., & Corral, A. G. (2007). Applications of Maximum Queue Length for Call Center Management. *Computers & Operations Research*, *34*(4), 983–996. doi:10.1016/j.cor.2005.05.020

Asai, K. (2005). Yashimagakuendaigaku Ni Okeru E-Learning Sisutemu No Genjou To Kadai [The Current Situation and Issues of e-Learning System at Yashima Gakuen University]. *Media Research, 1*(2), 59-71.

Ash, J., Stavre, Z., & Kuperman, G. J. (2003). A consensus statement on considerations for a successful CPOE implementation. *Journal of the American Medical Informatics Association, 10*(3), 229–234. doi:10.1197/jamia.M1204 PMID:12626376

Atkinson, R. D., & McKay, A. S. (2014). *Digital Prosperity – Understanding the Economic Benefits of the Information Technology Revolution.* Retrieved May 7, 2014 from http://www.itif.org/index.php?id=34

Auger, C., Forster, A. J., Oake, N., & Tamblyn, R. (2013). Usability of a computerised drug monitoring programme to detect adverse drug events and non-compliance in outpatient ambulatory care. *BMJ Quality & Safety, 22*(4), 306–316. doi:10.1136/bmjqs-2012-001492 PMID:23396853

Aversano, L., Grasso, C., & Tortorella, M. (2013). A Literature Review of Business/IT Alignment Strategies. *Lecture Notes in Business Information Processing, 141*, 471–488. doi:10.1007/978-3-642-40654-6_28

Avison, D. E., & Fitzgerald, G. (1995). Effective technical and human implementation of computer-based system (ETHICS). In Information system development: Methodologies, techniques and tools (pp. 353-364). Berkshire, UK: The McGraw-Hill Companies.

Azar, K. M., Lesser, L. I., Laing, B. Y., Stephens, J., Aurora, M. S., Burke, L. E., & Palaniapan, L. (2013). Mobile applications for weight management: Theory-based content analysis. *American Journal of Preventive Medicine, 45*(5), 583–589. doi:10.1016/j.amepre.2013.07.005 PMID:24139771

Babar, A., Wong, B., & Abedin, B. (2014). Investigating the role of business analysts competencies into strategic business requirements gathering. *The 18th Pacific Asia Conference on Information Systems (PACIS 2014).*

Bache, R., Miles, S, & Taweel, A. (2013). An adaptable architecture for patient cohort identification from diverse data sources. *J Am Med Inform Assoc, 20*(e2).

Bairi, J., & Manohar, M. (2011). Critical success factors in gaining user customer satisfaction in outsourced IT services. *Journal of Enterprise Information Management, 24*(6), 475–493. doi:10.1108/17410391111166530

Balas, E. A., Jaffrey, F., Kuperman, G. J., Boren, S. A., Brown, G. D., Pinciroli, F., & Mitchell, J. A. (1997). Electronic communication with patients. Evaluation of distance medicine technology. *Journal of the American Medical Association, 278*(2), 152–159. doi:10.1001/jama.1997.03550020084043 PMID:9214532

Balas, E. A., Krishna, S., Kretschmer, R. A., Cheek, T. R., Lobach, D. F., & Boren, S. A. (2004). Computerized knowledge management in diabetes care. *Medical Care, 42*(6), 610–621. doi:10.1097/01.mlr.0000128008.12117.f8 PMID:15167329

Ball, M. J., & Lillis, J. (2001). E-health: transforming the physician: patient relationship. *International Journal of Medical Informatics*, *61*(1), 1–10. doi:10.1016/S1386-5056(00)00130-1 PMID:11248599

Bano, M., & Zowghi, D. (2015). A systematic review on the relationship between user involvement and system success. *Information and Software Technology*, *58*, 148–169. doi:10.1016/j.infsof.2014.06.011

Bardram, J. E., Mihailidis, A., & Wan, D. (Eds.). (2006). *Pervasive Computing in Healthcare*. Boca Raton, FL: CRC.

Barlow, J., Bayer, S., & Curry, R. (2006). Implementing complex innovations in fluid multi-stakeholder environments: Experiences of 'telecare'. *Technovation*, *26*(3), 396–406. doi:10.1016/j.technovation.2005.06.010

Barr, J. L., Laufenberg, S., & Sieckman, B. L. (1997). Creating a vision for your medical call center. *Healthcare Information Management: Journal of the Healthcare Information and Management Systems Society of the American Hospital Association, 12*(2), 71-85.

Barry, M. J., & Edgman-Levitan, S. (2012). Shared decision making—the pinnacle of patient-centered care. *The New England Journal of Medicine*, *366*(9), 780–781. doi:10.1056/NEJMp1109283 PMID:22375967

Barua, A., Konana, P., & Whinston, A. B. (2004). An Empirical Investigation of Net-Enabled Business Value. *Management Information Systems Quarterly*, *28*(4), 585–620.

Bashshur, R., Shannon, G., Krupinski, E., & Grigsby, J. (2011). The taxonomy of telemedicine. *Telemedicine Journal and e-Health*, *17*(6), 484–494. doi:10.1089/tmj.2011.0103 PMID:21718114

Basili, V., Lindvall, M., Regardie, M., Seaman, C., Heidrich, J., Münch, J., & Trendowicz, A. et al. (2010). Linking Software Development and Business Strategy Through Measurement. *Computer*, *43*(4), 57–65. doi:10.1109/MC.2010.108

Bates, D. W., Cohen, M., Leape, L. L., Overhage, J. M., Shabot, M. M., & Sheridan, T. (2001). Reducing the frequency of errors in medicine using information technology. *Journal of the American Medical Informatics*, *8*(4), 299–308. doi:10.1136/jamia.2001.0080299 PMID:11418536

Bates, D. W., Leape, L. L., Cullen, D. J., Laird, N., Petersen, L. A., & Teich, J. M. et al. (1998). Effect of Computerized Physician Order Entry and a Team Intervention on Prevention of Serious Medication Errors. *Journal of the American Medical Association*, *280*(15), 1311–1316. doi:10.1001/jama.280.15.1311 PMID:9794308

Bayo-Moriones, A., Billón, M., & Lera-López, F. (2013). Perceived performance effects of ICT in manufacturing SMEs. *Industrial Management & Data Systems*, *113*(1), 117–135. doi:10.1108/02635571311289700

Bayo-Moriones, A., & Lera-López, F. (2007). A firm-level analysis of determinants of ICT adoption in Spain. *Technovation*, *27*(6-7), 352–366. doi:10.1016/j.technovation.2007.01.003

BBTU.com. (2014). *What's BBT University?* Retrieved from http://bbt.ac/about/

Beaulieu, R., & Humphreys, J. (2008). Evaluation of a telephone advice nurse in a nursing faculty managed pediatric community clinic. *Journal of Pediatric Health Care*, *22*(3), 175–181. doi:10.1016/j.pedhc.2007.05.006 PMID:18455066

Beimborn, D., Joachim, N., Schlosser, F., & Streicher, B. (2009). *The Role of IT/Business Alignment for Achieving SOA Business Value - Proposing a Research Model.* Paper presented at the 15th Americas Conference on Information Systems, San Francisco, CA.

Benevolo, C., & Spinelli, R. (2011). International service delivery and Internet-based technologies. *International Journal of Services. Economics and Management*, *3*(3), 251–266.

Berg, M. (2001). Implementing information systems in health care organizations: Myths and challenges. *International Journal of Medical Informatics*, *64*(2-3), 143–156. doi:10.1016/S1386-5056(01)00200-3 PMID:11734382

Berg, M., & Winthereik, B. R. (2004). Waiting for godot, episodes from the history of patient records. In M. Berg (Ed.), *Health information management: Integrating information technology in health care work* (pp. 11–44). London: Routledge.

Berman, A. H., Farzanfar, R., Kristiansson, M., Carlbring, P., & Friedman, R. H. (2012). Design and development of a telephone-linked care (TLC) system to reduce impulsivity among violent forensic outpatients and probationers. *Journal of Medical Systems*, *36*(3), 1031–1042. doi:10.1007/s10916-010-9565-1 PMID:20721686

Berner, E. S. (2008). Ethical and legal issues in the use of Health Information Technology to improve patient safety. *HEC Forum*, *20*(39), 243–258. doi:10.1007/s10730-008-9074-5 PMID:18803020

Berner, E. S., Ray, M. N., Panjamapirom, A., Maisiak, R. S., Willig, J. H., English, T. M., & Schiff, G. D. et al. (2014). Exploration of an automated approach for receiving feedback after outpatient acute care visits. *Journal of General Internal Medicine*, *29*(8), 1105–1112. doi:10.1007/s11606-014-2783-3 PMID:24610308

Bernstein, M. L., McCreless, T., & Côté, M. J. (2007). Five constants of Information technology Adoption in Healthcare. *Hospital Topics*, *85*(1), 17–25. doi:10.3200/HTPS.85.1.17-26 PMID:17405421

Bhagwati, J. (1987). International trade in services and its relevance for economic development. In O. Giarini (Ed.), *The Emerging Service Economy* (pp. 3–57). Oxford, UK: Pergamon Press.

Bhandari, G., & Snowdon, A. (2011). Design of a patient-centric, service-oriented health care navigation system for a local health integration network. *Behaviour & Information Technology*, 1–11. doi:10.1080/0144929x.2011.563798

Biem, H. J., Klimaszewski, A., & Florence, C. (2004). Computer Telephony in Healthcare. *ElectronicHealthcare*, *3*(2), 80–86. PMID:15540408

Biem, H. J., Turnell, R. W., & D'Arcy, C. (2003). Computer telephony: Automated calls for medical care. *Canadian Medical Association, 26*(5), 259–268. PMID:14596488

Bijker, W. E. (2009). How is technology made?—That is the question! *Cambridge Journal of Economics, 34*(1), 63–76. doi:10.1093/cje/bep068

Biske, T. (2008). *SOA Governance*. Birmingham, UK: Packt Publishing Ltd.

Bitner, M. J., Brown, S. W., Goul, M., & Urban, S. (2008). Services science journey: foundations, progress, and challenges. In B. Hefley & W. Murphy (Eds.), *Service science, management and engineering education for the 21st century* (pp. 227–233). Springer; doi:10.1007/978-0-387-76578-5_35

Black A.D., Car J., Pagliary C., Anadan C., Cresswell K., Bokun T., et al. (2011). The impact of eHealth on the quality and safety of health care: A systematic overview. *Public Library of Science (PLOS) in Medicine, 8*(1).

Black, A. D., Car, J., Pagliari, C., Anandan, C., Cresswell, K., Bokun, T., & Sheikh, A. et al. (2011). The impact of eHealth on the quality and safety of health care: A systematic overview. *PLoS Medicine, 8*(1), e1000387. PMID:21267058

Black, A. D., Car, J., Pagliari, C., Anandan, C., Cresswell, K., Bokun, T., & Sheikh, A. et al. (2011). The Impact of eHealth on the Quality and Safety of Health Care: A Systematic Overview. *PLoS Medicine, 8*(1), e1000387. PMID:21267058

Black, P., Marsh, C., & Ashworth, L. (2009). Assessment of customer satisfaction with verbal responses provided by a pharmaceutical company's third-party medical information call center. *Drug Information Journal, 43*(3), 263–271.

Bodenheimer, T., Lorig, K., Holman, H., & Grumbach, K. (2002). Patient self-management of chronic disease in primary care.[JAMA]. *Journal of the American Medical Association, 288*(19), 2469–2475. doi:10.1001/jama.288.19.2469 PMID:12435261

Bødker, K., Kensing, F., & Simonsen, J. (2004). *Participatory IT design. designing for business and workplace realities*. MIT Press.

Boulos, M. N., Wheeler, S., Tavares, C., & Jones, R. (2011). How smartphones are changing the face of mobile and participatory healthcare: An overview, with example from eCAALYX. *Biomedical Engineering Online, 10*(1), 24. PMID:21466669

Bourbeau, J., & van der Palen, J. (2009). Promoting effective self-management programmes to improve COPD. *The European Respiratory Journal, 33*(3), 461–463. doi:10.1183/09031936.00001309 PMID:19251792

Brandt, E. (2006). Designing exploratory design games: A framework for participation in participatory design?*Proceedings Participatory Design Conference*.

Brannigan, V. (1985). Acceptance Testing-The Critical Problem in Software Acquisition. *IEEE Transactions on Bio-Medical Engineering*, *BME-32*(4), 295–299. doi:10.1109/TBME.1985.325451 PMID:3838735

Brender, J. (1997). *Methodology for Assessment of Medical IT-Based Systems*. IOS Press.

Brender, J. (2006). Handbook of evaluation methods for health informatics. Burlington, MA: Academic Press; doi:10.1145/1147261.1147271

Breslin, E., & Denison, J. (2002). The development of telephone triage: Historical, professional and personal perspectives. *Journal of Orthopaedic Nursing*, *6*(4), 191–197. doi:10.1016/S1361-3111(02)00070-5

Briggs, J. K. (2007). *Telephone triage practices for nurses*. Lippincott Williams & Wilkins.

Britt, H., Miller, G. C., Charles, J., Pan, Y., Valenti, L., Henderson, J., ... Knox, S. (2007). General Practice Activity in Australia 2005-06, Cat. no. GEP 16. Canberra: AIHW.

Britz, B., Petri, G., Tramacere, G., Roy, A., Ng, F., & Blackmore, D. et al. (2014). Forecast Analysis: IT Outsourcing, Worldwide, 1Q14 Update. *Gartner Report*, *G00261935*, 14.

Brothers, K. B., & Rothstein, M. A. (2015). Ethical, legal and social implications of incorporating personalized medicine into healthcare. *Personalized Medicine*, *12*(1), 43–51. doi:10.2217/pme.14.65 PMID:25601880

Browne, G. J., & Ramesh, V. (2002). Improving Information Requirements Determination: A Cognitive Perspective. *Information & Management*, *39*(8), 625–645. doi:10.1016/S0378-7206(02)00014-9

Brynjolfsson, E., & Hitt, L. M. (2003). Computing Productivity: Firm-Level Evidence. *The Review of Economics and Statistics*, *85*(4), 793–808. doi:10.1162/003465303772815736

Budden, C. B., Anthony, J. F., Budden, M. C., & Jones, M. A. (2011). Managing the evolution of a revolution: Marketing implications of internet media usage among college students. *College Teaching Methods & Styles Journal (CTMS)*, *3*(3).

Bunik, M., Glazner, J. E., Chandramouli, V., Emsermann, C. B., Hegarty, T., & Kempe, A. (2007). Pediatric Telephone Call Centers: How do they affect health care use and costs? *Pediatrics*, *119*(2), 305–313. doi:10.1542/peds.2006-1511 PMID:17272593

Bunn, F., Byrne, G., & Kendall, S. (2005). The effects of telephone consultation and triage on healthcare use and patient satisfaction: A systematic review. *The British Journal of General Practice*, *55*(521), 956–961. PMID:16378566

Buntin, M. B., Burke, M. F., Hoaglin, M. C., & Blumenthal, D. (2011). The benefits of health information technology: A review of the recent literature shows predominantly positive results. *Health Affairs*, *30*(3), 464–471. doi:10.1377/hlthaff.2011.0178 PMID:21383365

Burman, E. (2003). *Shift!: The Unfolding Internet: Hype, Hope and History*. Chichester, UK: John Wiley & Sons.

Burney, A., Abbas, Z., Mahmood, N., & Arifeen, Q. U. (2013). Prospects for mobile health in Pakistan and other developing countries. *Advances in Internet of Things*, *3*(022A), 27–32. doi:10.4236/ait.2013.32A004

Byrd, T. A., Lewis, B. R., & Bryan, R. W. (2006). The Leveraging Influence of Strategic Alignment on IT Investment: An Empirical Examination. *Information & Management*, *43*(3), 308–321. doi:10.1016/j.im.2005.07.002

Cantu, R. V., Bell, J. E., Padula, W. V., Nahikian, K. R., & Pober, D. M. (2012). How do emergency department physicians rate their orthopaedic on-call coverage? *Journal of Orthopaedic Trauma*, *26*(1), 54–56. doi:10.1097/BOT.0b013e31821d7a81 PMID:21904223

Cao, Y., Lu, Y., Gupta, S., & Yang, S. (2015). The effects of differences between e–commerce and m–commerce on the consumers' usage transfer from online to mobile channel. *International Journal of Mobile Communications*, *13*(1), 51–70. doi:10.1504/IJMC.2015.065890

Carolan, M. C., Steele, C., & Margetts, H. (2010). Attitudes towards Gestational Diabetes among a multi-ethnic cohort in Australia. *Journal of Clinical Nursing*, *19*(17/18), 2446–2453. doi:10.1111/j.1365-2702.2010.03305.x PMID:20920072

Carter, O., Donovan, R. J., & Jalleh, G. (2011). Using Viral e-mails to Distribute Tobacco Control Advertisements to Young Adults: An Experimental Investigation. *Journal of Health Communication*, *16*(7), 698–707. doi:10.1080/10810730.2011.551998 PMID:21432712

Cassimatis, M., & Kavanagh, D. J. (2012). Effects of type 2 diabetes behavioural telehealth interventions on glycaemic control and adherence: A systematic review. *Journal of Telemedicine and Telecare*, *18*(8), 447–450. doi:10.1258/jtt.2012.GTH105 PMID:23209266

Castells, M. (2000). *The Rise of the Network Society*. Oxford, UK: Blackwell Publishers.

Castelnuovo, G., Manzoni, G. M., Corti, S., Cuzziol, P., Villa, V., & Molinari, E. (2011). Clinical psychology and medicine for the treatment of obesity in out-patient settings: the TECNOB project. *Telemedicine Techniques and Applications*, 257-268.

Castillejo, P., Martínez, J. F., Rodríguez-Molina, J., & Cuerva, A. (2013). Integration of wearable devices in a wireless sensor network for an E-health application. *IEEE Wireless Communicatons*, *20*(4), 38–49. doi:10.1109/MWC.2013.6590049

Catanzariti, L., Faulks, K., & Waters, A.-M. (2007). *National Diabetes Register: Statistical Profile 1999-2005, AIHW cat. no. CVD 39*. Canberra: AIHW.

Catwell, L., & Sheikh, A. (2009). Evaluating eHealth interventions: The need for continuous systemic evaluation. *PLoS Medicine*, *6*(8), 1–6. doi:10.1371/journal.pmed.1000126 PMID:19688038

Chanda, K. L., & Shaw, J. G. (2010). The development of telehealth as a strategy to improve health care services in Zambia. *Health Information and Libraries Journal*, *27*(2), 133–139. doi:10.1111/j.1471-1842.2010.00876.x PMID:20565554

Chang, M., He, J., Tsai, W., Xiao, B., & Chen, Y. (2006). *UCSOA: User-Centric Service-Oriented Architecture.* Paper presented at the IEEE International Conference on e-Business Engineering, Shanghai, China.

Chang, I., Hwang, H.-G., Hung, M.-C., Lin, M.-H., & Yen, D. C. (2007). Factors affecting the adoption of electronic signature: Executives' perspective of hospital information department. *Decision Support Systems*, *44*(1), 350–359. doi:10.1016/j.dss.2007.04.006

Chang, L., Kagaayi, J., Nakigozi, G., Packer, A., Serwadda, D., Quinn, T., & Reynolds, S. J. et al. (2008). Responding to the human resource crisis: Peer health workers, mobile phones, and HIV care in Rakai, Uganda. *AIDS Patient Care and STDs*, *22*(3), 173–174. doi:10.1089/apc.2007.0234 PMID:18290750

Chang, M.-Y., Pang, C., Tarn, J. M., Liu, T.-S., & Yen, D. C. (2015). Exploring user acceptance of an e-hospital service: An empirical study in Taiwan. *Computer Standards & Interfaces*, *38*, 35–43. doi:10.1016/j.csi.2014.08.004

Chan, Y. E., Huff, S. L., Barclay, D. W., & Copeland, D. G. (1997). Business strategy orientation. *Information Systems Research*, *8*(2), 125–150. doi:10.1287/isre.8.2.125

Chao, C. J., Lin, C., Lin, K., Shen, C. L., & Wang, C. H. (2012). Using the Analytic Hierarchy Process Methodology to Assess the Drivers Affecting the Implementation of Interactive Digital Television as a Commerce Platform. *International Journal of Wireless Networks and Broadband Technologies*, *2*(3), 42–51. doi:10.4018/ijwnbt.2012070104

Chase, R. B. (1978). Where does the customer fit in a service operation? *Harvard Business Review*, *56*(5), 137–142. PMID:10239167

Chatterjee, S., Chakraborty, S., Sarker, S., Sarker, S., & Lau, F. Y. (2009). Examining the success factors for mobile work in healthcare: A deductive study. *Decision Support Systems*, *46*(3), 620–633. doi:10.1016/j.dss.2008.11.003

Chau, P. Y. K., & Jim, C. C. F. (2002). Adoption of Electronic Data Interchange in Small & Medium Sized Enterprises. *Journal of Global Information Management*, *10*(4), 61–85. doi:10.4018/jgim.2002100104

Chau, S., & Turner, P. (2006). Utilisation of mobile handheld devices for care management at an Australian aged care facility. *Electronic Commerce Research and Applications*, *5*(4), 305–312. doi:10.1016/j.elerap.2006.04.005

Chávez, E., Krishnan, P., & Finnie, G. (2010). A taxonomy of e-health standards to assist system developers. In G. A. Papadopulos et al. (Eds.), *Information Systems Development. Towards a Service Provision Society* (pp. 737–745). New York, NY: Springer US.

Chen, C., Haddad, D., Selsky, J., Hoffman, J. E., Kravitz, R. L., Estrin, D. E., & Sim, I. (2012). Making sense of mobile health data: An open architecture to improve individual-and population-level health. *Journal of Medical Internet Research, 14*(4), e112. doi:10.2196/jmir.2152 PMID:22875563

Chesbrough, H. (2005). Toward a science of services. *Harvard Business Review, 83*(2), 16–17.

Chih, Y. Y., & Zwikael, O. (2015). Project benefit management: A conceptual framework of target benefit formulation. *International Journal of Project Management, 33*(2), 352–362. doi:10.1016/j.ijproman.2014.06.002

Chittleborough, C. R., Grant, J. F., Phillips, P. J., & Taylor, A. W. (2007). The increasing prevalence of diabetes in South Australia: The relationship with population ageing and obesity. *Public Health, 121*(2), 92–99. doi:10.1016/j.puhe.2006.09.017 PMID:17166533

Cho, S.-E. (2005). Developing new frameworks for operations strategy and service system design in electronic commerce. *International Journal of Service Industry Management, 16*(3), 294–314. doi:10.1108/09564230510601413

Clarke, K., O'Moore, R., Smeets, R., Talmon, J., Brender, J., & McNair, P. et al. (1994). A methodology for evaluation of knowledge-based systems in medicine. *Artificial Intelligence in Medicine, 6*(2), 107–121. doi:10.1016/0933-3657(94)90040-X PMID:8049752

Classen, D. C., Resar, R., Griffin, F., Federico, F., Frankel, T., & Kimmel, N. et al. (2011). 'Global trigger tool'shows that adverse events in hospitals may be ten times greater than previously measured. *Health Affairs, 30*(4), 581–589. doi:10.1377/hlthaff.2011.0190 PMID:21471476

Claxton, K., Paulden, M., Gravelle, H., Brouwer, W., & Culyer, A. J. (2011). Discounting & Decision Making in the Economic Evaluation of Health-Care Technologies. *Health Economics, 20*(1), 2–15. doi:10.1002/hec.1612 PMID:21154521

Clemensen, J., Rasmussen, J., Denning, A., & Craggs, M. (2011). *Patient Empowerment and New Citizen Roles through Telehealth Technologies - The Early Stage.* Paper presented at the Third International Conference on eHealth, Telemedicine, and Social Medicine, Gosier, France.

Coiera, E. (2003). *Guide to Health Informatics.* Hodder Arnold. doi:10.1201/b13618

Coiera, E. (2006). Communication systems in healthcare. *The Clinical Biochemist. Reviews / Australian Association of Clinical Biochemists, 27*(2), 89. PMID:17077879

Coile, R. C. Jr. (1999). Call centers: Phone lines, protocols, and patient care management in the 21st century. *Russ Coile's Health Trends, 11*(5), 1–4. PMID:10351310

Colagiuri, S., Colagiuri, R., & Ward, J. (1998). *National Diabetes Strategy and Implementation Plan.* Canberra: Diabetes Australia.

Commission of the European Communities. (2004). e-Health - making healthcare better for European citizens: An action plan for a European e-Health Area. Luxembourg: Commission of the European Communities.

Cook, J., Copeland, M., Hamilton, M., Jonikas, J., Razzano, L., Floyd, C., & Gray, D. D. et al. (2009). Initial outcomes of a mental illness self-management program based on wellness recovery action planning. *Psychiatric Services (Washington, D.C.)*, *60*(2), 246–249. doi:10.1176/ps.2009.60.2.246 PMID:19176420

Coombs, C. R. (2015). When planned IS/IT project benefits are not realized: A study of inhibitors and facilitators to benefits realization. *International Journal of Project Management*, *33*(2), 363–379. doi:10.1016/j.ijproman.2014.06.012

Coradeschi, S., Cesta, A., Cortellessa, G., Coraci, L., Gonzalez, J., Karlsson, L., . . . Otslund, B. (2013). Giraffplus: Combining social interaction and long term monitoring for promoting independent living. In *Human System Interaction (HSI), 2013 The 6th International Conference on*. IEEE.

Corkrey, R., & Parkinson, L. (2002). Interactive voice response: Review of studies 1989–2000. *Behavior Research Methods, Instruments, & Computers*, *34*(3), 342–353. doi:10.3758/BF03195462 PMID:12395550

Costa, F. F. (2013). Social networks, web-based tools and diseases: Implications for biomedical research. *Drug Discovery Today*, *18*(5), 272–281. doi:10.1016/j.drudis.2012.10.006 PMID:23103282

Cresswell, K., Bates, D. W., & Sheikh, A. (2013). Ten key considerations for the successful implementation and adoption of largescale health information technology. *Journal of the American Medical Informatics Association*, *20*(e1), 9–13. doi:10.1136/amiajnl-2013-001684 PMID:23599226

Croidieu, S., Charbotel, B., Vohito, M., Renaud, L., Jaussaud, J., Bourboul, C., & Bergeret, A. et al. (2008). Call-handlers' working conditions and their subjective experience of work: A transversal study. *International Archives of Occupational and Environmental Health*, *82*(1), 67–77. doi:10.1007/s00420-008-0308-2 PMID:18320205

Crouch, R., Patel, A., & Dale, J. (1996). Paediatric calls to inner city accident and emergency department: Service demand and advice given. *Accident and Emergency Nursing*, *4*(4), 170–174. doi:10.1016/S0965-2302(96)90072-7 PMID:8981836

Crowther, C. A., Hiller, J. E., Moss, J. R., McPhee, A. J., Jeffries, W. S., & Robinson, J. S. (2005). The effect of treatment of gestational diabetes mellitus on pregnancy outcomes. *The New England Journal of Medicine*, *352*(24), 2477–2486. doi:10.1056/NEJMoa042973 PMID:15951574

Cruz, I. F., & Xiao, H. (2009). Ontology Driven Data Integration in Heterogeneous Networks. *Complex Systems in Knowledge-based Environments: Theory, Models, and Applications*, *168*, 75–98.

Cutler, M., & Sterne, J. (2000). *E-Metrics: Business Metrics for the New Economy*. NetGenesis. Retrieved from http://www.netgen.com/emetrics/

Dale, J., Crouch, R., & Lloyd, D. (1998). Primary care: Nurse-led telephone triage and advice out of hours. *Nursing Standard*, *12*(47), 41–45. doi:10.7748/ns1998.08.12.47.39.c2520 PMID:9752159

Danvers, K., & Nikolov, P. (2010). Does Outsourcing Affect Hospital Profitability? *Journal of Health Care Finance*, *37*(1), 13–29. PMID:20973370

Darkins, A. W., & Carry, M. A. (2000). *Telemedicine and telehealth. Principles, policies, performance and pitfalls*. Springer Publishing Company.

Darkins, A., Foster, L., Anderson, C., Goldschmidt, L., & Selvin, G. (2013). The design, implementation, and operational management of a comprehensive quality management program to support national telehealth networks. *Telemedicine Journal and e-Health*, *19*(7), 557–564. doi:10.1089/tmj.2012.0263 PMID:23705961

Davis, F. D., Bagozzi, R. P., & Warshaw, P. R. (1989). User acceptance of computer technology: A comparison of two theoretical models. *Management Science*, *35*(8), 982–1003. doi:10.1287/mnsc.35.8.982

Davis, T. C., Jackson, R. H., George, R. B., Long, S. W., Talley, D., & Murphy, P. W. et al. (1993). Reading ability in patients in substance misuse treatment centers. *Substance Use & Misuse*, *28*(6), 571–582. doi:10.3109/10826089309039648 PMID:8098019

de Waal, B. M., & Batenburg, R. (2014). The process & structure of user participation: A BPM system implementation case study. *Business Process Management Journal*, *20*(1), 107–128. doi:10.1108/BPMJ-05-2012-0045

Delichatsios, H. K., Friedman, R. H., Glanz, K., Tennstedt, S., Smigelski, C., Pinto, B. M., & Killman, M. W. et al. (2001). Randomized trial of a talking computer to improve adults eating habits. *American Journal of Health Promotion*, *15*(4), 215–224. doi:10.4278/0890-1171-15.4.215 PMID:11349340

Demattè, C., Biffi, A., Mandelli, A., & Parolini, C. (2007). Firms and the Digital Technology in Italy: The Network Moves Forward. In U. Apte & U. Karmarkar (Eds.), *Managing in the Information Economy* (pp. 429–471). New York, NY: Springer. doi:10.1007/978-0-387-36892-4_18

Deslauriers, A., L'Ecuyer, P., Pichitlamken, J., Ingolfsson, A., & Avramidis, A. N. (2007). Markov chain models of a telephone call center with call blending. *Computers & Operations Research*, *34*(6), 1616–1645. doi:10.1016/j.cor.2005.06.019

Detmer, D., Bloomrosen, M., Raymond, B., & Tang, P. (2008). Integrated personal health records: Transformative tools for consumer-centric care. *BMC Medical Informatics and Decision Making*, *8*(1), 45. doi:10.1186/1472-6947-8-45 PMID:18837999

Devaraj, S., & Kohli, R. (2000). Information Technology payoff in the healthcare industry: A longitudinal study. *Journal of Management Information Systems*, *16*(4), 41–67. doi:10.1080/07421222.2000.11518265

DeVore, N. E. (1999). Telephone triage: A challenge for practicing midwives. *Journal of Nurse-Midwifery*, *44*(5), 471–479. doi:10.1016/S0091-2182(99)00087-7 PMID:10540521

Dewett, T., & Jones, G. R. (2001). The role of information technology in the organization: A review, model, and assessment. *Journal of Management*, *27*(3), 313–346. doi:10.1177/014920630102700306

Dhillon, J. S., Wünsche, B. C., & Lutteroth, C. (2013). *An online social-networking enabled telehealth system for seniors: a case study*. Paper presented at the Fourteenth Australasian User Interface Conference.

DiabCostAustralia. (2002). *Assessing the Burden of Type 2 Diabetes in Australia*. Adelaide: DiabCost Australia.

DiabetesAustralia. (2008). *Diabetes in Australia*. Retrieved from http://www.diabetesaustralia.com.au/Understanding-Diabetes/Diabetes-in-Australia/

Dini, E. F., Wilkins, R. W., & Sigafoos, J. (2000). The impact of computer-generated messages on childhood immunization coverage. *American Journal of Preventive Medicine*, *18*(2), 132–139. doi:10.1016/S0749-3797(99)00086-0 PMID:10698243

Dixon, B. E. (2007). A roadmap for the adoption of e-Health. *e-Service Journal*, *5*(3), 3–13. doi:10.2979/ESJ.2007.5.3.3

Dixon, T., & Webbie, K. (2006). *The National System for Monitoring Diabetes in Australia (AIHW Cat. No. CVD 32)*. Canberra: Australian Institute of Health and Wealfare.

Doherty, N. F. (2014). The Role of Socio-technical Principles in Leveraging Meaningful Benefits from IT Investments. *Applied Ergonomics*, *45*(2), 181–187. doi:10.1016/j.apergo.2012.11.012 PMID:23305923

Doherty, N. F., Ashurst, C., & Peppard, J. (2012). Factors Affecting the Successful Realisation of Benefits from Systems Development Projects: Findings from Three Case Studies. *Journal of Information Technology*, *27*(1), 1–16. doi:10.1057/jit.2011.8

Donovan, R. J., Boulter, J., Borland, B., Jalleh, G., & Carter, O. (2003). Continuous Tracking of the Australian National Tobacco Campaign: Advertising Effects on Recall, Recognition, Cognitions, & Behaviour. *Tobacco Control*, *12*(90002Suppl II), ii30–ii39. doi:10.1136/tc.12.suppl_2.ii30 PMID:12878771

Donovan, R. J., Jalleh, G., Clarkson, J., & Giles-Corti, B. (1999). Evidence for effectiveness of sponsorship as a health promotion tool. *Australian Journal of Primary Health*, *5*(3), 82–92.

Downer, S. R., Meara, J. G., Da Costa, A. C., & Sethuraman, K. (2006). SMS text messaging improves outpatient attendance. *Australian Health Review*, *30*(3), 389–396. doi:10.1071/AH060389 PMID:16879098

Drapeau, M., & Wells, I. (2009). *Social software and national security: An initial net assessment*. DTIC Document.

Duder, J. C., & Rosenwein, M. B. (2001). Towards "zero abandonments" in call center performance. *European Journal of Operational Research*, *135*(1), 50–56. doi:10.1016/S0377-2217(00)00289-7

Durugbo, C. (2012). Modelling User Participation in Organisations as Networks. *Expert Systems with Applications*, *39*(10), 9230–9245. doi:10.1016/j.eswa.2012.02.082

Dutot, V., Bergeron, F., & Raymond, L. (2014). Information management for the internationalization of SMEs: An exploratory study based on a strategic alignment perspective. *International Journal of Information Management*, *34*(5), 672–681. doi:10.1016/j.ijinfomgt.2014.06.006

Dwivedi, Y., Ravichandran, K., Williams, M., Miller, S., Lal, B., Antony, G., & Kartik, M. (2013). IS/IT Project Failures: A Review of the Extant Literature for Deriving a Taxonomy of Failure Factors. In Y. Dwivedi, H. Henriksen, D. Wastell, & R. De' (Eds.), *Grand Successes and Failures in IT. Public and Private Sectors* (Vol. 402, pp. 73–88). Springer Berlin Heidelberg. doi:10.1007/978-3-642-38862-0_5

Economic Research Office, General Policy Division, Information and Communications Policy Bureau, Ministry of Public Management, Home Affairs, Posts and Telecommunications. (2004). WHITE PAPER Information and Communications in Japan.

Economics, C. (2013). *IT Outsourcing Statistics: 2013/2014*. Irvine, CA: Computer Economics Inc.

Economo, K., Stewart, S., Sullivan, D., Jalleh, G., Carter, O., & Lin, C. (2010). The Importance of Public Education Campaigns in Raising Awareness & Support for Smoke-free Car Legislation in Western Australia. *Australian and New Zealand Journal of Public Health*, *34*(1), 92–93. doi:10.1111/j.1753-6405.2010.00483.x PMID:20920115

Eder, L. B., & Igbaria, M. (2001). Determinants of intranet diffusion and infusion. *Omega*, *29*(3), 233–242. doi:10.1016/S0305-0483(00)00044-X

Editors, P. M. (2013). A reality checkpoint for mobile health: Three challenges to overcome. *PLoS Medicine*, *10*(2), e1001395. doi:10.1371/journal.pmed.1001395 PMID:23468597

Edmondson, A. C. (2003). Framing for learning: Lessons in successfull technology implementation. *California Management Review*, *45*(2), 34–51. doi:10.2307/41166164

Edquist, C., & Edquist, O. (1979). Social carriers of techniques for development. *Journal of Peace Research*, *16*(4), 313–331. doi:10.1177/002234337901600403

Effing, T., Monninkhof, E., van der Valk, P., Zielhuis, G., Walters, E., van der Palen, J., & Zwerink, M. (2007). *Self-management education for patients with chronic obstructive pulmonary disease*. Academic Press.

Egea, J. M. O., González, M. V. R., & Menéndez, M. R. (2015). *E-Health Services Adoption by European General Practitioners Assessing the Different Roles of Marketing Theory and Practice in the Jaws of Economic Uncertainty*. Springer.

Eiglier, P., & Langeard, E. (1987). *Servuction. Le marketing des services*. Paris, France: McGraw-Hill.

Eikelboom, R. H., & Atlas, M. D. (2005). Attitude to telemedicine, and willingness to use it, in audiology patients. *Journal of Telemedicine and Telecare*, *11*(8), S22–S25. doi:10.1258/135763305775124920 PMID:16375788

Eisenhardt, K. M. (1989). Building Theories From Case Study Research. *Academy of Management Review*, *14*(4), 532–550.

Ekeland, A. G., Bowes, A., & Flottorp, S. (2010). Effectiveness of telemedicine: A systematic review of reviews. *International Journal of Medical Informatics*, *79*(11), 736–771. doi:10.1016/j.ijmedinf.2010.08.006 PMID:20884286

El-Khatib, H. T., Williams, M. H., MacKinnon, L. M., & Marwick, D. H. (2002). Using a Distributed Approach to Retrieve and Integrate Information from Heterogeneous Distributed Databases. *The Computer Journal*, *45*(4), 381–394. doi:10.1093/comjnl/45.4.381

eMarketer. (2014). *Global B2C Ecommerce Sales to Hit $1.5 Trillion This Year Driven by Growth in Emerging Markets: Asia-Pacific leapfrogs North America to become world's largest regional ecommerce market*. eMaketer Inc.

Eng, T. (2001). *The e-Health Landscape – a terrain map of emerging information and communication technologies in health and health care*. Princeton NJ: The Robert Wood Johnson Foundation. Retrieved May 23, 2014 from http://www.hetinitiative.org/media/pdf/eHealth.pdf

England, I., Steward, D., & Walker, S. (2000). Information technology adoption in health care: When organizations and technology collide. *Australian Health Review*, *23*(3), 176–185. doi:10.1071/AH000176 PMID:11186051

Ertogral, K., & Bamuqabel, B. (2008). Developing staff schedules for a bilingual telecommunication call center with flexible workers. *Computers & Industrial Engineering*, *54*(1), 118–127. doi:10.1016/j.cie.2007.06.040

Ethier, J. F., Dameron, O., Curcin, V., McGilchrist, M., Verheij, R. A., Arvanitis, T. A., & Burgun, A. et al. (2013). A unified structural/terminological interoperability framework based on LexEVS: Application to TRANSFoRm. *Journal of the American Medical Informatics Association*, *20*(5), 986–994. doi:10.1136/amiajnl-2012-001312 PMID:23571850

Evans, P., & Wurster, T. S. (2000). *Blown to bits. How the new economics of information transforms strategy*. Boston, MA: Harvard Business School Press.

Evenson, A., Harker, P. T., & Frei, F. X. (1999). *Effective Call Center Management: Evidence from Financial Services*. Working Paper 9925B. Wharton Financial Institutions Center.

Executive, N. H. S. (1999). Quality and Performance in the NHS: Clinical Indicators. Author.

Eysenbach, G. (2001). What is e-health? *Journal of Medical Internet Research*, *3*(2), e20. doi:10.2196/jmir.3.2.e20 PMID:11720962

Falch, A. M., & Jensen, F. (2005). *Erfaringer med udbudsformen "konkurrencepræget dialog" (the competitive dialogue process)*. Unpublished manuscript.

Fan, Z., Yang, H., Gao, H., Lintu, H., & Sun, W. (2006). Pregnancy outcome in gestational diabetes. *International Journal of Gynaecology and Obstetrics: the Official Organ of the International Federation of Gynaecology and Obstetrics*, *94*(1), 12–16. doi:10.1016/j.ijgo.2006.03.021 PMID:16733056

Faridi, Z., Liberti, L., Shuval, K., Northrup, V., Ali, A., & Katz, D. (2008). Evaluating the impact of mobile telephone technology on type 2 diabetic patients' self-management: The NICHE pilot study. *Journal of Evaluation in Clinical Practice*, *14*(3), 465–469. doi:10.1111/j.1365-2753.2007.00881.x PMID:18373577

Farmer, A., Gibson, O., Hayton, P., Bryden, K., Dudley, C., Neil, C., & Tarrassenko, L. (2005). A real-time, mobile phone-based telemedicine system to support young adults with type 1 diabetes. *Informatics in Primary Care*, *13*(3), 171–177. PMID:16259856

Farooq, A., & Shah, A. (2010). Similarity Identification and Measurement between Ontologies. *Journal of American Science*, *6*(4), 67–85.

Fatehi, F., & Wootton, R. (2012). Telemedicine, telehealth or e-health? A bibliometric analysis of the trends in the use of these terms. *Journal of Telemedicine and Telecare*, *18*(8), 460–464. doi:10.1258/jtt.2012.GTH108 PMID:23209265

Federspiel, C. C., Fisk, W. J., Price, P. N., Liu, G., Faulkner, D., Dibartolemeo, D. L., & Lahiff, M. et al. (2004). Worker performance and ventilation in a call center: Analyses of work performance data for registered nurses. *Indoor Air*, *14*(s8), 41–50. doi:10.1111/j.1600-0668.2004.00299.x PMID:15663459

Feldman-Naim, S., Myers, F. S., Clark, C. H., Turner, E. H., & Leibenluft, E. (1997). Agreement between face-to-face and telephone-administered mood ratings in patients with rapid cycling bipolar disorder. *Psychological Research*, *71*, 129–132. PMID:9255857

Ferdosi, M., Farahabadi, E., Mofid, M., Rejalian, F., Haghighat, M., & Naghdi, P. (2013). Evaluation of Outsourcing in Nursing Services: A Case Study of Kashani Hospital, Isfahan in 2011. *Materia Socio-Medica*, *25*(1), 37–39. PMID:23678338

Fickenscher, K., & Bakerman, M. (2011). Leadership and governance for IT projects. *Physician Executive*, *37*(1), 72–76. PMID:21302752

Fieschi, M. (2002). Information technology is changing the way society sees health care delivery. *International Journal of Medical Informatics*, *66*(1-3), 85–93. doi:10.1016/S1386-5056(02)00040-0 PMID:12453562

Finnegan, D., & Hamid, K. (2009). Information systems (IS) integration approaches in healthcare: a critical review. In W. Currie & D. Finnegan (Eds.), Integrating Healthcare With Information and Communications Technology. London: Radcliffe Publishing.

Firat, K., Moser, L., & Melliar-Smith, M. (2008). Building a Distributed E-Healthcare System Using SOA. *IT Professional*, *10*(2).

Fischer, S., & Soyez, K. (2015). *Trick or Treat: Assessing Health 2.0 and Its Prospects for Patients, Providers and Society Challenges and Opportunities in Health Care Management*. Springer.

Fitzgerald, G., & Russo, N. (2005). The turnaround of the London ambulance service computer-aided despatch system (LASCAD). *European Journal of Information Systems*, *14*(3), 244–257. doi:10.1057/palgrave.ejis.3000541

Fjeldsoe, B., Marshall, A., & Miller, Y. (2009). Behavior change interventions delivered by mobile telephone short-message service. *American Journal of Preventive Medicine*, *36*(2), 165–173. doi:10.1016/j.amepre.2008.09.040 PMID:19135907

Flagle, C., Grémy, F., & Perry, S. (1991). *Assessment of Medical Informatics Technology*. Paper presented at the Joint Working Conference.

Fossey, E., Harvey, C., McDermott, F., & Davidson, L. (2002). Understanding and evaluating qualitative research. *The Australian and New Zealand Journal of Psychiatry*, *36*(6), 717–732. doi:10.1046/j.1440-1614.2002.01100.x PMID:12406114

Fracolli, L. A., Gomes, M. F. P., Nabão, F. R. Z., Santos, M. S., Cappellini, V. K., & Almeida, A. C. C. (2014). Primary health care assessment tools: A literature review and metasynthesis. *Ciencia & Saude Coletiva*, *19*(12), 4851–4860. doi:10.1590/1413-812320141912.00572014 PMID:25388193

Franzini, L., Rosenthal, J., Spears, W., Martin, H. S., Balderas, L., Brown, M., & Hanson, C. et al. (2000). Cost effectiveness of childhood immunization reminder/recall systems in urban private practices. *Pediatrics*, *166*, 177–183. PMID:10888689

Free, C., Phillips, G., Galli, L., Watson, L., Felix, L., Edwards, P., & Haines, A. et al. (2013). The effectiveness of mobile-health technology-based health behaviour change or disease management interventions for health care consumers: A systematic review. *PLoS Medicine*, *10*(1), e1001362. doi:10.1371/journal.pmed.1001362 PMID:23349621

Freema, W. D., Vatz, K. A., & Demaerschalk, B. M. (2010). Telemedicine in 2010: Robotic caveats. *Lancet Neurology*, *9*(11), 1046. doi:10.1016/S1474-4422(10)70261-1 PMID:20965432

Frennert, S., & Östlund, B. (2014). Domestication of a telehealthcare system. *Gerontechnology (Valkenswaard)*, *13*(2), 197. doi:10.4017/gt.2014.13.02.105.00

Friedman, C. P., & Wyatt, J. C. (1997). *Evaluation Methods in Medical Informatics*. New York: Springer-Verlag. doi:10.1007/978-1-4757-2685-5

Friedman, R. H., Kazis, L. E., & Jette, A. (1996). A telecommunications system with monitoring and counseling patients with hypertension. Impact on medication adherence and blood pressure control. *American Journal of Hypertension*, *9*(4 pt 1), 285–292. doi:10.1016/0895-7061(95)00353-3 PMID:8722429

Frisse, M. E. (2009). Health Information Technology: One step at a time. *Health Affairs*, *28*(2), 379–w384. doi:10.1377/hlthaff.28.2.w379 PMID:19273814

FS. (2004). *Frost and Sullivan Country Industry Forecast.* Retrieved from http://www.news-medical.net/print_article.asp?id=1405

Fuchsia Howard, A., Smillie, K., Turnbull, K., Zirul, C., Munroe, D., Ward, A., & Olson, R. et al. (2014). Access to Medical and Supportive Care for Rural and Remote Cancer Survivors in Northern British Columbia. *The Journal of Rural Health, 30*(3), 311–321. doi:10.1111/jrh.12064 PMID:24483272

Funnell, M., Brown, T., Childs, B., Haas, L., Hosey, G., Jensen, B., & Weiss, M. et al. (2009). National standards for diabetes self-management education. *Diabetes Care, 32*(Supplement 1), S87–S94. doi:10.2337/dc09-S087 PMID:19118294

Fuwa, Y., Kunimune, H., Niimura, M., Wasaki, K., Shidama, Y., & Nakamura, Y. (2004). Shinshu-Daigaku Internet Daigakuin No Genjyo To Shorai-Keikaku[Current Status and Future Plan of the Graduate School on the Internet, Shinshu University]. *Media Research, 1*, 11–18.

Gaggioli, A., Di Carlo, S., Mantovani, F., Castelnuovo, G., & Riva, G. (2005). A telemedicine survey among Milan doctors. *Journal of Telemedicine and Telecare, 11*(1), 29–34. doi:10.1258/1357633053430476 PMID:15829041

Gagnon, M.-P., Lamothe, L., Fortin, J.-P., Cloutier, A., Godin, G., Gagné, C., & Reinharz, D. (2005). Telehealth adoption in hospitals: An organisational perspective. *Journal of Health Organization and Management, 19*(1), 32–56. doi:10.1108/14777260510592121 PMID:15938601

Ganapathy, K., & Ravindra, A. (2011). Telenursing in an emerging economy: An overview. In Telenursing (pp. 47-59). Springer London.

Gantz, J., & Reinsel, D. (2011). Extracting value from chaos. *IDC iview*, 1-12.

García, J. M., Junghans, M., Agarwal, S., & Ruiz-Cortés, A. (2013). Integrating semantic Web services ranking mechanisms using a common preference model. *Knowledge-Based Systems, 49*, 22–36. doi:10.1016/j.knosys.2013.04.007

Garde, S., Knaup, P., Hovenga, E., & Heard, S. (2007, December). Towards Semantic Interoperability for Electronic Health Records: Domain Knowledge Governance for *open*EHR Archetypes. *International Journal of Medical Informatics, 76*(Supplement 3), S334–S341. doi:10.1016/j.ijmedinf.2007.02.004 PMID:17392019

Garg, A. X., Adhikari, N. K. J., McDonald, H., Rosas-Arellano, M. P., Devereaux, P. J., Beyene, J., & Haynes, R. B. et al. (2005). Effects of Computerized Clinical Decision Support Systems on practitioner performance and patient outcomes: A systematic review. *Journal of the American Medical Association, 293*(10), 1223–1238. doi:10.1001/jama.293.10.1223 PMID:15755945

Garnet, O., Mandelbaum, A., & Reiman, M. (2002). Designing a call center with impatient customers. *Manufacturing & Service Operations Management, 4*(3), 208–227. doi:10.1287/msom.4.3.208.7753

Gefen, D., & Straub, D. W. (1997). Gender differences in the perception and use of e-mail: An extension to the technology acceptance model. *Management Information Systems Quarterly, 21*(4), 389–400. doi:10.2307/249720

Geng, W., Talwar, S., Johnsson, K., Himayat, N., & Johnson, K. D. (2011). M2M: From mobile to embedded internet. *IEEE Communications Magazine, 49*(4), 36–43. doi:10.1109/MCOM.2011.5741144

George, I. S. T., Cullen, M., Gardiner, L., Karabatsos, G., Ng, J. Y.-K., Patterson, A., & Wilson, A. (2007). Universal telenursing triage in Australia and New Zealand. *Australian Family Physician, 37*(6), 476–479. PMID:18523705

Gerber, T. (2009). Health Information Technology: Dispatches from the revolution. *Health Affairs, 28*(2), 390–w391. doi:10.1377/hlthaff.28.2.w390 PMID:19273816

Ghorai, K., Akter, S., Khatun, F., & Ray, P. (2014). mHealth for Smoking Cessation Programs: A Systematic Review. *Journal of Personalized Medicine, 4*(3), 412–423. doi:10.3390/jpm4030412 PMID:25563359

Giaglis, G. M., Paul, R. J., & Doukidis, G. I. (1999). Dynamic Modelling to Assess the Business Value of Electronic Commerce. *International Journal of Electronic Commerce, 3*(3), 35–51. doi:10.1080/10864415.1999.11518340

Gilmour, M. B. (2001). A model for a telephone response system to disaster and trauma. *Traumatology, 6*(3), 120–125. doi:10.1177/153476560100700304

Girling, D. (2000). Important issues in planning and conducting multi-centre randomised trials in cancer and publishing their results. *Critical Reviews in Oncology/Hematology, 36*(1), 13–25. doi:10.1016/S1040-8428(00)00095-0 PMID:10996520

Goldberg, S. (2009). *An Evolution of using social networks in chronic disease management.* Paper presented at the 22nd Bled eConference: Facilitating an Open, Effective and Representative Society, Bled, Slovenia.

Goldberg, S. a. (2002a). *Building the Evidence for a standardized Mobile Internet (wireless) Environment in Ontario, Canada, January Update, Internal INET Documentation.* Ontario, Canada: INET.

Goldberg, S. a. (2002b). *HTA Presentational Selection and Aggregation Component Summary. Internal INET Documentation.* Ontario, Canada: INET.

Goldberg, S. a. (2002c). *Wireless POC Device Component Summary, Internal INET documentation.* Ontario, Canada: INET.

Goldberg, S. a. (2002d). *HTA Presentation Rendering Component Summary, Internal INET documentation.* Ontario, Canada: INET.

Goldberg, S. a. (2002e). *HTA Quality Assurance Component Summary, Internal INET documentation.* Ontario, Canada: INET.

Gorla, N., & Somers, T. M. (2014). The Impact of IT Outsourcing on Information Systems Success. *Information & Management*, *51*(3), 320–335. doi:10.1016/j.im.2013.12.002

Gorschek, T., Svahnberg, M., Borg, A., Loconsole, A., & Sandahl, K. (2007). A controlled empirical evaluation of a requirements abstraction model. *Information and Software Technology*, *49*(7), 790–805. doi:10.1016/j.infsof.2006.09.003

Gottesman, O., Kuivaniemi, H., Tromp, G., Faucett, W. A., Li, R., Manolio, T. A., & …, eMERGE Network, T. (2013). The Electronic Medical Records and Genomics (eMERGE) network: Past, present, and future. *Genetics in Medicine*, *15*(10), 761–771. PMID:23743551

Graham, J., Tomcavage, J., Salek, D., Sciandra, J., Davis, D. E., & Stewart, W. F. (2012). Postdischarge monitoring using interactive voice response system reduces 30-day readmission rates in a case-managed Medicare population. *Medical Care*, *50*(1), 50–57. doi:10.1097/MLR.0b013e318229433e PMID:21822152

Green, L. (2006). Queueing analysis in healthcare. In Patient flow: Reducing delay in healthcare delivery (pp. 281-307). Springer US. doi:10.1007/978-0-387-33636-7_10

Gregoski, M. J., Mueller, M., Vertegel, A., Shaporev, A., Jackson, B. B., Frenzel, R. M., & Treiber, F. A. et al. (2012). Development and validation of a smartphone heart rate acquisition application for health promotion and wellness telehealth applications. *International Journal of Telemedicine and Applications*, *2012*, 696324. PMID:22272197

Grembergen, W., & Amelinckx, I. (2002). *Measuring and Managing E-business Projects through the Balanced Scorecard.* Paper presented at the 35th Hawaii International Conference on System Science, Hawaii, HI. doi:10.1109/HICSS.2002.994395

Grigsby, J., & Sanders, J. H. (1998). Telemedicine: Where it is and where it's going. *Annals of Internal Medicine*, *129*(2), 123–127. doi:10.7326/0003-4819-129-2-199807150-00012 PMID:9669971

Gritzalis, D. (1997). A baseline security policy for distributed healthcare information systems. *Computers & Security*, *16*(8), 709–719. doi:10.1016/S0167-4048(97)00009-6

Grönroos, C. (1990). *Service Management and Marketing: Managing the Moments of Truth in Service Competition.* New Britian, CT: Lexington Books.

Grosjean, V., & De Weerdt, C. R. V. (2005). Towards a psycho-ergonomics study of wellbeing and emotions: The effects of organisational control in call centers. *Le Travail Humain*, *68*(4), 355–378. doi:10.3917/th.684.0355

GS1 Australia. (2005). *Hospital Pharmaceutical eCommerce Looks Healthy.* Media Press Release. GS1 Australia.

Gunter, T. D., & Terry, N. P. (2005). The emergence of national electronic health record architectures in the United States and Australia: Models, costs, and questions. *Journal of Medical Internet Research*, *7*(1), e3. doi:10.2196/jmir.7.1.e3 PMID:15829475

Hadgkiss, E. J., & Renzaho, A. M. (2014). The physical health status, service utilisation and barriers to accessing care for asylum seekers residing in the community: A systematic review of the literature. *Australian Health Review*, *38*(2), 142–159. PMID:24679338

Haghighat, S., Yunesian, M., Akbari, M. E., Ansari, M., & Montezari, A. (2007). Telephone and face-to-face consultation in breast cancer diagnosis: A comparative study. *Patient Education and Counseling*, *67*(1-2), 39–43. doi:10.1016/j.pec.2007.01.015 PMID:17467949

Hahn, E. D., & Bunyaratavej, K. (2010). Services cultural alignment in offshoring: The impact of cultural dimensions on offshoring location choices. *Journal of Operations Management*, *28*(3), 186–193. doi:10.1016/j.jom.2009.10.005

Haidegger, T., Sándor, J., & Benyo, Z. (2011). Surgery in space: The future of robotic telesurgery. *Surgical Endoscopy*, *25*(3), 681–690. doi:10.1007/s00464-010-1243-3 PMID:20652320

Hair, J., Anderson, R., Tatham, R., & Black, W. (Eds.). (1998). *Multivariate Data Analysis*. Prentice Hall.

Halamka, J., Mandl, K., & Tang, P. (2008). Early Experiences with Personal Health Records. *Journal of the American Medical Informatics Association*, *15*(1), 1–7. doi:10.1197/jamia.M2562 PMID:17947615

Hall, J. A., & Dornan, M. C. (1988). Meta-analysis of satisfaction with medical care: Description of research domain and analysis of overall satisfaction levels. *Social Science & Medicine*, *27*(6), 637–644. doi:10.1016/0277-9536(88)90012-3 PMID:3067359

Hall, V., Gomez, C., & Fernandez-Llimos, F. (2006). Situation of drug information centers and services in Costa Rica. *Pharmacy Practice*, *4*(2), 83–87. PMID:25246999

Hamill, C. T., & Lorri, H.-S. (1998). 24-hour call centers and home health care. *Home Care Provider*, *3*(6), 324–325. doi:10.1016/S1084-628X(98)90012-0 PMID:10030213

Handley, S. M., & Angst, C. M. (2015). The Impact Of Culture On The Relationship Between Governance And Opportunism In Outsourcing Relationships. *Strategic Management Journal*, *36*(9), 1412–1434. doi:10.1002/smj.2300

Han, J., & Lee, S. T. (2012). Impact of Vendor Selection on Firms' IT Outsourcing: The Korea Experience. *Journal of Global Information Management*, *20*(2), 25–43. doi:10.4018/jgim.2012040102

Hattie, J., & Timperley, H. (2007). The power of feedback. *Review of Educational Research*, *77*(1), 81–112. doi:10.3102/003465430298487

Haux, R., Ammenwerth, E., Herzog, W., & Knaup, P. (2002). Health care in the information society. A prognosis for the year 2013. *International Journal of Medical Informatics*, *66*(1-3), 3–21. doi:10.1016/S1386-5056(02)00030-8 PMID:12453552

Health, I. T. (2014). Meaningful Use Definition & Objectives. *EHR Incentives & Certification*. Retrieved 04.05., 2014, from http://www.healthit.gov/providers-professionals/meaningful-use-definition-objectives

Heathfield, H., Pitty, D., & Hanka, R. (1998). Evaluating information technology in health care: Barriers and challenges. *BMJ (Clinical Research Ed.), 316*(7149), 1959–1961. doi:10.1136/bmj.316.7149.1959 PMID:9641938

Heeks, R. (1999). *Reinventing government in the information age: international practice in IT-enabled public sector reform.* London: Routledge. doi:10.4324/9780203204962

Heffner, R. (2009). *Forrester Report: Survey Results Show SOA Governance Improves SOA Benefit Realization.* Academic Press.

He, J., & King, W. R. (2008). The role of user participation in information systems development: Implications from a meta-analysis. *Journal of Management Information Systems, 25*(1), 301–331. doi:10.2753/MIS0742-1222250111

Hellang, Ø., Flak, L. S., & Päivärinta, T. (2013). Diverging Approaches to Benefits Realization from Public ICT Investments: A Study of Benefits Realization Methods in Norway. *Transforming Government: People. Process & Policy, 7*(1), 93–108.

Henderson, C., Knapp, M., Fernández, J.-L., Beecham, J., Hirani, S., Beynon, M., . . ., Doll, H. (2012). Cost-effectiveness of telehealth in people with social care needs: the Whole Systems Demonstrator cluster randomised trial. *International Journal of Integrated Care, 12*(Suppl1).

Heschong Mahone Group. (2003). *Windows and offices: A study of office workers performance and the indoor environment.* California Energy Commission. Retrieved from http://www.ecw.org/sites/default/files/HMG_Windows_Offices.pdf

Hesterly, W. S., Liebeskind, J., & Zenger, T. R. (1990). Organizational economics: An impeding revolution in organizational theory. *Academy of Management Review, 15*(3), 402–420. doi:10.2307/258016

Hesterly, W. S., & Zenger, T. R. (1993). The myth of a monolithic economics: Fundamental assumptions and the use of economic models in policy and strategy research. *Organization Science, 4*(3), 496–510. doi:10.1287/orsc.4.3.496

Heydon, N., Kennington, K. S., Jalleh, G., & Lin, C. (2012). Western Australian Smokers' Strongly Support Regulations on the Use of Chemicals and Additives in Cigarettes. *Tobacco Control, 21*(3), 381–382. doi:10.1136/tobaccocontrol-2011-050302 PMID:22170334

Heyworth, L., Kleinman, K., Oddleifson, S., Bernstein, L., Frampton, J., Lehrer, M., & Connelly, M. (2014). Comparison of interactive voice response, patient mailing, and mailed registry to encourage screening for osteoporosis: A randomized controlled trial. *Osteoporosis International, 25*(5), 1519–1526. doi:10.1007/s00198-014-2629-1 PMID:24566584

Hillestad, R., Bigelow, J., Bower, A., Girosi, F., Meili, R., Scoville, R., & Taylor, R. (2005). Can electronic medical record systems transform health care? Potential health benefits, savings, and costs. *Health Affairs, 24*(5), 1103–1117. doi:10.1377/hlthaff.24.5.1103 PMID:16162551

Hill, J. W., & Powell, P. (2009). The national healthcare crisis: Is eHealth a key solution? *Business Horizons, 52*(3), 265–277. doi:10.1016/j.bushor.2009.01.006

HIMSS – Healthcare Information and Management Systems Society. (2014). *Electronic health record (HER)*. Retrieved on May 16, 2014 from http://www.himss.org/ASP/topics_ehr.asp

Hippisley-Cox, J., Pringle, M., Cater, R., Wynn, A., Hammersley, V., & Coupland, C. et al. (2003). The electronic patient record in primary care-regression or progression? A cross sectional study. *British Medical Journal*, *326*(7407).

Hirsh, D. A., Massey, R., Simon, J., & Simon, H. (2004). Does use of a pediatric telephone triage system lead to appropriate pediatric ED utilization? *Pediatric Research*, *55*, 120A.

Hirsh, D. A., Simon, H. K., Massey, R., Thomton, L., & Simon, J. E. (2007). The Host Hospital 24-Hour Underreferral Rate: An Automated Measure of Call-Center Safety. *Pediatrics*, *119*(6), 1139–1144. doi:10.1542/peds.2006-1986 PMID:17545381

Hirzalla, M., Cleland-Huang, J., & Arsanjani, A. (2009). A Metrics Suite for Evaluating Flexibility and Complexity in Service Oriented Architectures. In G. Feuerlicht & W. Lamersdorf (Eds.), Service-Oriented Computing – ICSOC 2008 Workshops. Springer Berlin Heidelberg.

HL7/OMG. (2010). The Practical Guide for SOA in Health Care. *Healthcare Services Specification Project*. Retrieved 01.10.10, 1.0, from http://hssp.wikispaces.com/file/view/2008-12-29+SOA%2BHealthcare%2BPractical%2BGuide%2Bv1.0.pdf

Hoffman, L., Nola, C., Wilson, J. D., Oats, J. J. N., & Simmons, D. (1998). Gestational diabetes mellitus -- management guidelines. *The Medical Journal of Australia*, *169*, 93–97. PMID:9700346

Hofstede, G. H. (1997). *Cultures & organizations: Software of the mind*. New York, NY: McGraw-Hill.

Hogan, T. P., Wakefield, B., Nazi, K. M., Houston, T. K., & Weaver, F. M. (2011). Promoting access through complementary eHealth technologies: Recommendations for VA's Home Telehealth and personal health record programs. *Journal of General Internal Medicine*, *26*(2), 628–635. doi:10.1007/s11606-011-1765-y PMID:21989614

Holden, R. J., & Karsh, B. T. (2010). The technology acceptance model: Its past and its future in health care. *Journal of Biomedical Informatics*, *43*(1), 159–172. doi:10.1016/j.jbi.2009.07.002 PMID:19615467

Holler, J., Tsiatsis, V., Mulligan, C., Avesand, S., Karnouskos, S., & Boyle, D. (2014). *From Machine-to-machine to the Internet of Things: Introduction to a New Age of Intelligence*. Oxford, UK: Academic Press.

Horton, R. C., Minniti, A., Mireylees, S., & McEntegart, D. (2008). A randomized trial to determine the impact on compliance of a psychophysical peripheral cue based on the Elaboration Likelihood Model. *Contemporary Clinical Trials*, *29*(6), 823–828. doi:10.1016/j.cct.2008.08.005 PMID:18805509

Høstgaard, A. M. (2009). *Fryder forandring? casestudie af EPJ udbudsprocessen i region nord - belyst gennem en procesevaluering med fokus på lægerne som sociale bærere af den elektroniske patientjournal, EPJ* [change is the spice of life? process analysis case study of a region in Denmark]. (PhD Thesis). Aalborg Universitet.

Høstgaard, A. M. (2010). *Evaluering af præpilottest af "klinisk proces" på infektionsmedicinsk afd. aalborg sygehus syd* [evaluation of the pre-pilottest of "clinical process" at the department of infectious diseases]. Unpublished manuscript.

Høstgaard, A. M., Bertelsen, P., & Nøhr, C. (2010a). Evaluering af pilottest af klinisk proces "vieweren" [evaluation of the 'Clinical process' electronic health record (EHR) – evaluation report]. Aalborg University.

Høstgaard, A. M., Bertelsen, P., & Nøhr, C. (2011). Methods to identify, study and understand end-user involvement in HIT-development. *BioMedCentral: Medical Information and Decision Making, 11*(57).

Høstgaard, A. M., Bertelsen, P., Petersen, L. S., & Nøhr, C. (2013). *Constructive technology assessment for HIT development: Learning, feedback and user involvement.* Unpublished manuscript.

Høstgaard, A. M. (2012). End-user participation in health IT development: The EUPHIT method. In S. A. Zakariya Belkhamza (Ed.), *Measuring organizational information systems success: New technologies and practices* (pp. 318–340). Hershey, USA: IGI Global. doi:10.4018/978-1-4666-0170-3.ch016

Høstgaard, A. M., Bertelsen, P., & Nøhr, C. (2010b). How are clinicians involved in EHR planning?: A process analysis case study of a region in denmark. In C. Safran, S. Reti, & H.F. Marin (Eds.), *MEDINFO 2010: Proceedings of the 13th world congress on medical informatics* (pp. 121-125) IOS Press.

Høstgaard, A. M., & Nøhr, C. (2004a). Dealing with organizational change when implementing EHR systems. In *Medinfo 2004:Proceedings of the 11th World Congress on Medical Informatics*.

Høstgaard, A. M., & Nøhr, C. (2004b). *Metodehaandbog i forandringsparathed i forbindelse med udvikling og implementering af nye it-systemer indenfor sundhedsvæsnet [handbook in methods for change readiness in development and implementation of new IT-systems in healthcare].* Aalborg: Virtual Centre for Health Informatics.

Hsiao, C., Pai, J., & Chiu, H. (2009). The Study on the Outsourcing of Taiwan's Hospitals: A Questionnaire Survey Research. *BMC Health Services Research, 9*(1), 78. doi:10.1186/1472-6963-9-78 PMID:19435526

HSSP. (2013). *Healthcare Services Specification Program.* Retrieved 19.01.2013, from http://hssp.wikispaces.com/

Hsu, J. S., Lin, T., Zheng, G., & Hung, Y. (2012). Users as knowledge co-producers in the information system development project. *International Journal of Project Management, 30*(1), 27–36. doi:10.1016/j.ijproman.2011.05.008

Hsu, M. H., Chu, T. B., Yen, J. C., Chiu, W. T., Yeh, G. C., Chen, T. J., & Li, Y. C. J. (2010). Development and implementation of a national telehealth project for long-term care: A preliminary study. *Computer Methods and Programs in Biomedicine, 97*(3), 286–292. doi:10.1016/j.cmpb.2009.12.008 PMID:20092907

Huang, Y., Lin, C., Liu, Y., & Tung, M. (2013). The Effects of IT Resource Alignment and Organizational Dynamism on Alliance Performance in Hemodialysis Centers, *International Technology. Management Review, 3*(2), 105–115.

Huang, Y., Phau, I., & Lin, C. (2010). Consumer Animosity, Economic Hardship, & Normative Influence: How Do They Affect Consumer's Purchase Intention? *European Journal of Marketing, 44*(7/8), 909–937. doi:10.1108/03090561011047463

Huang, Y., Phau, I., Lin, C., Chung, H., & Lin, K. (2008). Allocentrism & Consumer Ethnocentrism: Social Identity on Purchase Intention, *Social Behavior & Personality. International Journal (Toronto, Ont.), 36*(8), 1097–1110.

Hung, S.-Y., Hung, W.-H., Tsai, C.-A., & Jiang, S.-C. (2010). Critical factors of hospital adoption on CRM system: Organizational and information system perspectives. *Decision Support Systems, 48*(4), 592–603. doi:10.1016/j.dss.2009.11.009

Hunt, D. (2007). *Urgent health system reform needed to tackle disease epidemic, says head of new University of Melbourne centre*. Retrieved 25 November, 2008, from http://uninews.unimelb.edu.au/view.php?articleID=4615

Hunt, D. L., Haynes, R. B., Hanna, S. E., & Smith, K. (1998). Effects of computer-based clinical decision support systems on physician performance and patient outcomes. *Journal of the American Medical Association, 280*(15), 1339. doi:10.1001/jama.280.15.1339 PMID:9794315

Hu, P. J., Chau, P. Y. K., Sheng, O. R. L., & Tam, K. Y. (1999). Examining the technology acceptance model using physician acceptance of telemedicine technology. *Journal of Management Information Systems, 16*(2), 91–112. doi:10.1080/07421222.1999.11518247

Hyman, D. J., Ho, K. S., Dunn, J. K., & Simons-Morton, D. (1998). Dietary intervention for cholesterol reduction in public clinic patients. *American Journal of Preventive Medicine, 15*(2), 139–145. doi:10.1016/S0749-3797(98)00038-5 PMID:9713670

ICIC. (2008). *Improving Chronic Illness Care: The Chronic Care Model*. Retrieved from http://www.improvingchroniccare.org/indix.php?p=The_Chronic_Care_Model&s=2

IHE. (2012). *Integrating the Healthcare Enterprise*. Retrieved 01.03.2011, 2011., from http://www.ihe.net/

Informa. (2005a). *Mobile Content and Services: Worldwide Market Analysis & Strategic Outlook*. London: Informa Telecoms & Media.

Informa. (2005b). *Global Mobile Forecasts to 2010: Worldwide Market Analysis & Strategic Outlook 2005-2010* (5th ed.). London: Informa Telecoms & Media.

Inklaar, R., O'Mahony, M., & Timmer, M. (2005). ICT and Europe's productivity performance. industry level growth account comparisons with the United States. *Review of Income and Wealth*, *51*(4), 505–536. doi:10.1111/j.1475-4991.2005.00166.x

IOM – Institute of Medicine. (2001). *Crossing the Quality Chasm: A New Health System for the 21st Century*. Washington, DC: National Academy Press.

Irvine, A. B., Ary, D. V., Grove, D. A., & Gilfillan-Morton, L. (2004). The effectiveness of an interactive multimedia program to influence eating habits. *Health Education Research*, *19*(3), 290–305. doi:10.1093/her/cyg027 PMID:15140849

Isenberg, S. F., Davis, C. L., Adams, C. E., Isenberg, J. S., & Isenberg, M. A. (2001). Incentivized Digital Outcomes Collection. *American Journal of Medical Quality*, *16*(6), 202–211. doi:10.1177/106286060101600604 PMID:11816851

Issarny, V., & Bennaceur, A. (2013). Composing Distributed Systems: Overcoming the Interoperability Challenge. *Lecture Notes in Computer Science*, *7866*, 168–196. doi:10.1007/978-3-642-40615-7_6

ITGI. (2011). Global Status Report on the Governance of Enterprise I.T. (GEIT). In Global Status Research. Rolling Meadows, IL: IT Governance Institute.

Jack, E. P., Bedics, T. A., & McCary, C. E. (2006). Operational challenges in the call center industry: A case study and resource-based framework. *Managing Service Quality*, *16*(5), 477–500. doi:10.1108/09604520610686142

Jakobovits, R. (1997). Integrating Autonomous Heterogeneous Information Sources. *Principles for Digital Library Development Communications of the ACM*, *44*(5), 49–54.

Jalleh, G., Donovan, R. J., Lin, C., & Slevin, T. (2008). Changing Perceptions of Solaria & Cancer Risk: The Role of the Media. *The Medical Journal of Australia*, *188*(12), 735–735. PMID:18558905

Jalleh, G., Donovan, R. J., Lin, C., Slevin, T., Clayforth, C., Pratt, S., & Ledger, M. (2010). Beliefs about Bowel Cancer among the Target Group for the National Bowel Cancer Screening Program in Australia. *Australian and New Zealand Journal of Public Health*, *34*(2), 187–192. doi:10.1111/j.1753-6405.2010.00505.x PMID:23331364

Janson, S. L., McGrath, K. W., Covington, J. K., Cheng, S. C., & Boushey, H. A. (2009). Individualized asthma self-management improves medication adherence and markers of asthma control. *The Journal of Allergy and Clinical Immunology*, *123*(4), 840–846. doi:10.1016/j.jaci.2009.01.053 PMID:19348923

Javalgi, R. G., Martin, C. L., & Todd, P. R. (2004). The export of e-services in the age of technology transformation: Challenges and implications for international service providers. *Journal of Services Marketing*, *18*(7), 560–573. doi:10.1108/08876040410561884

Jennett, P., & Watanabe, M. (2006). Healthcare and Telemedicine: Ongoing and Evolving Challenges. *Disease Management & Health Outcomes*, *14*(1).

Jennings, N., Clifford, S., Fox, A. R., O'Connell, J., & Gardner, G. (2015). The impact of nurse practitioner services on cost, quality of care, satisfaction and waiting times in the emergency department: A systematic review. *International Journal of Nursing Studies*, *52*(1), 421–435. doi:10.1016/j.ijnurstu.2014.07.006 PMID:25443302

Jensen, J., Tøndel, I. A., Jaatun, M. G., Meland, P. H., & Andresen, H. (2009). *Reusable Security Requirements for Healthcare Applications*. Academic Press.

Johnson, N., Murphy, A., McNeese, N., Reddy, M., & Purao, S. (2013). A Survey of Rural Hospitals' Perspectives on Health Information Technology Outsourcing. In *AMIA Annual Symposium Proceedings*. American Medical Informatics Association.

Johnson, C. W. (2006). Why did that happen? exploring the proliferation of barely usable software in healthcare systems. *Quality & Safety in Health Care*, *15*(supplement 1), i76–i81. doi:10.1136/qshc.2005.016105 PMID:17142614

Johnson, C. W. (2011). Identifying common problems in the acquisition and deployment of large-scale, safety–critical, software projects in the US and UK healthcare systems. *Safety Science*, *49*(5), 735–745.

Johnson, R., Jalleh, G., Pratt, I. S., Donovan, R. J., Lin, C., Saunders, C., & Slevin, T. (2013). Online advertising by three commercial breast imaging services: Message takeout and effectiveness. *The Breast*, *22*(5), 780–786. doi:10.1016/j.breast.2013.01.013 PMID:23422256

Jones, C., Hesterly, W. S., & Borgatti, S. P. (1997). A general theory of network governance: Exchange conditions and social mechanisms. *Academy of Management Review*, *22*(4), 911–945.

Joshi, A., Rane, M., Roy, D., Emmadi, N., Srinivasan, P., Kumarasamy, N., & Rutten, R. et al. (2014, April). Supporting treatment of people living with HIV/AIDS in resource limited settings with IVRs. In *Proceedings of the 32nd annual ACM conference on Human Factors in Computing Systems* (pp. 1595-1604). ACM. doi:10.1145/2556288.2557236

Jouini, O., Koole, G., & Roubos, A. (2013). Performance indicators for call centers with impatient customers. *IIE Transactions*, *45*(3), 341–354. doi:10.1080/0740817X.2012.712241

Kahn, J. G., Yang, J., & Kahn, J. S. (2010). 'Mobile' health needs and opportunities in developing countries. *Health Affairs*, *29*(2), 252–258. doi:10.1377/hlthaff.2009.0965 PMID:20348069

Kaipio, J. (2011). *Usability in healthcare: Overcoming the mismatch between information systems and clinical work*. Aalto University, School of Science, Department of Computer Science and Engineering.

Kamei, T., Yamamoto, Y., Kajii, F., Nakayama, Y., & Kawakami, C. (2013). Systematic review and meta-analysis of studies involving telehome monitoring-based telenursing for patients with chronic obstructive pulmonary disease. *Japan Journal of Nursing Science*, *10*(2), 180–192. doi:10.1111/j.1742-7924.2012.00228.x PMID:24373441

Kandpal, A., Goudar, R. H., Chauhan, R., Garg, S., & Joshi, K. (2014). Effective Ontology Alignment: An Approach for Resolving the Ontology Heterogeneity Problem for Semantic Information Retrieval. *Advances in Intelligent Systems and Computing*, *243*, 1077–1087. doi:10.1007/978-81-322-1665-0_110

Kanstrup, A. M., & Bertelsen, P. (2006). Participatory IT-support.*Participatory Design Conference*, pp. 87-94.

Kanstrup, A. M., & Bertelsen, P. (2011). *User innovation management.* Aalborg: Aalborg University Press.

Kaplan, B., & Maxwell, J. (2005). Qualitative Research Methods for Evaluating Computer Information Systems: Evaluating the Organizational Impact of Healthcare Information Systems. Springer New York.

Kaplan, B., & Harris-Salamone, K. (2009). Health IT success and failure: Recommendations from literature and an AMIA workshop. *Journal of the American Medical Informatics Association*, *16*(3), 291–299. doi:10.1197/jamia.M2997 PMID:19261935

Karimi, S., Agharahimi, Z., & Yaghoubi, M. (2012). Impacts of Outsourcing in Educational Hospitals in Iran: A Study on Isfahan University of Medical Sciences-2010. *Journal of Education & Health Promotion*, *1*(1), 25. doi:10.4103/2277-9531.99959 PMID:23555128

Karsh, B. T., Weinger, M. B., Abbott, P. A., & Wears, R. L. (2010). Health information technology: Fallacies and sober realities. *Journal of the American Medical Informatics Association*, *17*(6), 617–623. doi:10.1136/jamia.2010.005637 PMID:20962121

Karthik, V., & Kumar, S. (2013). Investigating 'Degree of Adoption' Effects on e–procurement Benefits. *International Journal of Procurement Management*, *6*(2), 211–234. doi:10.1504/IJPM.2013.052470

Kathryn, A., Cull, A., & Sharpe, M. (2003). Diagnosing medical depression in medical outpatient: Acceptability of telephone interviews. *Journal of Psychosomatic Research*, *55*(4), 385–387. doi:10.1016/S0022-3999(02)00637-2 PMID:14507551

Kaufman, D., Roberts, W. D., Merrill, J., Lai, T. Y., & Bakken, S. (2006). Applying an evaluation framework for health information system design, development, and implementation. *Nursing Research*, *55*(2Suppl), S37–S42. doi:10.1097/00006199-200603001-00007 PMID:16601633

Kawahara, H. (2010). Student Authentication for Course Credit in Distance Learning. *Journal of Multimedia Education Research.*, *7*(1), 57–63.

Kaye, R., Kokia, E., Shalev, V., Idar, D., & Chinitz, D. (2010). Barriers and success factors in health information technology: A practitioner's perspective. *Journal of Management & Marketing in Healthcare*, *3*(2), 163–175. doi:10.1179/175330310X12736577732764

Kempe, A., Bunik, M., Ellis, J., Magid, D., Hegarty, T., Dickinson, L. M., & Steiner, J. F. (2006). How safe is triage by an after-hours telephone call center? *Pediatrics*, *118*(2), 457–463. doi:10.1542/peds.2005-3073 PMID:16882795

Kempe, A., Dempsey, C., Hegarty, T., Frei, N., Chandramouli, V., & Poole, S. R. (2000a). Reducing after-hours referrals by an after-hours call center with second-level physician triage. *Pediatrics*, *106*(1), 226–230. PMID:10888697

Kempe, A., Dempsey, C., Whitefield, C., Bothner, T., Mackenzie, T., & Poole, S. (2000b). Appropriateness of urgent referrals by nurses at a hospital-based pediatric call center. *Archives of Pediatrics & Adolescent Medicine*, *154*(4), 355–360. doi:10.1001/archpedi.154.4.355 PMID:10768672

Kempe, A., Luberti, A. A., Hertz, A. R., Sherman, H. B., Amin, H. B., Dempsey, C., & Hegarthy, T. W. et al. (2001). Delivery of pediatric after-hours care by call centers: A multicenter study of parental perceptions and compliance. *Pediatrics*, *108*(6), 111–117. doi:10.1542/peds.108.6.e111 PMID:11731638

Kennedy, S., & Berk, B. (2011), Enabling E-Health: A revolution for informatics in health care. *BCG Perspectives*. Retrieved on June 17, 2011 from www.bcgperspectives.com

Kensing, F., & Blomberg, J. (1998). Participatory design; issues and concerns. *Computer Supported Cooperative Work*, *7*(3-4), 167–185. doi:10.1023/A:1008689307411

Kensing, F., Simonsen, J., & Bødker, K. (1996). MUST - a method for participatory design.*The Fourth Biennial Conference on Participatory Design.*

Khalil, O. E. M., & Elkordy, M. M. (2005). EIS Information: Use & Quality Determination. *Information Resources Management Journal*, *18*(2), 68–93. doi:10.4018/irmj.2005040104

Kidd, L., Cayless, S., Johnston, B., & Wengstrom, Y. (2010). Telehealth in palliative care in the UK: A review of the evidence. *Journal of Telemedicine and Telecare*, *16*(7), 394–402. PMID:20813893

Kim, C. S., Spahlinger, D. A., Kin, J. M., & Billi, J. E. (2006). Lean health care: What can hospitals learn from a world-class automaker? *Journal of Hospital Medicine*, *1*(3), 191–199. doi:10.1002/jhm.68 PMID:17219493

Kim, C., Berger, D. K., & Chamany, S. (2007). Recurrence of gestational diabetes mellitus: A systematic review. *Diabetes Care*, *30*(5), 1314–1319. doi:10.2337/dc06-2517 PMID:17290037

Kim, H., Bracha, A., & Tipnis, A. (2007). Automated depression screening in disadvantaged pregnant women in an urban obstetric clinic. *Archives of Women's Mental Health*, *10*(4), 163–169. doi:10.1007/s00737-007-0189-5 PMID:17593320

King, W. R., & He, J. (2006). A meta-analysis of the technology acceptance model. *Information & Management*, *43*(6), 740–755. doi:10.1016/j.im.2006.05.003

Knuiman, M. W., Welborn, T. A., & Bartholomew, H. C. (1996). Self-reported health and use of health services: A comparison of diabetic and nondiabetic persons from a national sample. *Australian and New Zealand Journal of Public Health*, *20*(3), 241–247. doi:10.1111/j.1467-842X.1996.tb01023.x PMID:8768412

Kocher, M. G., & Sutter, M. (2006). Time is Money: Time Pressure, Incentives, & the Quality of Decision Making. *Journal of Economic Behavior & Organization*, *61*(3), 375–392. doi:10.1016/j.jebo.2004.11.013

Koch, S. (2006). Home telehealth-Current state and future trends. *International Journal of Medical Informatics*, *75*(8), 565–576. doi:10.1016/j.ijmedinf.2005.09.002 PMID:16298545

Kogo, C. (2003). Daigaku Ni Okeru Web Base Kobetsu-Ka Kyojyu Shisutemu[Conducting Classes through Web-based Personalized System of Instruction (PSI) in Universities]. *Annual Journal of Educational Psychology*, *42*, 182–192. doi:10.5926/arepj1962.42.0_182

Korcz, I. P., & Moreland, S. (1998). Telephone prescreening: Enhancing a model for proactive healthcare practice. *Cancer Practice*, *6*(5), 270–275. doi:10.1046/j.1523-5394.1998.00021.x PMID:9767345

Kørnøv, L. (2007). Public participation. In L. Kørnøv, M. Thrane, A. Remmen, & H. Lund (Eds.), *Tools for sustainable development* (pp. 721–738). Aalborg, Denmark: Aalborg Universitetsforlag.

Koufi, V., Malamateniou, F., Papakonstantinou, D., & Vassilacopoulos, G. (2010). In G. A. Papadopoulos, W. Wojtkowski, G. Wojtkowski, S. Wrycza, & J. Zupancic (Eds.), *Using ESB and BPEL for Evolving Healthcare Systems Towards Pervasive, Grid-Enabled SOA Information Systems Development* (pp. 167–175). Springer, US.

Koumaditis, K., & Themistocleous, M. (2013). *SOA Governance from a Healthcare Perspective*. Paper presented at the IADIS International Conference e-Health 2013, Prague, Czech Republic.

Koumaditis, K., Themistocleous, M., & Morabito, V. (2013). New Trends in Healthcare Information Systems (HIS) Integration. In I. M. Miranda & M. M. Cruz-Cunha (Eds.), Handbook of Research on ICTs for Healthcare and Social Services: Developments and Applications (Vol. 1). IGI Global.

Koumaditis, K., Themistocleous, M., Mantzana, V., & Souliotis, K. (2012). *A Proposition of Critical Sucess Factors Influencing SOA Implementation in Healthcare*. Paper presented at the European Conference on Information Systems, Barcelona, Spain.

Kreps, G. L., & Neuhauser, L. (2010). New directions in eHealth communication: Opportunities and challenges. *Patient Education and Counseling*, *78*(3), 329–336. doi:10.1016/j.pec.2010.01.013 PMID:20202779

Krishna, S., Balas, E. A., Francisco, B. D., Konig, P., Graff, G. R., & Madsen, R. W. (2003). Internet-enabled interactive multimedia asthma education program: A randomized trial. *Pediatrics*, *111*(3), 503–510. doi:10.1542/peds.111.3.503 PMID:12612228

Kuanda, J. (2003). Culture and technological transformation in the south. Danmark: Samfundslitteratur Press.

Kuhn, K. A., Giuse, D. A., & Talmon, J. L. (2003). The Heidelberg Conference: Setting an Agenda for the IMIA Working Group on Health Information Systems. *International Journal of Medical Informatics*, *69*(2–3), 77–82. doi:10.1016/S1386-5056(02)00097-7 PMID:12810112

Kulkarni, R., & Nathanson, L. A. (2005). *Medicine Informatics in Medicine.* Retrieved from http://www.emedicine.com/emerg/topic879.htm

Kumar, R., Novak, J., & Tomkins, A. (2010). Structure and evolution of online social networks. *Link Mining: Models, Algorithms, and Applications*, 337-357.

Kumar, S., Nilsen, W. J., Abernethy, A., Atienza, A., Patrick, K., Pavel, M., & Swendeman, D. et al. (2013). Mobile health technology evaluation: The mHealth evidence workshop. *American Journal of Preventive Medicine*, *45*(2), 228–236. doi:10.1016/j.amepre.2013.03.017 PMID:23867031

Kuo, W., Lin, C., Hsu, G., & Huang, Y. (2006). An Empirical Study of Resource Contribution in SMEs Alliance. *Journal of Global Business Management*, *2*(2), 103–111.

Kushniruk, A., & Turner, P. (2011). Who's users? participation and empowerment in socio-technical approaches to health IT development. *International Perspectives in Health Informatics*, 280-285.

Kwan, S. K., Davis, M. M., & Greenwood, A. G. (1988). A simulation model for determining variable worker requirements in a service operation with time-dependent customer demand. *Queueing Systems*, *3*(3), 265–276. doi:10.1007/BF01161218

Lacroix, A. (1999). International concerted action on collaboration in telemedicine: G8sub-project 4. *Studies in Health Technology and Informatics*, *64*, 12–19. PMID:10747530

Lai, L. S., & Turban, E. (2008). Groups formation and operations in the Web 2.0 environment and social networks. *Group Decision and Negotiation*, *17*(5), 387–402. doi:10.1007/s10726-008-9113-2

Lander, E., & Liker, J. K. (2007). The Toyota production system and art: Making highly customized and creative products the Toyota way. *International Journal of Production Research*, *45*(16), 3681–3698. doi:10.1080/00207540701223519

Land, F. (1987). Adapting to Changing User Requirements. In R. D. Galliers (Ed.), *Information Analysis: Selected Readings*. Sydney: Addison - Wesley.

Landon, M. B., Spong, C. Y., Thom, E., Carpenter, M. W., Ramin, S. M., Casey, B., & Anderson, G. B. et al. (2009). A multicenter, randomized trial of treatment for mild gestational diabetes. *The New England Journal of Medicine*, *361*(14), 1339–1348. doi:10.1056/NEJMoa0902430 PMID:19797280

Lapointe, L., & Rivard, S. (2006). Getting physicians to accept new information technology: Insights from case studies. *Canadian Medical Association Journal*, *174*(11), 1573–1578. doi:10.1503/cmaj.050281 PMID:16717265

Lateef, F. (2011). The practice of telemedicine: Medicolegal and ethical issues. *Ethics & Medicine*, *27*(1), 17–25.

Lau, A. S. (2011). Hospital-based nurses' perceptions of the adoption of Web 2.0 tools for knowledge sharing, learning, social interaction and the production of collective intelligence. *Journal of Medical Internet Research*, *13*(4), e92. doi:10.2196/jmir.1398 PMID:22079851

Lawrence, C., & Firth, D. (2013). Improving Healthcare Administration: Real Time Locations Systems or Outsourcing? *Information Systems Education Journal*, *11*(5), 49.

Lee, W., Lee, M., Choi, Y., Choi, D., Cho, M., Song, S., . . . Yoon, H. (2013). ETL-based interoperable data management system. In Multimedia Tools and Applications. Springer.

Lee, H. J., Lee, S. H., Ha, K.-S., Jang, H. C., Chung, H. C., Kim, H. C., & Yoo, D. H. et al. (2009). Ubiquitous healthcare service using Zigbee and mobile phone for elderly patients. *International Journal of Medical Informatics*, *78*(3), 193–198. doi:10.1016/j.ijmedinf.2008.07.005 PMID:18760959

Lee, H., Friedman, M. E., Cukor, P., & Ahern, D. (2003). Interactive Voice Response System (IVRS) in Health Care Services. *Nursing Outlook*, *51*(6), 277–283. doi:10.1016/S0029-6554(03)00161-1 PMID:14688763

Lee, J., & Runge, J. (2001). Adoption of Information Technology in Small Business: Testing Drivers of Adoption for Entrepreneurs. *Journal of Computer Information Systems*, *42*(1), 44–57.

Lee, K. S., Lim, G. H., & Tan, S. J. (1999). Dealing with Resource Disadvantage: Generic Strategies for SMEs. *Small Business Economics*, *12*(4), 299–311. doi:10.1023/A:1008085310245

Lee, M. A., & Yom, Y. H. (2007). A comparative study of patients' and nurses' perceptions of the quality of nursing services, satisfaction and intent to revisit the hospital: A questionnaire survey. *International Journal of Nursing Studies*, *44*(4), 545–555. doi:10.1016/j.ijnurstu.2006.03.006 PMID:16687147

Lee, M., & Jones, A. M. (2004). How Did Dentists Respond to the Introduction of Global Budgets in Taiwan? An Evaluation Using Individual Panel Data. *International Journal of Health Care Finance and Economics*, *4*(4), 307–326. doi:10.1023/B:IHFE.0000043760.57999.36 PMID:15467407

Lee, S., & Kim, K.-J. (2007). Factors affecting the implementation success of Internet-based information systems. *Computers in Human Behavior*, *23*(4), 1853–1880. doi:10.1016/j.chb.2005.12.001

Lee, T. J., Baraff, L. J., Guzy, J., Johnson, D., & Woo, H. (2003b). Does telephone triage delay significant medical treatment? *Archives of Pediatrics & Adolescent Medicine*, *157*(7), 635–641. doi:10.1001/archpedi.157.7.635 PMID:12860783

Lenhart, A., Purcell, K., Smith, A., & Zickuhr, K. (2010). *Social media & mobile Internet use among teens and young adults*. Pew Internet and American Life Project.

Lenz, R., & Manfred, R. (2006). IT support for healthcare processes– premises, challenges, perspectives. *Data & Knowledge Engineering*, *61*(1), 39–58. doi:10.1016/j.datak.2006.04.007

Leventhal, T., Taliaferro, P., Wong, K., Hughes, C., & Mun, S. (2012). The Patient-Centered Medical Home and Health Information Technology. *Telemedicine Journal and e-Health*, *18*(2), 145–149. doi:10.1089/tmj.2011.0130 PMID:22304440

Levin, L. S., & Idler, E. L. (1983). Self-care in health. *Annual Review of Public Health*, *4*(1), 181–201. doi:10.1146/annurev.pu.04.050183.001145 PMID:6860437

Levy, Y., & Ellis, T. J. (2006). A Systems Approach to Conduct an Effective Literature Review in Support of Information Systems Research. *Informing Science Journal*, *9*(9), 181–212.

Leydon, G. M., Ekberg, K., Kelly, M., & Drew, P. (2013). Improving ethnic monitoring for telephone-based healthcare: A conversation analytic study. *BMJ Open*, *3*(6e002676), 1–7. doi:10.1136/bmjopen-2013-002676 PMID:23811170

Liao, S. H. (2003). Knowledge management technologies and applications - literature review from 1995 to 2002. *Expert Systems with Applications*, *25*(2), 155–164. doi:10.1016/S0957-4174(03)00043-5

Licht, A. N. (2004). Legal plug-Ins: Cultural distance, cross-listing, & corporate governance reform. *Berkeley Journal of International Law*, *22*, 195–239.

Li, J. J. (2012). The alignment between organizational control mechanisms & outsourcing strategies: A commentary essay. *Journal of Business Research*, *65*(9), 1384–1386. doi:10.1016/j.jbusres.2011.09.020

Lin, C. (2002). *An Investigation of the Process of IS/IT Investment Evaluation & Benefits Realisation in Large Australian Organisations*. (PhD Thesis). Curtin University of Technology, Perth, Western Australia. Retrieved from http://adt.curtin.edu.au/theses/available/adt-WCU20030826.094151/

Lin, C., & Lin, K. (2011). A Study of Information Requirement Determination Process of an Executive Information System. In Enterprise Information Systems: Concepts, Methodologies, Tools & Applications. IGI Publishing.

Lin, C., Lin, H. K., Huang, Y., Jalleh, G., Liu, Y. C., Huang, Y-H., … Chao, C. (2014). Towards a B2B E-Commerce Evaluation Management Model to Assess Organizational Drivers in Hospitals. *International Technology Management Review*, *4*(3), 115-132.

Lin, C. W., Pan, C. J., Paranjape, K., Yu, C., & Feng, P. (2014). Taipei Citizen Telecare Service System for Hypertension Management in Elders. In *2014 Annual SRII Global Conference (SRII)* (pp. 157-180). IEEE.

Lin, C., & Huang, Y. (2007). An Integrated Framework for Managing eCRM Evaluation Process. *International Journal of Electronic Business*, *5*(4), 340–359. doi:10.1504/IJEB.2007.014782

Lin, C., Huang, Y., & Burn, J. (2007). Realising B2B e-Commerce Benefits: The Link with IT Maturity, Evaluation Practices, & B2B e-Commerce Adoption Readiness. *European Journal of Information Systems*, *16*(6), 806–819. doi:10.1057/palgrave.ejis.3000724

Lin, C., Huang, Y., Jalleh, G., Liu, Y., & Tung, M. (2010). An Exploratory Study of Factors Affecting Adoption & Implementation of B2B E-Commerce in Australian Health Care Organizations. *International Journal of Electronic Commerce Studies*, *1*(2), 77–96.

Lin, C., Huang, Y., & Stockdale, R. (2011). Developing a B2B Website Effectiveness Model for SMEs. *Internet Research, 21*(3), 304–325. doi:10.1108/10662241111139327

Lin, C., Lin, K., Huang, Y., & Kuo, W. (2006). Evaluation of Electronic Customer Relationship Management: The Critical Success Factors. *The Business Review, Cambridge, 6*(2), 206–212.

Lin, C., & Pervan, G. (2000) Realising the Benefits of IS/IT Investments in Australian Organisations. *Proceedings of the Eleventh Australasian Conference on Information Systems (ACIS 2000).*

Lin, C., & Pervan, G. (2001) IS/IT Investment Evaluation & Benefits Realisation Issues in a Government Organisation. *Proceedings of the Twelfth Australasian Conference on Information Systems (ACIS 2001).*

Lin, C., Pervan, G., Lin, K., & Tsao, H. (2008). An Investigation into Business-to-Business Electronic Commerce Organizations. *Journal of Research & Practice in Information Technology, 40*(1), 3–18.

Lin, C., Pervan, G., & McDermid, D. (2002). Research on IS/IT Investment Evaluation & Benefits Realization in Australia. In W. Van Grembergen (Ed.), *Information Systems Evaluation Management* (pp. 244–254). Hershey, PA: IRM Press. doi:10.4018/978-1-931777-18-6.ch015

Lindsay, J. A., Minard, C. G., Hudson, S., Green, C. E., & Schmitz, J. M. (2014). Using prize-based incentives to enhance daily interactive voice response (IVR) compliance: A feasibility study. *Journal of Substance Abuse Treatment, 46*(1), 74–77. doi:10.1016/j.jsat.2013.08.003 PMID:24029622

Lin, J., Zou, J., & Yao, G. (2013). Application Discovery of Semantic Web Service Based on Qos Ontology. *Information Technology Journal, 12*(20), 5501–5504. doi:10.3923/itj.2013.5501.5504

Liu, W., & Park, E. K. (2014). Big Data as an e-Health Service. In *Computing, Networking and Communications (ICNC), 2014 International Conference on*. IEEE. doi:10.1109/ICCNC.2014.6785471

Liu, C. H., Chen, S. L., & Huang, T. Y. (2013). Data flow analysis and testing for OWL-S semantic web service compositions. *International Journal on Computer Science and Engineering, 8*(4), 349–360. doi:10.1504/IJCSE.2013.057299

Liu, J. Y., Chen, H., Chen, C., & Sheu, T. S. (2011). Relationships among Interpersonal Conflict, Requirements Uncertainty, & Software Project Performance. *International Journal of Project Management, 29*(5), 547–556. doi:10.1016/j.ijproman.2010.04.007

Liu, M.-S., & Liu, N.-C. (2008). Sources of knowledge acquisition and patterns of knowledge-sharing behaviors--An empirical study of Taiwanese high-tech firms. *International Journal of Information Management, 28*(5), 423–432. doi:10.1016/j.ijinfomgt.2008.01.005

Liu, Y., Huang, Y., & Lin, C. (2012). Organizational Factors' Effects on The Success of E-Learning System & Organizational Benefits - An Empirical Study in Taiwan. *International Review of Research in Open and Distance Learning, 13*(4), 130–151.

Lizcano, D., Soriano, J., Reyes, M., & Hierro, J. (2009). A user-centric approach for developing and deploying service front-ends in the future internet of services. *Int. J. Web Grid Serv.*, *5*(2), 155–191. doi:10.1504/IJWGS.2009.027572

Logan, A. G. (2013). Transforming hypertension management using mobile health technology for telemonitoring and self-care support. *The Canadian Journal of Cardiology*, *29*(5), 579–585. doi:10.1016/j.cjca.2013.02.024 PMID:23618506

Lorentzen, A. (1994). Teknologi og udvikling i den nordjyske maskinindustri [technology and development in engineering in the northern part of Denmark]. Aalborg: Aalborg Universitetsforlag.

Lorig, K., Ritter, P., Laurent, D., & Plant, K. (2008). The Internet-based arthritis self-management program: A one-year randomized trial for patients with arthritis or fibromyalgia. *Arthritis Care and Research*, *59*(7), 1009–1017. doi:10.1002/art.23817 PMID:18576310

Lorig, K., Sobel, D., Stewart, A., Brown, B. Jr, Bandura, A., Ritter, P., & Halstead, R. et al. (1999). Evidence suggesting that a chronic disease self-management program can improve health status while reducing hospitalization: A randomized trial. *Medical Care*, *37*(1), 5–14. doi:10.1097/00005650-199901000-00003 PMID:10413387

Lovelock, C. H. (1983). Classifying services to gain strategic marketing insights. *Journal of Marketing*, *3*(47), 9–20. doi:10.2307/1251193

Lovelock, C. H. (1996). *Service Marketing* (3rd ed.). London: Prentice Hall International.

Lovelock, C. H., & Wirtz, J. (2004). *Services Marketing: People, Technology, Strategy* (5th ed.). Upper Saddle River, NJ: Prentice Hall.

Love, P. E. D., Irani, Z., Standing, C., Lin, C., & Burn, J. (2005). The Enigma of Evaluation: Benefits, Costs & Risks of IT in Small-Medium Sized Enterprises. *Information & Management*, *42*(7), 947–964. doi:10.1016/j.im.2004.10.004

Low, C., & Chen, Y. H. (2012). Criteria for the Evaluation of a Cloud-based Hospital Information System Outsourcing Provider. *Journal of Medical Systems*, *36*(6), 3543–3553. doi:10.1007/s10916-012-9829-z PMID:22366976

Lucas, H. (2008). Information and communications technology for future health systems in developing countries. *Social Science & Medicine*, *66*(10), 2122–2132. doi:10.1016/j.socscimed.2008.01.033 PMID:18343005

Lu, J., Yu, C. S., Liu, C., & Yao, J. E. (2003). Technology acceptance model for wireless Internet. *Internet Research*, *13*(3), 206–222. doi:10.1108/10662240310478222

Lunt, N., Smith, R., Exworthy, M., Green, S., Horsfal, D., & Mannion, R. (2011). Medical Tourism: Treatments, markets and health system implications: A scoping review. In OECD (Ed.), *International Trade in Health Services* (Vol. 1, p. 55). Paris, France: Directorate for Employment,Labour and Social Affairs.

Luxton, D. D., Kayl, R. A., & Mishkind, M. C. (2012). mHealth data security: The need for HIPAA-compliant standardization. *Telemedicine Journal and e-Health*, *18*(4), 284–288. doi:10.1089/tmj.2011.0180 PMID:22400974

Macedo, M., & Isaías, P. (2009). Patient Standardization Identification as a Healthcare Issue. *Human Interface and the Management of Information. Information and Interaction*, 566-575.

Mackay, M. M., & Weidlich, O. (2007, March). *Australian Mobile Phone Lifestyle Index* (3rd ed.). Australian Interactive Media Industry Association (AIMIA), Mobile Content Industry Development Group (MCIDG). Retrieved 8 April, 2007, from http://www.aimia.com.au/mobile

Maglio, P. P., & Spohrer, J. (2008). Fundamentals of service science. *Journal of the Academy of Marketing Science*, *36*(1), 18–20. doi:10.1007/s11747-007-0058-9

Mahesh, V. S., & Kasturi, A. (2006). Improving call centre agent performance - A UK-India study based on the agents' point of view. *International Journal of Service Industry Management*, *17*(2), 136–157. doi:10.1108/09564230610656971

Maibach, E., & Parrott, R. (1995). *Designing health messages: approaches from communication theory and public health practice*. Thousand Oaks, CA: Sage Publications.

Malecki, E. J., & Moriset, B. (2008). *The Digital Economy: Business Organization, Production Processes, and Regional Developments*. Oxon, UK: Routledge.

Mancini, M. (2014). Exploiting big data for improving healthcare services. *Journal of e-Learning and Knowledge Society, 10*(2), 23-33.

Mantzana, V., Koumaditis, K., & Themistocleous, M. (2011). *Healthcare IS Interoperability: Challenges and Solutions.* Paper presented at the HEALTHINF 2011: International Conference on Health Informatics, Rome, Italy.

Mariño, R., Clarke, K., Manton, D. J., Stranieri, A., Collmann, R., Kellet, H., & Borda, A. (2015). Teleconsultation and Telediagnosis for Oral Health Assessment: An Australian Perspective. In Teledentistry (pp. 101-112). Springer International Publishing.

Marks, E. (2008). *Service-Oriented Architecture (SOA) Governance for the Services Driven Enterprise*. Wiley.

Marques, A., Oliveira, T., Dias, S. S., & Martins, M. F. O. (2011). Medical Records System Adoption in European Hospitals. *The Electronic Journal Information Systems Evaluation*, *14*(1), 89–99.

Martin, A. C. (2013). Legal, clinical, and ethical issues in teletherapy.*Psychoanalysis Online: Mental Health, Teletherapy, and Training*, 75.

Martin, D., Burstein, M., & Hobbs, J. R. (2004). *Website.* Available at http://www.w3.org/Submission/OWL-S/

Martin, D., Burstein, M., McDermott, D., McIlraith, S., Paolucci, M., Sycara, K, McGuinness, D., Sirin, E. & Srinivasan, N. (2007), Bringing Semantics to Web Services with OWL-S. *Journal of World Wide Web, 10*(3).

Martínez-Pérez, B., de la Torre-Díez, I., & López-Coronado, M. (2014). Privacy and security in mobile health apps: A review and recommendations. *Journal of Medical Systems, 39*(1). PMID:25486895

Martin, L., Anguita, A., & Graf, N. (2011). ACGT: Advancing clinico-genomic trials on cancer—four years of experience. *Studies in Health Technology and Informatics, 169*, 734–738. PMID:21893844

Masys, D. (1998). Advances in Information Technology. Implications for medical education. *The Western Journal of Medicine, 168*(5), 341–347. PMID:9614791

Mathieson, K. (1991). Predicting user intentions: Comparing the technology acceptance model with the theory of planned behavior. *Information Systems Research, 2*(3), 173–191. doi:10.1287/isre.2.3.173

Matsuoka, I. (2001). *Dejitaru Kyanpasu* [Digital Campus]. Tokyo: Toyo Keizai Inc.

McBride, C. M., & Rimer, B. K. (1999). Using the telephone to improve health behavior and health service delivery. *Patient Education and Counseling, 37*(1), 3–18. doi:10.1016/S0738-3991(98)00098-6 PMID:10640115

McConnell, K. J., Johnson, L. A., Arab, N., Richards, C. F., Newgard, C. D., & Edlund, T. (2007). The on-call crisis: A statewide assessment of the costs of providing on-call specialist coverage. *Annals of Emergency Medicine, 49*(6), 727–733. doi:10.1016/j.annemergmed.2006.10.017 PMID:17210209

McDaniel, J. G. (1995). Discrete event simulation of a wide area health care network. *Journal of the American Medical Informatics Association, 2*(4), 220–237. doi:10.1136/jamia.1995.96010391 PMID:7583646

McGaughey, R. E. (2002). Benchmarking Business-to-business Electronic Commerce, *Benchmarking. International Journal (Toronto, Ont.), 9*(5), 471–484.

McGowan, B. S., Wasko, M., Vartabedian, B. S., Miller, R. S., Freiherr, D. D., & Abdolrasulnia, M. (2012). Understanding the factors that influence the adoption and meaningful use of social media by physicians to share medical information. *Journal of Medical Internet Research, 14*(5), e117. doi:10.2196/jmir.2138 PMID:23006336

McIvor, R. (2000). A practical framework for understanding the outsourcing process. *Supply Chain Management: An International Journal, 5*(1), 22–36. doi:10.1108/13598540010312945

McKay, J., & Marshall, P. (2004). Strategic Management of eBusiness, John Wiley & Sons Australia, Ltd, Queensland.

McKee, D. O., Varadarajan, P. R., & Pride, W. M. (1989). Strategic Adaptability and Firm Performance: A Market-Contingent Perspective. *Journal of Marketing*, *53*(3), 21–35. doi:10.2307/1251340

McKinstry, B., Walker, J., Campbell, C., Heaney, D., & Wyke, S. (2002). Telephone consultations to manage requests for same-day appointments: A randomized controlled trial in two practices. *The British Journal of General Practice*, *52*(477), 306–310. PMID:11942448

McNall, L. A., & Roch, S. G. (2009). A social exchange model of employee reactions to electronic performance monitoring. *Human Performance*, *22*(3), 204–224. doi:10.1080/08959280902970385

McNemish, J., Lyle, D., McCowan, M., Emmerson, S., McAuley, S., & Reilly, J. (2007). Post-discharge surgical site infection surveillance by automated telephony. *Journal of Hospital Telephony*, *66*(3), 232–236. doi:10.1016/j.jhin.2007.04.003 PMID:17544545

MEDgle Inc. (2014). *The details*. Retrieved on May 15, 2014 from http://www.medgle.com/front.jsp?task=technology&section=details

Melville, N., Kraemer, K., & Gurbaxani, V. (2004). Review: Information Technology & Organizational Performance: An integrative Model of IT Business Value. *Management Information Systems Quarterly*, *28*(2), 283–322.

Menachemi, N., Burke, D., & Diana, M. (2007). Characteristics of Hospitals that Outsource Information. System Functions. *Journal of Healthcare Information Management*, *19*(1), 63–69. PMID:15682678

MeriTalk. (2014). *The Big Data Cure*. Retrieved on January 25, 2015 from http://www.meritalk.com/bigdatacure

Mettler, T., Fitterer, R., Rohner, P., & Winter, R. (2014). Does a hospital's IT architecture fit with its strategy? An approach to measure the alignment of health information technology. *Health Systems*, *3*(1), 29–42.

Metzger, B. E. (2008). Hyperglycemia and adverse pregnancy outcomes. *The New England Journal of Medicine*, *358*(19), 1191–2002. PMID:18463375

Miciak, A., & Desmarais, M. (2001). Benchmarking service quality performance at business-to-business and business-to-consumer call centers. *Journal of Business and Industrial Marketing*, *16*(5), 340–353. doi:10.1108/08858620110400205

Miles, A. (2009). Complexity in medicine and healthcare: People and systems, theory and practice. *Journal of Evaluation in Clinical Practice*, *15*(3), 409–410. doi:10.1111/j.1365-2753.2009.01204.x PMID:19522904

Miles, M. B., & Huberman, A. M. (1994). *Qualitative Data Analysis: An Expanded Sourcebook*. California: Sage Publications.

Miller, D. I., Bruce, H., Gagnon, M., Talbot, V., & Messier, C. (2011). Improving older adults' experience with interactive voice response systems. *Telemedicine Journal and e-Health*, *17*(6), 452–455. doi:10.1089/tmj.2010.0204 PMID:21631386

Milliken, F. J. (1987). Three types of perceived uncertainty about the environment: State, effect, and response uncertainty. *Academy of Management Review*, *12*(1), 133–143.

Mirza, F., Norris, T., & Stockdale, R. (2008). Mobile technologies and the holistic management of chronic diseases. *Health Informatics Journal*, *14*(4), 309–321. doi:10.1177/1460458208096559 PMID:19008280

Misra, R. B. (2004). Global IT Outsourcing: Metrics for Success of All Parties. *Journal of Information Technology Cases & Applications*, *6*(3), 21–34. doi:10.1080/15228053.2004.10856047

Mitchell, R., Agle, B., & Wood, D. (1997). Towards a therory of stakeholder identification and salience: Defining the principles of who and what really counts. *Academy of Management Review*, *22*(4), 853–886.

Mitra, S., Sambamurthy, V., & Westerman, G. (2011). Measuring IT Performance & Communicating Value. *MIS Quarterly Executive*, *10*(1), 47–59.

Mitseva, A., Kyriazakos, S., Litke, A., Papadakis, N., & Prasad, N. (2009). ISISEMD: Intelligent System for Independent living and self-care of SEniors with mild cognitive impairment or Mild Dementia. *The Journal on Information Technology in Healthcare*, *7*(6), 383–399.

Moghaddasi, H., Asadi, F., Hosseini, A., & Ebnehoseini, Z. (2012). E-health: A global approach with extensive semantic variation. *Journal of Medical Systems*, *36*(5), 3173–3176. doi:10.1007/s10916-011-9805-z PMID:22113437

Mohan, J., Razali, R., & Yaacob, R. (2003). The Malaysian telehealth flagship application: A national approach to health data protection and utilisation and consumer rights. *International Journal of Medical Informatics*, *73*(3), 217–227. doi:10.1016/j.ijmedinf.2003.11.023 PMID:15066550

Mohanty, S. A., Donna, L., Washington, S., Lambe, S., Fink, A., & Asch, S. M. (2006). Predictors of on-call specialist response times in California emergency departments. *Academic Emergency Medicine*, *13*(5), 505–512. doi:10.1111/j.1553-2712.2006.tb01000.x PMID:16609102

Moon, J., Choe, Y. C., Chung, M., Jung, G. H., & Swar, B. (2014). IT outsourcing success in the public sector lessons from e-government practices in Korea. *Information Development*, *0266666914528930*, 1–19.

Moran, M. (2014). Rule change on emergency care could reduce specialty coverage. *Psychiatr News*, *38*, 10-28. Retrieved from http://pn.psychiatryonline.org/cgi/content/full/38/22/10?etoc

More, E., & McGrath, M. (2002). An Australian Case in e-Health Communication & Change. *Journal of Management Development*, *21*(7/8), 612–632.

Morrissey, J. (1999). FHS hooks up with Access Health Group. Calif. HMO will outsource its telephone medical advice services to Colo. Company. *Modern Healthcare*, *29*(4), 36. PMID:10345464

Morton, J. M., Baker, C. C., Farrell, T. M., Yohe, M. H., Kimple, R. J., Herman, D. C., & Meyer, A. et al. (2004). What do surgery residents do on their call nights? *American Journal of Surgery*, *188*(3), 225–229. doi:10.1016/j.amjsurg.2004.06.011 PMID:15450824

Moruzzi, M. (2009). *E-health e fascicolo sanitario elettronico*. Milano, Italy: Il Sole 24 Ore.

Mudambi, S. M., & Tallman, S. (2010). Make, buy or ally? Theoretical perspectives on knowledge process outsourcing through alliances. *Journal of Management Studies*, *47*(8), 1434–1456. doi:10.1111/j.1467-6486.2010.00944.x

Muhr, T. (2004). ATLAS the knowledge workbench. V5.0 user's guide and reference. Berlin: ATLAS.ti.Scientific Software Development GmbH.

Muir, J., Xu, C., Paul, S., Staib, A., McNeill, I., Singh, P., & Sinnott, M. (2011). Incorporating teledermatology into emergency medicine. *Emergency Medicine Australasia*, *23*(5), 562–568. doi:10.1111/j.1742-6723.2011.01443.x PMID:21995470

Mukhopadhyay, S. (2015). Wearable sensors for human activity monitoring: A review. *IEEE Sensors Journal*, *15*(3), 1321–1330. doi:10.1109/JSEN.2014.2370945

Müller, J. (1990). Teknologivurdering og trovaerdighed [technology assessment and credibility]. In Cronberg T., & Friis D. (Eds.), Metoder i teknologivurdering. erfaring og fornyelse (pp. 267-279). Kobenhavn: Blytmanns forlag.

Müller, J. (1991). Hvad er teknologi? (what is technology?). In M. Rostgaard, A. Remmen, & J. Christensen (Eds.), *Samfundet i teknologien* (pp. 27–47). Aalborg: Aalborg Universitetsforlag.

Müller, J., Kjaer-Rasmussen, J., & Nøhr, C. (1988). *Perspektiver for EDB-teknologi i sygehusvaesenet* [perspectives for IT-technology in the hospital sector]. Aalborg: Institut for Samfundsudvikling og Planlaegning, Aalborg Universitetscenter.

Müller, J., Kjaer-Rasmussen, J., & Nohr, C. (1989). *Proactive technology assessment as a tool in HIS development*. North Holland.

Mumford, E. (1983). *Designing human systems for new technology - the ETHICS method*. Manchester, UK: Manchester Business Schol.

Mumford, E., & Weir, M. (1979). *Computer systems in work design: The ETHICS method*. London: Associated Business Press.

Mundt, J. C., Katzelnick, D. J., Kennedy, S. H., Eisfeld, B. S., Bouffard, B. B., & Greist, J. H. (2006). Validation of an IVRS version of the MADRS. *Journal of Psychiatric Research*, *40*(3), 243–246. doi:10.1016/j.jpsychires.2005.05.002 PMID:15979643

Murphy, G. D. (2010). *Using Web 2.0 tools to facilitate knowledge transfer in complex organisational environments: a primer*. Academic Press.

Musen, M. A. (1998). Domain ontologies in software engineering: Use of Protégé with the EON architecture. *Methods of Information in Medicine*, (37): 540–550. PMID:9865052

Nakatsu, R. T., & Iacovou, C. L. (2009). A Comparative Study of Important Risk Factors Involved in Offshore & Domestic Outsourcing of Software Development Projects: A Two-Panel Delphi Study. *Information & Management*, *46*(1), 57–68. doi:10.1016/j.im.2008.11.005

Naml, T., Aluc, G., & Dogac, A. (2009). An Interoperability Test Framework for HL7-Based Systems. *IEEE Transactions on Information Technology in Biomedicine, 13*(3), 389–399. doi:10.1109/TITB.2009.2016086 PMID:19304492

Narayan, M. C. (2001). Oasis Voice Mailbox InServices. *Home Healthcare Nurse, 19*(9), 542–548. doi:10.1097/00004045-200109000-00011 PMID:11982193

Nazareth, I., & Murray, E. (2010). Promoting self care for minor illness. *British Medical Journal, 340*, c2913.

NCI. (2014). Available at https://wiki.nci.nih.gov/display/LexEVS/LexEVS+6.0

NEHTA. (2010). *Australia Launches Leading Edge e-Health Supply Chain Location Directory – NEHTA*. National E-Health Transition Authority, Media Press Release. Retrieved from http://www.nehta.gov.au/

Netsize. (2009). *Netsize Guide 2009 Edition: Mobile Society and Me: When worlds combine.* Levallois-Perret: Netsize.

Nicholls, W. L. (1988). Computer-assisted telephone interviewing: A general introduction. In R. M. Groves, P. P. Biemer, L. E. Lyberg, J. T. Massey, W. L. Nicholls, & J. Waksberg (Eds.), *Telephone Survey Methodology* (pp. 377–385). New York: Wiley.

Nielsen, J. (2005). *Ten usabiligy heuristics.* Retrieved December, 2012, from http://zonecours.hec.ca/documents/H2010-1-2357287.portionOK.pdf

Niemann, M., Miede, A., Wolfgang, J., Repp, N., & Steinmetz, R. (2010). Structuring SOA Governance. *International Journal of IT/Business Alignment and Governance, 1*(1), 58–75.

Nishimura, S., Asada, T., Kogo, C., Kikuchi, H., Jin, Q., Matsui, T., & Nojima, E. (2004). *Kyampus Moderu e-Learning No Jissen: Waseda Daigaku Ningen Kagakubu e-School No Torikumi* [The "Campus Model" of e-Learning in Practice: A Case Study of Waseda University's School of Human Sciences' "e-School."]. Paper presented at Japan Society for Educational Technology Annual Conferenc.

Nøhr, C., & Bernstein, K. (1992). Implementation and diffusion of medical informatics; the case of electronic prescription communication. between practitioners and pharmacies. Primary Health Care Specialist Group of the British Computer Society.

Nøhr, C., Høstgaard, A. M., Botin, L., & Kjær-Andersen, S. (2004). *Evaluering af GEPKA-projektet, delrapport 2, klinisk afprovning* [evaluation of the GEPKA-project, report 2, clinical testing]. Unpublished manuscript.

Nøhr, C., & Høstgaard, A. M. (2011). *Evaluering af ABT-projektet: Genanvendelse af administrative patientdata til måling af den sundhedsfaglige kvalitet [evaluation af the ABT-project: Recycling of administrative patient data to measure health professional quality].* Denmark: Virtuel Centre for Health Informatics.

Nordjyllands Amt (The County of North Jutland). (2000). *IT-handlingsplan for sundhedsomraa-det i nordjyllands amt 2002-2004* [IT-plan for the healthcare area in the county of north jutland 2002-2004]. Academic Press.

Normann, R. (1984). *Service Management Strategy and Leadership in Service Business*. Chichester, UK: John Wiley & Sons.

Norton, A. L., Coulson-Thomas, Y. M., Coulson-Thomas, C. J., & Ashurst, C. (2013). Ensuring Benefits Realisation from ERP II: The CSF Phasing Model. *Journal of Enterprise Information Management*, *26*(3), 218–234. doi:10.1108/17410391311325207

Norum, J., Grev, A., Moen, M. A., Balteskard, L., & Holthe, K. (2003). Information and communication technology (ICT) in oncology. Patients' and relatives' experiences and suggestions. *Supportive Care in Cancer*, *11*(5), 286–293. PMID:12690539

Nykänen, P., Brender, J., Talmon, J. D. K., de Keizer, N., Rigby, M., Beuscart-Zephir, M.-C., & Ammenwerth, E. (2011). Guideline for good evaluation practice in health informatics (GEP-HI). *International Journal of Medical Informatics*, *80*(12), 815–927. doi:10.1016/j.ijmedinf.2011.08.004 PMID:21920809

O'Brien, J. A., Ward, A. J., Jones, M. K. C., McMillan, C., & Lordan, L. (2003). Utilization of health care services by patients with chronic obstructive pulmonary disease. *Respiratory Medicine*, *97*(S1), S53–S58. doi:10.1016/S0954-6111(03)80015-X PMID:12564611

Oake, N., Jennings, A., van Walrayen, C., & Forster, A. J. (2009). Interactive Voice Response Systems for Improving Delivery of Ambulatory Care. *The American Journal of Managed Care*, *15*(6), 283–291. PMID:19514804

O'Doherty, K., Rao Hill, S., Mackay, M. M., & McPherson, J. (2010). Mobile Data Service usage and preference: An investigation of Australian consumers. *International Journal of Mobile Communications*, *8*(1), 106–127. doi:10.1504/IJMC.2010.030523

OECD – Organisation for Economic Co-operation and Development. (2010). *Improving Health Sector Efficiency. The Role of Information and Communication Technologies*. Paris, France: OECD.

Oh, H., Rizo, C., Enkin, M., Jadad, A., Powell, J., & Pagliari, C. (2005). What is eHealth (3): A systematic review of published definitions. *Journal of Medical Internet Research*, *7*(1), e1. doi:10.2196/jmir.7.1.e1 PMID:15829471

Oh, S., Yang, S., Kurnia, S., Lee, H., Mackay, M. M., & O'Doherty, K. (2008). The characteristics of mobile data users in Australia. *International Journal of Mobile Communications*, *8*(2), 217–230. doi:10.1504/IJMC.2008.016578

Ōmae, K. (2012). *Shinka Suru Kyōiku: Anata No Nōryoku Wa Shinka Suru* [Evolving education: Evolve your brainpower]. Tokyo: Business Breakthrough Publishing.

O'Malley, A. S. (2011). Tapping the unmet potential of health information technology. *The New England Journal of Medicine*, *364*(12), 1090–1091. doi:10.1056/NEJMp1011227 PMID:21428764

Ondo, K., & Smith, M. (2006). Outside IT the Case for Full IT Outsourcing: Study Findings Indicate Many Hospitals Are Turning to Full IT Outsourcing to Achieve IT Excellence. What's the Best Approach for Your Organization? *Healthcare Financial Management*, (February): 1–3.

Opie, A. (1998). Nobody's asked me for my view: Users' empowerment by multidisciplinary health teams. *Qualitative Health Research*, *18*(2), 188–206. doi:10.1177/104973239800800204

Orguna, B., & Vub, J. (2006). HL7 ontology and mobile agents for interoperability in heterogeneous medical information systems. *Computers in Biology and Medicine*, *36*(7–8), 817–836. doi:10.1016/j.compbiomed.2005.04.010 PMID:16139263

Osservatorio ICT in Sanità – School of Management of the Politecnico di Milano. (2008). *ICT e innovazione in sanità: nuove sfide e opportunità per i CIO*. Milano: Politecnico di Milano, Dipartimento di Ingegneria gestionale.

Osservatorio ICT in Sanità – School of Management of the Politecnico di Milano. (2013). *ICT in sanità: perché il digitale non rimanga solo in agenda*. Milano: Politecnico di Milano, Dipartimento di Ingegneria gestionale.

Ozkan, S., Baykal, N., & Sincan, M. (2012). *Process-Based Evaluation of Hospital Information Systems: Application of an Information System Success Model (PRISE) in the Healthcare Domain. In Health Information Systems: Concepts, Methodologies, Tools, and Applications* (pp. 339–355). Hershey, PA: IGI Global.

Oztas, M. O., Calikoglu, E., Baz, K., Birol, A., Onder, M., Calikoglu, T., & Kitapci, M. T. (2004). Reliability of Web-based teledermatology consultations. *Journal of Telemedicine and Telecare*, *10*(1), 25–28. doi:10.1258/135763304322764158 PMID:15006212

Pagliari, C. (2007). Design and evaluation in eHealth: Challenges and implications for an interdisciplinary field. *Journal of Medical Internet Research*, *9*(15). PMID:17537718

Pagliari, C., Sloan, D., Gregor, P., Sullivan, F., Detmer, D., Kahan, J. P., & Mac Gillivray, S. et al. (2005). What is eHealth (4): A scoping exercise to map the field. *Journal of Medical Internet Research*, *7*(1), e9. doi:10.2196/jmir.7.1.e9 PMID:15829481

Papakonstantinou, D., Malamateniou, F., & Vassilacopoulos, G. (2010). A SOA approach to the implementation of an electronic medical record. *International Journal of Applied Systemic Studies*, *3*(3), 343–352. doi:10.1504/IJASS.2010.034626

Papastathopoulou, P., Avlonitis, G. J., & Panagopoulos, N. G. (2007). Intraorganizational information and communication technology diffusion: Implications for industrial sellers and buyers. *Industrial Marketing Management*, *36*(3), 322–336. doi:10.1016/j.indmarman.2005.10.002

Pape-Haugaard, L., Haugaard, K., Carøe, P., & Høstgaard, A. (2013). *Exploring barriers for health visitors' adaption of the danish children's database through an empirical study*. LiU Electronic Press.

Pare, G., Sicotte, C., & Jacques, H. (2006). The effects of creating psychological ownership on physicians' acceptance of clinical information systems. *Journal of the American Medical Informatics Association, 13*(2), 197–205.

Parker, M. M. (1996). *Strategic Transformation & Information Technology*. Upper Saddle River, NJ: Prentice-Hall.

Patrick, K., Griswold, W., Raab, F., & Intille, S. (2008). Health and the mobile phone. *American Journal of Preventive Medicine, 35*(2), 177–181. doi:10.1016/j.amepre.2008.05.001 PMID:18550322

Paul, S., & Nazareth, D. L. (2010). Input information complexity, perceived time pressure, & information processing in GSS-based work groups: An experimental investigation using a decision schema to alleviate information overload conditions. *Decision Support Systems, 49*(1), 31–40. doi:10.1016/j.dss.2009.12.007

Peansupap, V., & Walker, D. (2005). Factors enabling information and communication technology diffusion and actual implementation in construction organisations. *Electronic Journal of Information Technology in Construction, 10*, 193–218.

Peirce, L., & Bakke, E. (2010, June21). Healthcare perceptions and mobile phone use: a predictive model of text-based health communication.*Annual meeting of the International Communication Association, Suntec,* Singapore.

Petersen, J. A., Mackel, R., Antonsen, K., & Rasmussen, L. S. (2014). Serious adverse events in a hospital using *early warning score*–What went wrong? *Resuscitation, 85*(12), 1699–1703. doi:10.1016/j.resuscitation.2014.08.037 PMID:25238741

Petter, S., DeLone, W., & McLean, E. R. (2013). Information Systems Success: The Quest for the Independent Variables. *Journal of Management Information Systems, 29*(4), 7–62. doi:10.2753/MIS0742-1222290401

Peute, L. W., Aarts, J., Bakker, P. J., & Jaspers, M. W. (2010). Anatomy of a failure: A sociotechnical evaluation of a laboratory physician order entry system implementation. *International Journal of Medical Informatics, 79*(4), e58–e70. doi:10.1016/j.ijmedinf.2009.06.008 PMID:19640778

Pfeffer, J., & Salancik, G. R. (1978). *The external control of organizations: a resource dependence perspective*. New York: Harper & Row.

Piette, J. D. (2000). Perceived Access Problems among patients with diabetes in two public systems of care. *Journal of General Internal Medicine, 15*(11), 797–804. doi:10.1046/j.1525-1497.2000.91107.x PMID:11119172

Piette, J. D., & Schilinger, D. (2007). *Medical management of vulnerable and underserved patients. Principles, practices and populations. Mc* Graw Hill Companies.

Pike, J. H. (2003). Nature of After-Hours Calls at a Tertiary-Level Rehabilitation Center. *Archives of Physical Medicine and Rehabilitation, 84*(7), 1039–1042. doi:10.1016/S0003-9993(03)00028-5 PMID:12881831

Pilat, D. (2004). The ICT productivity paradox: Insights from micro data. *OECD Economic Studies*, *38*(1), 37–65.

Pinto, B. M., Friedman, R., Marcus, B. H., Kelley, H., Tennstedt, S., & Gillman, M. W. (2002). Effects of a computer based telephone-counseling system on physical activity. *American Journal of Preventive Medicine*, *23*(2), 113–120. doi:10.1016/S0749-3797(02)00441-5 PMID:12121799

Pirnejad, H., Bal, R., Stoop, A. P., & Berg, M. (2007). Inter-organisational communication networks in healthcare: Centralised versus decentralised approaches. *International Journal of Integrated Care*, *7*(2). PMID:17627296

Pohjanoksa-Mantyla, M. K., Antila, J., Eerikainen, S., Enakoski, M., Hannuksela, O., Pietila, K., & Airaksinen, M. (2008). Utilization of a community pharmacy-operated national drug information call center in Finland. *Research in Social & Administrative Pharmacy*, *4*(2), 144–152. doi:10.1016/j.sapharm.2007.05.001 PMID:18555967

Poole, S. R., Schmitt, B. D., Carruth, T., Peterson-Smith, A., & Slusarski, M. (1993). After-hours telephone coverage: The application of an area-wide telephone triage and advice system for pediatric practices. *Pediatrics*, *92*(5), 670–679. PMID:8414853

Porter, M. (2001). Strategy and the Internet. *Harvard Business Review*, *79*(2), 63–78. PMID:11246925

Porter, M., & Tiesberg, E. (2006). *Re-defining health care delivery*. Boston: Harvard Business Press.

Poster, W. R. (2007). Who's On the Line? Indian Call Center Agents Pose as Americans for US-Outsourced Firms. *Industrial Relations*, *46*(2), 271–304. doi:10.1111/j.1468-232X.2007.00468.x

Poulton, B. C. (1999). User involvement in identifying health needs and shaping and evaluating services: Is it being raised? *Journal of Advanced Nursing*, *30*(6), 1289–1296. doi:10.1046/j.1365-2648.1999.01224.x PMID:10583638

Prasad, M. K. S., Mahmood, S., Gregson, B. A., & Mitchell, P. (2012). Telephone logs of neurosurgery specialty trainees: A time study. *British Journal of Neurosurgery*, *26*(2), 195–198. doi:10.3109/02688697.2011.633643 PMID:22149539

Pratt, S. I., Naslund, J. A., Wolfe, R. S., Santos, M., & Bartels, S. J. (2014). Automated telehealth for managing psychiatric instability in people with serious mental illness. *Journal of Mental Health*, 1-5.

Preuveneers, D., & Berbers, Y. (2008). Mobile phones assisting with health self-care: a diabetes case study. *10th Annual Conference on Human Computer Interaction with Mobile Devices and Services.*

PricewaterhouseCoopers. (2007). *The Economics of IT and Hospital Performance*. Retrieved July 14, 2011 from http://www.pwc.com/us/en/healthcare/publications/the-economics-of-it-and-hospital-performance.jhtml

Prince, S. B., & Herrin, D. M. (2007). The role of information technology in healthcare communications, efficiency, and patient safety. *The Journal of Nursing Administration, 37*(4), 184–187. doi:10.1097/01.NNA.0000266841.46684.50 PMID:17415105

Protti, D. (2002). What can the american electronic health record (EHR) pioneers tell us about what it takes to be successful? *Health Management Forum, 15*(2), 33–35. doi:10.1016/S0840-4704(10)60578-9 PMID:12078354

Public Relations Office, Government of Japan. (2009). *Flexible Education, 20*(11). Retrieved from https://www.gov-online.go.jp/pdf/hlj_ar/vol_0020e/14-15.pdf

Rachlis, M. (2006). *Key to sustainable healthcare system.* Retrieved 21 June, 2008, from http://www.improveinchroniccare.org

Radin, P. (2006). To me, it's my life: Medical communication, trust, and activism in cyberspace. *Social Science & Medicine, 6*(3), 591–601. doi:10.1016/j.socscimed.2005.06.022 PMID:16039031

Ragu-Nathana, B. S., Apigian, C. H., Ragu-Nathana, T. S., & Tu, Q. (2004). A path analytic study of the effect of top management support for information systems performance. *Omega, 32*(6), 459–471. doi:10.1016/j.omega.2004.03.001

Rahim, M. M., Kurnia, S., Samson, D., & Singh, P. (2014). Developing an IT Maturity Model for Sustainable Supply Chain Management Implementation. *The 18th Pacific Asia Conference on Information Systems (PACIS 2014).*

Rahimi, B., & Vimarlund, V. (2007). Methods to evaluate health information systems in healthcare settings: A literature review. *Journal of Medical Systems, 31*(5), 397–432. doi:10.1007/s10916-007-9082-z PMID:17918694

Rahman, Z. (2004). E-commerce solution for services. *European Business Review, 16*(6), 564–576. doi:10.1108/09555340410565396

Raisinghani, M. S., Melemez, T., Zhou, L., Paslowski, C., Kikvidze, I., Taha, S., & Simons, K. (2005). E-Business Models in B2B: Process Based Categorization & Analysis of B2B Models. *International Journal of E-Business Research, 1*(1), 16–36. doi:10.4018/jebr.2005010102

Raitoharju, R. (2005). *When Acceptance is not Enough-Taking TAM-Model into Healthcare.* Academic Press.

Ralston, D. A., Holt, D. H., Terpstra, R. H., & Kai-Cheng, Y. (2008). The impact of national culture & economic ideology on managerial work values: A study of the United States, Russia, Japan, & China. *Journal of International Business Studies, 39*(1), 8–26. doi:10.1057/palgrave.jibs.8400330

Ramezan, M. (2011). Intellectual capital & organizational organic structure in knowledge society:How are these concepts related? *International Journal of Information Management, 31*(1), 88–95. doi:10.1016/j.ijinfomgt.2010.10.004

Randi, P. (2004). Web-Assisted Courses for Business Education: An Examination of Two Sections of Principles of Marketing. *Journal of Marketing Education*, *26*(2), 161–173. doi:10.1177/0273475304265635

Rao, S., & Troshani, I. (2006). AMC-ER Preliminary Research Report: Understanding Market and Mobile Content Selection for Distribution. Adelaide, South Australia: Australian Mobile Content – Export Research Initiative, m.Net Corporation Ltd.

Rao, M. B., Lerro, C., & Gross, C. P. (2010). The Shortage of On-call Surgical Specialist Coverage: A National Survey of Emergency Department Directors. *Academic Emergency Medicine*, *17*(12), 1374–1382. doi:10.1111/j.1553-2712.2010.00927.x PMID:21091822

Rask, K. J., LeBaron, C. W., & Starnes, D. M. (2001). The Cost of Registry-Based Immunization Based Interventions. *American Journal of Preventive Medicine*, *21*(4), 267–271. doi:10.1016/S0749-3797(01)00370-1 PMID:11701296

Rasmussen, B., Wellard, S., & Nankervis, A. (2001). Consumer issues in navigating health care services for type I diabetes. *Journal of Clinical Nursing*, *10*(5), 628–634. doi:10.1046/j.1365-2702.2001.00550.x PMID:11822513

Rateb, S. A. H., El Nouman, A. A. R., Rateb, M. A. H., Asar, M. N., El Amin, A. M., & Mohamed, M. S. E. (2011). Re-engineering pre-employment check-up systems: A model for improving health services. *International Journal of Health Care Quality Assurance*, *24*(6), 484–497. doi:10.1108/09526861111150734 PMID:21916149

Reach, G., Zerrouki, D., Leclercq, D., & d'Ivernois, J. F. (2005). Adjusting insulin doses: From knowledge to decision. *Patient Education and Counseling*, *56*(1), 98–103. doi:10.1016/j.pec.2004.01.001 PMID:15590229

Reardon, G. T., Blumenfield, S., Weissman, A., & Rosenberg, G. (1988). Findings and implications from preadmission screening of elderly patients waiting for elective surgery. *Social Work in Health Care*, *13*(3), 51–63. doi:10.1300/J010v13n03_05 PMID:2852851

Remenyi, D., & Whittaker, L. (1996). The Evaluation of Business Process Re-engineering Projects. In L. Willcocks (Ed.), *Investing in information systems: evaluation & management* (pp. 143–167). Chapman & Hall.

Remschmidt, H., Hirsch, O., & Mattejat, F. (2003). Reliability and validity of evaluation data collected by telephone. *Zeitschrift fur Kinder- und Jugendpsychiatrie und Psychotherapie*, *31*(1), 35–49. doi:10.1024/1422-4917.31.1.35 PMID:12616747

Reti, S. R., Feldman, H. J., & Safran, C. (2009). Governance for Personal Health Records. *Journal of the American Medical Informatics Association*, *16*(1), 14–17. doi:10.1197/jamia.M2854 PMID:18952939

Revicki, D. A., Tohen, M., Gyulai, L., Thompson, C., Pike, S., Davis-Vogel, A., & Zarate, C. (1997). Telephone versus in-person clinical and health assessment interviews in patients with bipolar disorder. *Harvard Review of Psychiatry*, *5*(2), 75–81. doi:10.3109/10673229709034730 PMID:9385024

Rhoads, J., Cooper, T., Fuchs, K., Schluter, P., & Zambuto, R. P. (2010). Medical device interoperability and the Integrating the Healthcare Enterprise (IHE) initiative. *Biomedical Instrumentation & Technology,* 21-27.

Richter, A., Stocker, A., Müller, S., & Avram, G. (2013). Knowledge management goals revisited: A cross-sectional analysis of social software adoption in corporate environments. *Vine*, *43*(2), 132–148. doi:10.1108/03055721311329927

Riley, W. T., Rivera, D. E., Atienza, A. A., Nilsen, W., Allison, S. M., & Mermelstein, R. (2011). Health behavior models in the age of mobile interventions: Are our theories up to the task? *Translational Behavioral Medicine*, *1*(1), 53–71. doi:10.1007/s13142-011-0021-7 PMID:21796270

Rimner, T., Blozik, E., Begley, C., Grandchamp, C., & von Overbeck, J. (2011). Patient adherence to recommendations after teleconsultation: Survey of patients from a telemedicine centre in Switzerland. *Journal of Telemedicine and Telecare*, *17*(5), 235–239. doi:10.1258/jtt.2011.101013 PMID:21565847

Rise, M. B., Solbjør, M., & Steinsbekk, A. (2014). Experiences from the implementation of a comprehensive development plan for user involvement in a mental health hospital: A qualitative case study. *The International Journal of Social Psychiatry*, *60*(4), 387–395. doi:10.1177/0020764013491739 PMID:23812411

Rissler, A. (1994). Extended periods of challenging demands in high tech work. Consequences for efficiency, quality of life & health. In G. E. Bradley & H. W. Hendrick (Eds.), *Human factors in organizational design & management* (vol. 4, pp. 727–732). Amsterdam: Elsevier.

Ritchie, C., Richman, J., Sobko, H., Bodner, E., Phillips, B., & Houston, T. (2012). The E-Coach transition support computer telephony implementation study: Protocol of a randomized trial. *Contemporary Clinical Trials*, *33*(6), 1172–1179. doi:10.1016/j.cct.2012.08.007 PMID:22922245

Robertson, A. et al. (2010). *Implementation and adaption of nationwide electronic health records in secondary care in England: Qualitative analysis of interim results from a prospective national evaluation*. Academic Press.

Robinson, G., & Morley, C. (2006). Call centre management: Responsibilities and performance. *International Journal of Service Industry Management*, *17*(3), 284–300. doi:10.1108/09564230610667122

Rohde, P., Lewinsohn, P. M., & Seeley, J. R. (1997). Comparability of telephone and face-to-face interviews in assessing axis I and II disorders. *The American Journal of Psychiatry*, *154*(11), 1593–1598. doi:10.1176/ajp.154.11.1593 PMID:9356570

Rohleder, T., Bailey, B., Crum, B., Faber, T., Johnson, B., Montgomery, L., & Pringnitz, R. (2013). Improving a patient appointment call center at Mayo Clinic. *International Journal of Health Care Quality Assurance*, *26*(8), 714–728. doi:10.1108/IJHCQA-11-2011-0068 PMID:24422261

Röing, M., & Holmström, I. K. (2015). Malpractice Claims in Swedish Telenursing: Lessons Learned From Interviews With Telenurses and Managers. *Nursing Research*, *64*(1), 35–43. doi:10.1097/NNR.0000000000000063 PMID:25502059

Romano, M. J., & Stafford, R. S. (2011). Electronic health records and clinical decision support systems: Impact on national ambulatory care quality. *Archives of Internal Medicine*, *171*(10), 897–903. doi:10.1001/archinternmed.2010.527 PMID:21263077

Romano, N. C. Jr, & Fjermestad, J. (2001). Electronic commerce customer relationship management: An assessment of research. *International Journal of Electronic Commerce*, *6*(2), 61–113.

Rubin, G., Cleare, A., & Wessely, S. (2008). Psychological factors associated with self-reported sensitivity to mobile phones. *Journal of Psychosomatic Research*, *64*(1), 1–9. doi:10.1016/j.jpsychores.2007.05.006 PMID:18157992

Rudi, R., & Celler, B. G. (2006). *Design and implementation of expert-telemedicine system for diabetes management at home.* Paper presented at the International Conference on Biomedical and Pharmaceutical Enginering 2006 (ICBPE2006), Singapore.

Rudkin, S. E., Langdorf, M. I., Oman, J. A., Kahn, C. A., White, H., & Anderson, C. L. (2009). The worsening of ED on-call coverage in California: 6-year trend. *The American Journal of Emergency Medicine*, *27*(7), 785–791. doi:10.1016/j.ajem.2008.06.012 PMID:19683105

Rudkin, S. E., Oman, J., Langdorf, M. I., Hill, M., Bauche, J., Kivela, P., & Johnson, L. (2004). The state of ED on-call coverage in California. *The American Journal of Emergency Medicine*, *22*(7), 578–581. doi:10.1016/j.ajem.2004.08.001 PMID:15666264

Ruland, C. M., & Ravn, I. H. (2003). Usefulness and effects on costs and staff management of a nursing resource management information system. *Journal of Nursing Management*, *11*(3), 208–215. doi:10.1046/j.1365-2834.2003.00381.x PMID:12694368

Rumbold, A. R., & Crowther, C. A. (2001). Guideline use for gestational diabetes mellitus and current screening, diagnostic and management practices in Australian hospitals. *Australian and New Zealand Journal of Obstetrics and Gynaecology*, *41*(1), 86–90. doi:10.1111/j.1479-828X.2001.tb01301.x PMID:11284655

Rumbold, A. R., & Crowther, C. A. (2002). Women's experiences of being screened for gestational diabetes mellitus. *Australian and New Zealand Journal of Obstetrics and Gynaecology*, *42*(2), 131–137. doi:10.1111/j.0004-8666.2002.00131.x PMID:12069138

Ruotsalainen, P., Iivari, A., & Doupi, P. (2008). Finland's strategy and implementation of citizens' access to health information. *Studies in Health Technology and Informatics*, *137*, 379–385. PMID:18560100

Russell, B. (2012). Professional call centres, professional workers and the paradox of the algorithm: The case of telenursing. *Work, Employment and Society*, *26*(2), 195–210. doi:10.1177/0950017011433155

Russell, L. B., Churl Suh, D., & Safford, M. M. (2005). Time requirements for diabetes management: Too much for many? *The Journal of Family Practice*, *54*(1), 52–56. PMID:15623407

Sadoughi, F., & Aminpour, F. (2011). A Review on the Evaluation Methods of Health Information Systems. *Indian Journal of Medical Education*, *10*(5), 1077–1086.

Safavi, S., & Shukur, Z. (2014). Conceptual privacy framework for health information on wearable device. *PLoS ONE*, *9*(12), e114306. doi:10.1371/journal.pone.0114306 PMID:25478915

Safran, C. (2003). The collaborative edge: Patient empowerment for vulnerable populations. *International Journal of Medical Informatics*, *69*(2), 185–190. doi:10.1016/S1386-5056(02)00130-2 PMID:12810122

Sahoo, P. K. (2012). Efficient security mechanisms for mHealth applications using wireless body sensor networks. *Sensors (Basel, Switzerland)*, *12*(9), 12606–12633. doi:10.3390/s120912606 PMID:23112734

Sakar, C. O., & Kursun, O. (2010). Telediagnosis of Parkinson's disease using measurements of dysphonia. *Journal of Medical Systems*, *34*(4), 591–599. doi:10.1007/s10916-009-9272-y PMID:20703913

Salomann, H., Kolbe, L., & Brenner, W. (2006). Self-services in customer relationships: Balancing high-tech and high-touch today and tomorrow. *E-Service Journal*, *4*(2), 65–84. doi:10.2979/ESJ.2006.4.2.65

Samantra, C., Datta, S., & Mahapatra, S. S. (2014). Risk Assessment in IT Outsourcing using Fuzzy Decision-making Approach: An Indian Perspective. *Expert Systems with Applications*, *41*(8), 4010–4022. doi:10.1016/j.eswa.2013.12.024

Santana, M. A. S., Aupet, J. B., Betbeder, M. L., Lapayre, J. C., & Ibarrola, J. A. C. (2012). Adaptive collaborative environment for vascular problems telediagnosis. In *Ambient Assisted Living and Home Care* (pp. 1–8). Springer Berlin Heidelberg. doi:10.1007/978-3-642-35395-6_1

Saorín-Iborra, M. C., Redondo-Cano, A., Revuelto-Taboada, L., & Vogler, É. (2015). Negotiating behavior in service outsourcing. An exploratory case study analysis. *Service Business*, 1–31. doi:10.1007/s11628-014-0259-5

Sarasohn-Kahn, J. (2010). *How smartphones are changing health care for consumers and providers*. California HealthCare Foundation. Retrieved from http://www.chcf.org/

Saraux, A., Guillemin, F., Fardellone, P., Guggenbuhl, P., Behier, J. M., Cantagrel, A., & Coste, J. et al. (2004). Agreement between rheumatologist visit and lay interviewer telephone survey for screening for rheumatoid arthritis and spondyloarthropathy. *Joint, Bone, Spine*, *71*(1), 44–50. doi:10.1016/S1297-319X(03)00092-7 PMID:14769520

Sarkar, U., Piette, J. D., Gonzales, R., Lessler, D., Chew, L. D., Reilly, B., & Schillin.ger, D. et al. (2008). Prefere.nces for self-management support: Findings from a survey of diabetes patients in safety-net health systems. *Patient Education and Counseling*, *70*(1), 102–110. doi:10.1016/j.pec.2007.09.008 PMID:17997264

Scalone, L., Mantovani, L. G., Krol, M., Rofail, D., Ravera, S., & Grazia Bisconte, M. et al. (2008). Costs, quality of life, treatment satisfaction and compliance in patients with -thalassemia major undergoing iron chelation therapy: The ITHACA study. *Current Medical Research and Opinion*, *24*(7), 1905–1917. PMID:18507891

Schick, A. G., Gordon, L. A., & Haka, S. (1990). Information overload: A temporal approach. *Accounting, Organizations and Society*, *15*(3), 199–220. doi:10.1016/0361-3682(90)90005-F

Schillewaert, N., Ahearne, M. J., Frambach, R. T., & Moenaert, R. K. (2005). The adoption of information technology in the sales force. *Industrial Marketing Management*, *34*(4), 323–336. doi:10.1016/j.indmarman.2004.09.013

Schot, J., & Rip, A. (1997). The past and future of constructive technology assessment. *Technological Forecasting and Social Change*, *54*, 251–268.

Schultze, U., & Vandenbosch, B. (1998). Information overload in a groupware environment: Now you see it, now you don't. *Journal of Organizational Computing and Electronic Commerce*, *8*(2), 127–148. doi:10.1207/s15327744joce0802_3

Schweiger, A., Sunyaev, A., Leimeister, J. M., & Krcmar, H. (2007). Information systems and healthcare XX: Toward seamless healthcare with software agents. *Communications of the Association for Information Systems*, *19*(1), 33.

Seemann, J. (2013). Interorganizational innovation in systemic networks. *The Innovation Journal: The Public Sector Innovation Journal, 18*(3), 1-1-18.

Sekaran, U. (2006). *Research methods for business*. Wiley India Pvt. Ltd.

Shani, A. B., & Sena, J. A. (1994). Information technology & the integration of change: Sociotechnical system approach. *The Journal of Applied Behavioral Science*, *30*(2), 247–261. doi:10.1177/0021886394302007

Shapiro, D. (2009). Examining Taiwan's hospitals. *Topics*, *39*(3).

Shapiro, C., & Varian, H. R. (1999). *Information Rules: A Strategic Guide to the Network Economy*. Boston, MA: Harvard Business School Press.

Sharma, S., Kilian, R., & Leung, F.-H. (2014). Health 2.0—Lessons Learned Social Networking With Patients for Health Promotion. *Journal of Primary Care & Community Health*.

Sheikh, A., Cornford, T., & Barber, N. (2011). Implementation and adoption of nationwide electronic health record in secondary care in England: Final qualitative results from prospective national evaluation in "eraly adopter"hospitals. *British Medical Journal, 343*(d6054).

Shekelle, P., & Goldzweig, C. L. (2009). *Costs and Benefits of Health Information Technology: An Updated Systematic Review*. London, UK: The Health Foundation.

Sheng, M., Chang, S.-Y., Teo, T. S., & Lin, Y.-F. (2013). Knowledge Barriers, Knowledge Transfer, and Innovation Competitive Advantage in Healthcare Settings. *Management Decision, 51*(3), 1–1. doi:10.1108/00251741311309607

Sheth, A. P. (1998). Changing Focus on Interoperability in Information Systems: From System, Syntax, Structure to Semantics. In M. F. Goodchild, M. J. Egenhofer, R. Fegeas, & C. A. Kottman (Eds.), *Interoperating Geographic Information Systems*. Kluwer.

Shi, J., Peng, Y., Erdem, E., & Woodbridge, P. (2014, September). Simulation analysis on patient visit efficiency of a typical VA primary care clinic with complex characteristics. *Simulation Modelling Practice and Theory*, *47*, 165–181. doi:10.1016/j.simpat.2014.06.003

Shimizu, Y. (2004). Koto-Kyoiku Ni Okeru E-Learning No Shien To Kyoiku Kontentsu No Kyoyu [Support by e-Learning in Higher Education and Sharing of Educational Contents]. *Media Research, 1*, 1-10.

Shimizu, Y. (2002). E-Learning Wo Sasaeru Seisaku To Kongo No Tembo[Polices to Support e-Learning and Foresight Thereof]. *Information Processing*, *43*, 421–426.

Shokrollahi, K., Tadiparthi, S., & Jayagopal, S. (2008). How fast is fast enough? An audit and league table of response times of acute hospital NHS Trust switchboards in England. *Journal of the Royal Society of Medicine*, *101*(7), 364–371. doi:10.1258/jrsm.2008.080006 PMID:18591690

Showell, C., & Nohr, C. (2012). How should we define eHealth, and does the definition matter?. *Quality of Life through Quality of Information, 180*, 881-884.

Shuraida, S., & Barki, H. (2013). The Influence of Analyst Communication in IS Projects. *Journal of the Association for Information Systems*, *14*(9), 482–520.

Shvaiko, P., & Euzenat, J. (2013). Ontology Matching: State of the Art and Future Challenges. *IEEE Transactions on Knowledge and Data Engineering*, *25*(1), 158–176. doi:10.1109/TKDE.2011.253

Silverman, D. (2001). *Interpreting qualitative data* (2nd ed.). London: Sage.

Silvestro, R., Fitzgerald, L., Johnston, R., & Voss, C. (1992). Towards a classification of service processes. *International Journal of Service Industry Management*, *3*(3), 62–75. doi:10.1108/09564239210015175

Silvestro, R., & Silvestro, C. (2003). New service design in NHS: An evaluation of the strategic alignment of NHS Direct. *International Journal of Operations & Production Management*, *23*(4), 401–417. doi:10.1108/01443570310467320

Simonsen, J., & Hertzum, J. (2006). A regional PD strategy for EPR systems: Evidence-based IT development.*Ninth Biennial Conference on Participatory Design, 2,*125-128.

Simonsen, J., & Hertzum, J. (2008). Participative design and the challenges of large-scale systems: Estending the itereative PD approach.*Proceedings Participatory Design Conference.*

Sinaiko, J. E. (1999). The danger of being too lean. Warning signs that your health care organization has cut too much. *Cost & Quality: CQ*, *5*(4), 29–31. PMID:11066613

Singer, S., Burgers, J., Friedberg, M., Rosenthal, M., Leape, L., & Schneider, E. (2011). Defining and measuring integrated patient care: Promoting the next frontier in health care delivery. *Medical Care Research and Review*, *68*(1), 112–127. doi:10.1177/1077558710371485 PMID:20555018

Slack, C. (2007). The robot surgeon. *Proto Magazine*. Retrieved May 17, 2014 from: http://www.protomag.com/assets/the-robot-surgeon?page=1

Snooks, H. A., Williams, A. M., Griffiths, L. J., Peconi, J., Rance, J., Snelgrove, S., & Cheung, W. Y. et al. (2008). Real nursing? The development of telenursing. *Journal of Advanced Nursing*, *62*(6), 631–640. doi:10.1111/j.1365-2648.2007.04546.x PMID:18302604

Sood, S., Mbarika, V., Jugoo, S., Dookhy, R., Doarn, C. R., Prakash, N., & Merrell, R. C. (2007). What is telemedicine? A collection of 104 peer-reviewed perspectives and theoretical underpinnings. *Telemedicine Journal and e-Health*, *13*(5), 573–590. doi:10.1089/tmj.2006.0073 PMID:17999619

Spear, S. J. (2005). Fixing health care from inside. *Harvard Business Review*, *83*(9), 78–91. PMID:16171213

Spears, J. L., & Barki, H. (2010). User Participation in Information Systems Security Risk Management. *Management Information Systems Quarterly*, *34*(3), 503–528.

Sperling, J. (2000). *Rebel with a Cause: The Entrepreneur Who Created the University of Phoenix and the For-Profit Revolution in Higher Education*. New York: John Wiley & Sons.

Spinelli, R. (2008). The digital economy: A conceptual framework for a new economic paradigm. *The Journal of Business*, *8*(1/2), 53–59.

Spohrer, J., & Maglio, P. P. (2008). The emergence of service science: Toward systematic service innovations to accelerate co-creation of value. *Production and Operations Management*, *17*(3), 238–246. doi:10.3401/poms.1080.0027

Sprivulis, P., Walker, J., Johnston, D., Pan, E., Adler-Milstein, J., Middleton, B., & Bates, D. W. (2007). The economic benefits of health information exchange interoperability. *Australian Health Review*, *31*(4), 531–539. doi:10.1071/AH070531 PMID:17973611

Srinivasan, U., & Arunasalam, B. (2013). Leveraging big data analytics to reduce healthcare costs. *IT Professional*, *15*(6), 21–28. doi:10.1109/MITP.2013.55

Stanberry, B. (2001). Legal and Ethical Issues in Telemedicine. *Computer Methods and Programs in Telemedicine*, *64*(3), 225–233. doi:10.1016/S0169-2607(00)00142-5 PMID:11226620

Standing, C., & Lin, C. (2007). Organizational Evaluation of the Benefits, Constraints & Satisfaction with Business-To-Business Electronic Commerce. *International Journal of Electronic Commerce, 11*(3), 107–153. doi:10.2753/JEC1086-4415110304

Standing, S., Standing, C., & Lin, C. (2008). A Framework for Managing Knowledge in Strategic Alliances in the Biotechnology Sector. *Systems Research and Behavioral Science, 25*(6), 783–796. doi:10.1002/sres.861

Stead W., Miller R., Musen M. & Hersh, W. (2000), Integration and Beyond: Linking Information from Disparate Sources and into Workflow. *AMIA*, (7), 135-145.

Stead, W. W. (1994). Designing medical informatics research and library: Resource projects to increase what is learned. *Journal of the American Medical Association, 1*(1), 27–33.

Steinhubl, S. R., Muse, E. D., & Topol, E. J. (2013). Can mobile health technologies transform health care? *Journal of the American Medical Association, 310*(22), 2395–2396. doi:10.1001/jama.2013.281078 PMID:24158428

Stephens, E. (2008). *Managing IT investment - The role of EA and SOA with governance.* Paper presented at the SOA in Healthcare realizing quality-of-care, Chicago, IL.

Steventon, A., Bardsley, M., Billings, J., Dixon, J., Doll, H., Hirani, S., . . . Henderson, C. (2012). Effect of telehealth on use of secondary care and mortality: findings from the Whole System Demonstrator cluster randomised trial. *BMJ: British Medical Journal, 344.*

Stewart, J. I., Moyle, S., Criner, G. J., Wilson, C., Tanner, R., Bowler, R. P., & Regan, E. A et al.. (2012). Automated telecommunication to obtain longitudinal follow-up in a multicenter cross-sectional COPD study. *COPD: Journal of Chronic Obstructive Pulmonary Disease, 9*(5), 466–472. doi:10.3109/15412555.2012.690010 PMID:22676387

Stier, R. D. (1999). The medical call center. *Marketing Health Services, 19*(2), 25–28. PMID:10557751

Stiglitz, J. E., Sen, A., & Fitoussi, J.-P. (2009). *Report by the Commission on the Measurement of Economic Performance and Social Progress.* Retrieved on January 25, 2015 from http://www.stiglitz-sen-fitoussi.fr/en/index.htm

Stirewalt, C. F., Linn, M. W., Godoy, G., Knopka, F., & Linn, B. S. (1982). Effectiveness of an ambulatory care telephone service in reducing drop-in visits and improving satisfaction with care. *Medical Care, 20*(7), 739–748. doi:10.1097/00005650-198207000-00009 PMID:7121093

Stratopoulos, T., & Dehning, B. (2000). Does Successful Investments in Information Technology Solve the Productivity Paradox? *Information & Management, 38*(2), 103–117. doi:10.1016/S0378-7206(00)00058-6

Stringham, B. B., & Gerdes, J. Jr. (2010). An Analysis of Word-of-Mouse Ratings & Guest Comments of Online Hotel Distribution Sites. *Journal of Hospitality Marketing & Management, 19*(7), 773–796. doi:10.1080/19368623.2010.508009

Stritzke, W. G. K., Dandy, J., Durkin, K., & Houghton, S. (2005). Use of interactive voice response (IVR) technology in health research with children. *Behavior Research Methods*, *37*(1), 119–126. doi:10.3758/BF03206405 PMID:16097351

Strnadl, C. (2007). Bridging Architectural Boundaries Design and Implementation of a Semantic BPM and SOA Governance Tool Service-Oriented Computing – ICSOC 2007 (Vol. 4749, pp. 518-529). Springer Berlin / Heidelberg.

Stroetmann, K. A., Jones, T., Dobrev, A., & Stroetmann, V. N. (2006). eHealth is Worth it. The Economic Benefits of Implemented eHealth Solutions at Ten European Sites. Luxembourg: Commission of the European Communities.

Suggs, L. (2006). A 10-year retrospective of research in new technologies for health communication. *Journal of Health Communication*, *11*(1), 61–74. doi:10.1080/10810730500461083 PMID:16546919

Sugumaran, V., & Arogyaswamy, B. (2004). Measuring IT Performance: "Contingency" Variables & Value Modes. *Journal of Computer Information Systems*, *44*(2), 79–86.

Sujata, T. L., Reddy, B. K., & Jayalakshmi, C. (2013). Hospitals Outsourcing Complete Departments: A Study. *International Journal of Research in Commerce & Management*, *4*(9), 1–4.

Suleiman, A. B. (2001). The untapped potential of tele-health. *International Journal of Medical Informatics*, *61*(2-3), 103–112. doi:10.1016/S1386-5056(01)00132-0 PMID:11311664

Suomi, R., Serkkola, A., & Mikkonen, M. (2010). Automated Telephone Services in Dentist Appointment Management. *Informatics in Oral Medicine: Advanced Techniques in Clinical and Diagnostic Technologies*, 269-276.

Swanepoel, D. W., & Hall, J. W. III. (2010). A systematic review of telehealth applications in audiology. *Telemedicine Journal and e-Health*, *16*(2), 181–200. doi:10.1089/tmj.2009.0111 PMID:20187743

Swerissen, H., & Taylor, M. J. (2008). Reforming funding for chronic illness: Medicare-CDM. *Australian Health Review*, *32*(1), 76–84. doi:10.1071/AH080076 PMID:18241151

Syrek, C. J., Apostel, E., & Antoni, C. H. (2013). Stress in Highly Demanding IT Jobs: Transformational Leadership Moderates the Impact of Time Pressure on Exhaustion & Work–life Balance. *Journal of Occupational Health Psychology*, *18*(3), 252–261. doi:10.1037/a0033085 PMID:23834443

Tallon, P. P., Kraemer, K. L., & Gurbaxani, V. (2000). Executives' Perceptions of the Business Value of Information Technology: A Process-Oriented Approach. *Journal of Management Information Systems*, *16*(4), 145–173. doi:10.1080/07421222.2000.11518269

Tang, P., Ash, J., Bates, D., Overhage, J., & Sands, D. (2006). Personal Health Records: Definitions, Benefits, and Strategies for Overcoming Barriers to Adoption. *Journal of the American Medical Informatics Association*, *13*(2), 121–126. doi:10.1197/jamia.M2025 PMID:16357345

Taweel, A., Rector, A., et al. (2006). Grid-based Collaborative Secure Distributed Biomedical Research System. *The Universal Computer Science Journal, 12*(1), 80-98.

Taweel, A., Rector, A., Kalra, D., Rogers, J., et al. (2004). Joining up Healthcare with Clinical and Post-Genomic Research. In *Proceedings of Health Computing 2004*.

Taylor, J., Dearnley, C., Laxton, J., Coates, C., Treasure-Jones, T., Campbell, R., & Hall, I. (2010). Developing a mobile learning solution for health and social care practice. *Distance Education, 31*(2), 175–192. doi:10.1080/01587919.2010.503343

Taylor, R., Bower, A., Girosi, F., Bigelow, J., Fonkych, K., & Hillestad, R. (2005). Promoting Health Information Technology: Is there a case for more-aggressive government action? *Health Affairs, 24*(5), 1234–1345. doi:10.1377/hlthaff.24.5.1234 PMID:16162568

Tekli, J., Rjeily, A. A., Chbeir, R., Tekli, G., Houngue, P., Yetongnon, K., et al. (2013). *Semantic to intelligent web era: building blocks, applications, and current trends*. Paper presented at the Fifth International Conference on Management of Emergent Digital EcoSystems.

Tham, K. W., & Willem, H. C. (2004). *Effects of reported neurobehavioral symptoms on call center operator performance in the tropics*. In RoomVentilation Conference, Coimbra, Portugal

Tham, K. W. (2004). Effects of temperature and outdoor air supply rate on the performance of call center operators in the tropics. *Indoor Air, 14*(s7), 119–125. doi:10.1111/j.1600-0668.2004.00280.x PMID:15330779

Thatcher, M. D., & Pingry, D. E. (2004). Understanding the Business Value of Information Technology Investments: Theoretical Evidence from Alternative Market & Cost Structure. *Journal of Management Information Systems, 21*(2), 61–85.

The European Union. (2012). *Redesigning health in Europe in 2020*. Belgium: The European Union.

Themistocleous, M., Azab, N., Kamal, M., Ali, M., & Morabito, V. (2012). Location-Based Services for Public Policy Making: The Direct and Indirect Way to e-Participation. *Information Systems Management, 29*(4), 269–283. doi:10.1080/10580530.2012.716743

Thomas, D. R. E. (1978). Strategy is different in service businesses. *Harvard Business Review, 56*(4), 158–165.

Thomas, J., & Kumar, P. (2013). The scope of teledermatology in India. *Indian Dermatology Online Journal, 4*(2), 82. doi:10.4103/2229-5178.110579 PMID:23741661

Thomas, R. W., Fugate, B. S., & Koukova, N. T. (2011). Coping with Time Pressure & Knowledge Sharing in Buyer-Supplier Relationships. *Journal of Supply Chain Management, 47*(3), 22–42. doi:10.1111/j.1745-493X.2011.03229.x

THRF. (2011). *Hospital Finance: The Financial Supervision for the Health Institutions in Taiwan*. Taipei, Taiwan: Taiwan Healthcare Reform Foundation.

Tiago, M. B., & Tiago, F. (2013). *Roadmaps for Future ICT Use in the Health Sector Handbook of Research on ICTs and Management Systems for Improving Efficiency in Healthcare and Social Care*. IGI Global. doi:10.4018/978-1-4666-3990-4.ch035

Tiago, M. T. B., Couto, J. P. A., Tiago, F. G., & Vieira, J. A. C. (2008). The missing link between virtual CRM and e-business performance1. *International Journal of Business and Management*, *2*(1).

Tiago, M. T. B., Couto, J. P., Tiago, F., & Vieira, A. C. (2007). Knowledge management: An overview of European reality. *Management Research News*, *30*(2), 100–114. doi:10.1108/01409170710722946

Tiago, T., & Verı́ssimo, J. (2014). Digital marketing and social media: Why bother? *Business Horizons*, *57*(6), 703–708. doi:10.1016/j.bushor.2014.07.002

Tocci, R. (1988). *Digital System- Principles and Applications* (4th ed.). Englewood Cliffs, NJ: Prentice-Hall International.

Torkzadeh, G., & Dhillon, G. (2002). Measuring Factors that Influence the Success of Internet Commerce. *Information Systems Research*, *13*(2), 187–204. doi:10.1287/isre.13.2.187.87

Tornatzky, L. G., & Fleischer, M. (1990). *The processes of technological innovation*. Lexington Books.

Toverud, E. L., Pike, E., & Walloe, E. (2009). The national poison center in Norway: User satisfaction and health economic evaluation. *European Journal of Clinical Pharmacology*, *65*(9), 935–940. doi:10.1007/s00228-009-0693-9 PMID:19590863

Trist, E. H., Murray, B. J., & Pollack, A. (1963). *Organizational Choice*. London: Tavistock.

Troshani, I. & Rao, S. (2007a). The diffusion of mobile services in Australia: an evaluation using stakeholder and transaction cost economics theories. *IADIS International Journal of WWW/Internet*, *5*(2), 40-57.

Tsao, H., Lin, K., & Lin, C. (2004). An Investigation of Critical Success Factors in the Adoption of B2BEC by Taiwanese Companies. *The Journal of American Academy of Business, Cambridge*, *5*(1/2), 198–202.

Tsiknakis, M., & Kouroubali, A. (2009). Organizational factors affecting successful adoption of innovative eHealth services: A case study employing the FITT framework. *International Journal of Medical Informatics*, *78*(1), 39–52. doi:10.1016/j.ijmedinf.2008.07.001 PMID:18723389

Tulu, B., Chatterjee, S., & Laxminarayan, S. (2005). A taxonomy of telemedicine efforts with respect to applications, infrastructure, delivery tools, type of setting and purpose. In *Proceedings of the 38th Hawaii International Conference on System Sciences*. IEEE. doi:10.1109/HICSS.2005.56

Tulu, B., Chatterjee, S., & Maheshwari, M. (2007). Telemedicine taxonomy: A classification tool. *Telemedicine Journal and e-Health*, *13*(3), 349–358. doi:10.1089/tmj.2006.0055 PMID:17603838

Ueno, M. (2004). Kompakuto Na E-Learning Keiei [Small Scaled e-Learning Management]. *Articles Compiled for* the *29th National Conference of* the *Japanese Society for Information and Systems in Education.*

Urquhart, C. (2001). Analysts & Clients in Organizational Context: A Conversational Perspective. *The Journal of Strategic Information Systems, 10*(3), 243–262. doi:10.1016/S0963-8687(01)00046-4

Van Ark, B., Inklaar, R., & McGuckin, R. H. (2003). ICT and productivity in Europe and the United States Where do the differences come from? *CESifo Economic Studies, 49*(3), 295–318. doi:10.1093/cesifo/49.3.295

van der Marck, M. A., Overeem, S., Klok, P., Bloem, B. R., & Munneke, M. (2011). Evaluation of the falls telephone: An automated system for enduring assessment of falls. *Journal of the American Geriatrics Society, 59*(2), 340–344. doi:10.1111/j.1532-5415.2010.03263.x PMID:21314652

Van der Meijden, M. J., Tange, H., Troost, J., & Hasman, A. (2001). Development and implementation of an EPR: How to encourage the user. *International Journal of Medical Informatics, 64*(2-3), 173–185. doi:10.1016/S1386-5056(01)00208-8 PMID:11734384

Van der Meijden, M. J., Tange, H., Troost, J., & Hasman, A. (2003). Determinants of success of inpatient clinical information systems: A literature review. *Journal of the American Medical Informatics Association, 10*(3), 235–243. doi:10.1197/jamia.M1094 PMID:12626373

Van Eyk, H., & Baum, F. (2002). Learning about interagency collaboration: Trialling collaborative projects between hospitals and community health services. *Health & Social Care in the Community, 10*(4), 262–269. doi:10.1046/j.1365-2524.2002.00369.x PMID:12193170

van Gemert-Pijnen, J. E. W. C., Nijland, N., van Limburg, M., Ossebaard, H. C., Kelders, S. M., Eysenbach, G., & Seydel, E. R. (2011). A holistic framework to improve the uptake and impact of eHealth technologies. *Journal of Medical Internet Research, 13*(4), e111–e111. doi:10.2196/jmir.1672 PMID:22155738

Van Halteren, A., Bults, R., Wac, K., Konstantas, D., Widya, I., Dokovsky, N., & Herzog, R. et al. (2004). Mobile patient monitoring: The MobiHealth system. *The Journal on Information Technology in Healthcare, 2*(5), 365–373.

van Velsen, L., Beaujean, D. J., & van Gemert-Pijnen, J. E. (2013). Why mobile health app overload drives us crazy, and how to restore the sanity. *BMC Medical Informatics and Decision Making, 13*(1), 23. doi:10.1186/1472-6947-13-23 PMID:23399513

Venkatesh, V., & Morris, M. G. (2000). Why don't men ever stop to ask for directions? Gender, social influence, and their role in technology acceptance and usage behavior. *Management Information Systems Quarterly, 24*(1), 115–139. doi:10.2307/3250981

Verdegem, P., & Verhoest, P. (2009). Profiling the non-user: Rethinking policy initiatives stimulating ICT acceptance. *Telecommunications Policy, 33*(10-11), 642–652. doi:10.1016/j.telpol.2009.08.009

Vincent, A., Cusack, C. M., Pan, E., Hook, J. M., Kaelber, D. C., & Middleton, B. (2007). A new taxonomy for telehealth technologies. In *AMIA Annual Symposium Proceedings*.

Visser, P. R. S., Jones, D. M., Bench-Capon, T. J. M., & Shave, M. J. R. (1997, March). *An analysis of ontology mismatches; heterogeneity versus interoperability.* AAAI 1997 Spring Symposium on Ontology Engineering, Stanford, CA.

vom Brocke, J., Simons, A., Niehaves, B., Riemer, K., Plattfaut, R., & Cleven, A. (2009). *Reconstructing the Giant: On the Importance of Rigour in Documenting the Literature Search Process.* Paper presented at the ECIS 2009, Verona, Italy.

Wache, H., Wache, T., Vögele, U., Visser, H., Stuckenschmidt, G., Schuster, N. H., & Hübner, S. (2001), Ontology-based Integration of Information - A Survey of Existing Approaches. In *Proceedings of IJCAI-01 Workshop: Ontologies and Information Sharing*.

Wagner, E., & McCorkle, R. (2010). Self-management support. In *Psycho-Oncology*. London: Oxford University Press. doi:10.1093/med/9780195367430.003.0063

Wahlberg, A., Anna, C., Cedersund, E., & Wredling, R. (2003). Telephone nurses' experience of problems with telephone advice in Sweden. *Journal of Clinical Nursing*, *12*(1), 37–45. doi:10.1046/j.1365-2702.2003.00702.x PMID:12519248

Walston, S. L., Bennett, C. J., & Al-Harbi, A. (2014). Understanding the Factors Affecting Employees' Perceived Benefits of Healthcare Information Technology. *International Journal of Healthcare Management*, *7*(1), 35–44. doi:10.1179/2047971913Y.0000000051

Wan, Y. N. (2012). *Call centre communication: an analysis of interpersonal meaning*. (Master's thesis). The Hong Kong Polytechnic University.

Wang, S. J., Middleton, B., Prosser, L. A., Bardon, C. G., Spurr, C. D., & Carchidi, P. J. et al. (2003). A cost-benefit analysis of electronic medical records in primary care. *The American Journal of Medicine*, *114*(5), 397–403. doi:10.1016/S0002-9343(03)00057-3 PMID:12714130

Ward, J., & Griffiths, P. (1996). *Strategic Planning For Information Systems*. Chichester, UK: John Wiley & Sons Ltd.

Ware, J. E., Davies, A. R., & Stewart, A. L. (1977). *The measurement and meaning of patient satisfaction: a review of the literature*. Rand Corporation.

Wargocki, P., Wyon, D. P., & Fanger, P. O. (2004). The performance and subjective responses of call-center operators with new and used supply air filters at two outdoor air supply rates. *Indoor Air*, *14*(s8Suppl. 8), 7–16. doi:10.1111/j.1600-0668.2004.00304.x PMID:15663456

Waseda Daigaku. (1972). *Kōhon Waseda Daigaku Hyakunenshi* (Vol. 1). Waseda University Press.

Waseda University. (2002). Waseda-Daigaku Ningenkagakbu Setsurisu Shui Oyobi Tokuni Secchiwo Hituyou To Sururiyu [Intent and purpose of Establishing the School of Human Sciences, Waseda University]. Unpublished application submitted to the Ministry of Education, Culture, Sports, Science, and Technology, Government of Japan.

Wears, R. L., & Berg, M. (2005). Computer technology and clinical work. still waiting for godot. *Journal of the American Medical Association, 293*(10), 1261–1263. doi:10.1001/jama.293.10.1261 PMID:15755949

Weir, H., & Waddington, K. (2008). Continuities in caring? Emotion work in a NHS Direct call centre. *Nursing Inquiry, 15*(1), 67–77. doi:10.1111/j.1440-1800.2008.00391.x PMID:18271792

Wellard, S. J., Rennie, S., & King, R. (2008). Perceptions of people with type 2 diabetes about self-management and the efficiency of community based services. *Contemporary Nurse, 29*(2), 218–226. doi:10.5172/conu.673.29.2.218 PMID:18844535

Whitmore, A., Agarwal, A., & Da Xu, L. (2014). The Internet of Things—A survey of topics and trends. *Information Systems Frontiers*, 1–14.

Whittaker, R., Merry, S., Dorey, E., & Maddison, R. (2012). A development and evaluation process for mHealth interventions: examples from New Zealand. *Journal of Health Communication, 17*(sup1), 11-21.

Whitten, P., & Love, B. (2005). Patient and provider satisfaction with the use of telemedicine: Overview and rationale for cautious enthusiasm. *Journal of Postgraduate Medicine, 51*(4), 294–299. PMID:16388172

WHO – World Health Organisation. (2006a). eHealth Tools and Services. Needs of the Member States. Geneva, Switzerland: WHO.

WHO – World Health Organisation. (2006b). *Building Foundations for eHealth. Progress of Member States*. Geneva, Switzerland: WHO.

Wickramasinghe, N., & Goldberg, S. (2003). *The wireless panacea for healthcare*. Paper presented at the 36th Hawaii International Conference on System Sciences, Hawaii, HI.

Wickramasinghe, N., & Goldberg, S. (2006). M-health: A New Paradigm for Mobilizing Healthcare Delivery. IGI Global.

Wickramasinghe, N. (2007). Fostering knowledge assets in healthcare with the KMI model. *International Journal of Management and Enterprise Development, 4*(1), 52–65. doi:10.1504/IJMED.2007.011455

Wickramasinghe, N., & Goldberg, S. (2004). How M=EC2 in healthcare. *International Journal of Mobile Communications, 2*(2), 140–156. doi:10.1504/IJMC.2004.004664

Wickramasinghe, N., & Goldberg, S. (2007). Adaptive mapping to realisation methodology (AMR) to facilitate mobile initiatives in healthcare. *International Journal of Mobile Communications, 5*(3), 300–318. doi:10.1504/IJMC.2007.012396

Wickramasinghe, N., Goldberg, S., & Bali, R. (2007). Enabling superior m-health project success: A tri-country validation. *International Journal of Services and Standards, 4*(1), 97–117. doi:10.1504/IJSS.2008.016087

Wickramasinghe, N., & Schaffer, J. (2006). Creating knowledge driven healthcare processes with the intelligence continuum. *International Journal of Electronic Healthcare*, *2*(2), 164–174. doi:10.1504/IJEH.2006.008830 PMID:18048242

Wickramasinghe, N., Troshani, I., & Goldberg, S. (2009). Supporting diabetes self-management with pervasive wireless technology solutions. *International Journal of Healthcare Delivery Reform Initiatives*, *1*(4), 17–31. doi:10.4018/jhdri.2009100102

Wickramasinghe, N., Troshani, I., & Goldberg, S. (2010). An investigation into the use of pervasive wireless technologies to support diabetes healthcare. In A. Coronato & G. De Pietro (Eds.), *Pervasive and Smart Technologies for Healthcare: Ubiquitous Methodologies and Tools* (Vol. 114-129). New York: IGI Global. doi:10.4018/978-1-61520-765-7.ch006

Wild, R., & Griggs, K. (2008). A model of information technology opportunities for facilitating the practice of knowledge management. *Vine*, *38*(4), 490–506. doi:10.1108/03055720810917732

Wild, S., Roglic, G., Green, A., Sicree, R., & King, H. (2004). Global prevalence of diabetes: Estimates for the year 2000 and projections for 2030. *Diabetes Care*, *27*(5), 1047–1053. doi:10.2337/diacare.27.5.1047 PMID:15111519

Williams, B., Warren, S., McKim, R., & Janzen, W. (2012). Caller self-care decisions following teletriage advice. *Journal of Clinical Nursing*, *21*(7-8), 1041–1050. doi:10.1111/j.1365-2702.2011.03986.x PMID:22283747

Williamson, O. E. (1985). *The Economic Institutions of Capitalism: Firms, Markets, and Relational Contracting*. New York: Free Press.

Williamson, O. E. (1991). Comparative economic organization: The analysis of discrete structural alternatives. *Administrative Science Quarterly*, *36*(2), 269–296. doi:10.2307/2393356

Wilson, V., & Strong, D. (2014). Editors' Introduction to the Special Section on Patient-centered e-Health: Research Opportunities and Challenges. *Communications of the Association for Information Systems*, *34*(15).

Witt, L. A., Andrews, M. C., & Carlson, D. S. (2004). When conscientiousness isn't enough: Emotional exhaustion and performance among call center customer service representatives. *Journal of Management*, *30*(1), 149–160. doi:10.1016/j.jm.2003.01.007

Wolf, M. S., Seligman, H., Davis, T. C., Fleming, D. A., Curtis, L. M., & Pandit, A. U. et al. (2014). Clinic-Based Versus Outsourced Implementation of a Diabetes Health Literacy Intervention. *Journal of General Internal Medicine*, *29*(1), 59–67. doi:10.1007/s11606-013-2582-2 PMID:24002623

Wu, I., & Shen, Y. (2006). A Model for Exploring the Impact of Purchasing Strategies on User Requirements determination of e-SRM. *Information & Management*, *43*(4), 411–422. doi:10.1016/j.im.2004.11.004

Wu, M., Wang, Z., Zhang, A., & Yang, H. (2009). Ontology-driven Heterogeneous Geographic Data Set Integration. In *Proceedings of the 2009 WRI Global Congress on Intelligent Systems*. doi:10.1109/GCIS.2009.347

Yayla, A. A., & Hu, Q. (2012). The impact of IT-business strategic alignment on firm performance in a developing country setting: Exploring moderating roles of environmental uncertainty & strategic orientation. *European Journal of Information Systems*, *21*(4), 373–387. doi:10.1057/ejis.2011.52

Yeh, C. H., Lee, G. G., & Pai, J. C. (2014). Using a technology-organization-environment framework to investigate the factors influencing e-business information technology capabilities. *Information Development*.

Yi, M. Y., & Hwang, Y. (2003). Predictingthe use of web-based information systems: Self-efficacy, enjoyment, learning goal orientation, and the technology acceptance model. Int. *J. Human-Computer Studies*, *59*(4), 431–449. doi:10.1016/S1071-5819(03)00114-9

Yin, R. K. (2002). *Case Study Research, Design & Methods* (3rd ed.). Newbury Park, CA: Sage Publications.

Yoon, Y., Guimaraes, T., & O'Neal, Q. (1995). Exploring the factors associated with expert systems success. *Management Information Systems Quarterly*, *19*(1), 83–106. doi:10.2307/249712

Yoshida, A. (2002). Koto-Kyoiku Ni Okeru E-Learning - Virtual University No Tojyo[e-Learning in Higher Education - the Advent of the Virtual University]. *Information Processing*, *43*, 407–413.

Young, M., Sparrow, D., Gottlieb, D., Selim, A., & Friedman, R. (2001). A telephone linked computer system for COPD care. *Chest*, *119*(5), 1565–1575. doi:10.1378/chest.119.5.1565 PMID:11348968

Young, R. J., Taylor, J., Friede, T., Hollis, S., Mason, J. M., Lee, P., & Gibson, J. M. et al. (2005). Pro-active call centre treatment support (PACCTS) to improve glucose control in type 2 diabetes: A randomized controlled trial. *Diabetes Care*, *28*(2), 278–282. doi:10.2337/diacare.28.2.278 PMID:15677779

Young, R., & Jordan, E. (2008). Top management support: Mantra or necessity. *International Journal of Project Management*, *26*(7), 713–725. doi:10.1016/j.ijproman.2008.06.001

Yu, P. (2010). A multi-method approach to evaluate health information systems.*World Congress on Medical Informatics* (pp. 1231-1235). Amsterdam: IOS Press.

Yusof, M. M., Kuljis, J., Papazafeiropoulou, A., & Stergioulas, L. K. (2008b). An Evaluation Framework for Health Information Systems: Human, Organization & Technology-fit Factors (HOT-fit). *International Journal of Medical Informatics*, *77*(6), 386–398. doi:10.1016/j.ijmedinf.2007.08.011 PMID:17964851

Yusof, M. M., Papazafeiropoulou, A., Paul, R. J., & Stergioulas, L. K. (2008). Investigating evaluation frameworks for health information systems. *International Journal of Medical Informatics*, *77*(6), 377–385. doi:10.1016/j.ijmedinf.2007.08.004 PMID:17904898

Zanaboni, P., Scalvini, S., Bernocchi, P., Borghi, G., Tridico, C., & Masella, C. (2009). Teleconsultation service to improve healthcare in rural areas: Acceptance, organizational impact and appropriateness. *BMC Health Services Research*, *9*(1), 238. doi:10.1186/1472-6963-9-238 PMID:20021651

Zeithaml, V. A., & Bitner, M. J. (2000). *Service Marketing: Integrating Customer Focus across the Firm*. New York, NY: McGraw Hill.

Zeng, Y. E., Wen, H. J., & Yen, D. C. (2003). Customer Relationship Management (CRM) in Business-to-business (B2B) E-commerce. *Information Management & Computer Security*, *11*(1), 39–44. doi:10.1108/09685220310463722

Zhijiang, D., Zhiheng, J., & Minxiu, K. (2006). Virtual reality-based telesurgery via teleprogramming scheme combined with semi-autonomous control.*Proceedings of the 27th Annual International Conference*. Engineering in Medicine and Biology Society.

Zhou, F., Yang, H., Álamo, J., Wong, J., & Chang, C. (2010). Mobile Personal Health Care System for Patients with Diabetes. In Y. Lee, Z. Z. Bien, M. Mokhtari, J. Kim, M. Park, J. Kim, H. Lee, & I. Khalil (Eds.), Aging Friendly Technology for Health and Independence. Springer Berlin Heidelberg.

Zhuang, Y. (2005). Does Electronic Business Create Value For Firms? An Organizational Innovation Perspective. *Journal of Electronic Commerce Research*, *6*(2), 146–159.

Zhu, K., & Kraemer, K. (2002). E-commerce Metrics for Net-enhanced Organizations: Assessing the Value of e-commerce to Firm Performance in the Manufacturing Sector. *Information Systems Research*, *13*(3), 275–295. doi:10.1287/isre.13.3.275.82

Zhu, K., Kraemer, K., & Dedrick, J. (2004). Information Technology payoff in e-business environments: Na international perspective of value creation of e-business in the financial service industry. *Journal of Management Information Systems*, *21*(1), 17–54.

Zigbor, J. C., & Songer, T. J. (2001). External barriers to diabetes care: Addressing personal and health systems issues. *Diabetes Spectrum*, *14*(1), 23–28. doi:10.2337/diaspect.14.1.23

Zika-Viktorsson, A., Sundstrom, P., & Engwall, M. (2006). Project overload: An exploratory study of work & management in multi-project settings. *International Journal of Project Management*, *24*(5), 385–394. doi:10.1016/j.ijproman.2006.02.010

About the Contributors

Ashish Dwivedi is the Deputy Director of the Centre for Systems Studies at Hull University Business School, UK. Previously, he was the Deputy Graduate Research Director at Hull University Business School, and was also associated with the management of the high-tech Management Learning Laboratory. His primary research interests are in knowledge management (in which he obtained his PhD), supply chain management, healthcare management and information, and communication technologies. He has published 4 books, and over 50 journal and conference papers. He has served as an Invited reviewer and Guest Editor for several journals, including the IEEE Transactions on Information Technology in Biomedicine.

* * *

Clara Benevolo holds a degree in Business and Economics from the University of Genoa (Italy). She is an Associate Professor in Management at the same institution. She teaches management, international management and marketing, e-business. Her research interests include service firms, global strategies, internationalization processes and entry modes to foreign markets, relationships between internationalization and adoption of ICT. She published in international journals such as *Social Science Computer Review* and the *International Journal of Services, Economics and Management*; she presented her research in national and international conferences such as AEDEM, ICIME, iCETS and ItAIS.

Steve Goldberg has a B.A. (Economics) from the University of Western Ontario. He is also a program committee member, International Conference on Electronic Commerce Research (ICECR), SMU, Dallas, Texas, and he found and served as the Chair of the Wireless IT Committee, ITAC Ontario. Mr. Goldberg gives talks in Canada and United States on wireless technology in Healthcare. He has several papers accepted under peer review for presentation at international conferences, and his work is published in leading international journals.

Konstantinos Koumaditis is an assistant professor at the department of Business Development and Technology of Aarhus University. He holds a bachelor degree on Electrical/Electronic Engineering from the University of Portsmouth UK, Masters degree with specialization in Electronics, Digital Systems, University of Hertfordshire UK, Masters degree on Engineering Management with honors from Brunel University, UK and a PhD from University of Piraeus, Greece. His last post was as a Research Associate at University of Piraeus in the Department of Digital Systems with research focus on Service Oriented Architecture (SOA) and especially SOA Governance in Healthcare Information Systems (HIS).In the past he has worked as an educator of new technologies/ICT and as a seminar trainer in various management/IS/HIS subjects. Also, he participated as a researcher in European research projects. He has published research articles in international scientific conferences/ journals and chapters in books with focus on: IS, SOA, SOA Governance, HIS. His research interests include amongst other: digital health services, HIS, EHR, SOA, SOA & Cloud Computing Governance, IS and project management.

Rupananda Misra has more than 19 years of teaching experience in higher education, including interactive digital media, health communication, and learning technologies. He has completed a two-year, NIH-funded postdoctoral fellowship at Columbia University in health informatics focused on exploring technology-mediated information interventions to promote healthy behavioral choices. His doctoral research at Columbia University, focused on understanding design issues of government and non-government educational HIV/AIDS Web sites. From a broader perspective, his fields of interest include the study of the design of the Public Health Message from a semiotic perspective, that is, exploring the study of signs and how the public health sector uses them to construct its message and how users interpret the health message. Signs can mean words, images, sounds, and gestures. Chandler posits meanings are not transmitted to us, but we actively create them according to the complex interplay of codes and conventions that we are usually not aware of. Another interest is in understanding the communicative aspect of emerging media and how public health messages use them, that is, both how the sector uses media in representation as well as how the user assigns meaning based on its interpretation.

Riccardo Spinelli received his PhD in Service Management and Economics from the University of Genoa (Italy). He is an Assistant Professor in Management at the same institution, where he teaches marketing and international management. His research interests include the foundations of the digital economy, the relationship between the development of e-business and the internationalization of firms, the application of ICT in SMEs and the management of SMEs. He published in international journals such as *Industrial Management & Data Systems*, the *Journal of*

Small Business and Enterprise Development, the *International Journal of Services, Economics and Management*; he presented his research in national and international conferences such as ECIME, ICE-B, ISBE and ItAIS.

Marinos Themistocleous is an Associate Professor at the Department of Digital Systems at University of Piraeus, Greece. He holds a B.Sc. in Computer Science, a Postgraduate Degree in Teaching and Learning in Higher Education, a M.Sc. in Information Systems Management and Ph.D. in Informatics. Before joining University of Piraeus, he worked as a Lecturer and a Senior Lecturer at Brunel University, UK. He has close relationships with industry and has worked as a consultant for the Greek Ministry of Finance, the Bank of Greece, the Greek Standardization body, the Greek Federation of SMEs, ORACLE UK, Havering Council, BTO Research etc. He has authored several teaching textbooks, internationally refereed journal papers and conference articles and has received many citations and awards of excellence. His research has attracted funding from various funding bodies. He acts as an international reviewer for research proposals submitted to the European Union and other funding bodies. His current research interests include Information Systems, Information Systems Management, Service-Oriented Architectures, cloud computing, e-business, e-health and e-government.

Indrit Troshani is a senior lecturer in accounting information systems at the University of Adelaide Business School. He holds a Ph.D. (computer science), an M.Sc. (computer-based information systems), and a Bachelor of Business Administration (Hons). His research interests include digital business reporting (e.g. XBRL), impact of information and communications technology (ICT) on accounting, adoption, and diffusion of innovations (e.g. XBRL, Green IS/IT, e-health, and mobile services). His work has been published in several journals including *Accounting and Business Research, Journal of Contemporary Accounting and Economics, Information Technology & People, Electronic Markets, Journal of Computer Information Systems, Journal of Engineering and Technology Management, European Journal of Innovation Management*, and *Industrial Management & Data Systems*.

Nilmini Wickramasinghe (PhD, MBA, BSc.) is the Professor of Health Informatics Management at Deakin University and the Professor-Director of Health Informatics Management at Epworth HealthCare, Melbourne, Australia. She researches and teaches in various aspects of using technology solutions to provide superior and sustainable patient centric healthcare delivery scenarios. She is well published with over 300 peer reviewed articles, numerous book chapters, books and encyclopaedia entries. Professor Wickramasinghe regularly presents her work in Asia, Europe and North America and the editor in chief of 2 international journals.

Index

A

Assessment 3, 14, 18, 19, 49, 57-60, 81-84, 96-99, 105, 113, 115, 122, 123, 126, 130, 156, 166, 171, 173, 228, 232, 273, 287, 293, 297, 313, 317
Asset-Specific Exchanges 19, 42

B

Benefits Realization 132-138, 143-146, 151-157, 160, 163, 171
Big Data 231-234, 241-245, 292, 296, 308

C

Connected Health 246, 247

D

Data Integration 249, 262
Data Protection 42, 123, 297
Degree Program 175, 176
Demand Uncertainty 19, 26, 42
Diabetes 2-4, 9-43, 92, 100, 115, 125, 169, 213, 214, 228, 286, 321
Diabetes Self-Management 3, 10, 14-20, 26, 27, 34, 41, 42
Digital Economy 205-209, 219, 222, 225, 227, 241-245
Distance Education 13, 173, 174

E

E-Commerce 28, 35, 132-155, 159, 162-164, 167, 170-172, 237, 317
E-Health 12, 22, 37, 39, 105, 114, 123, 129, 164, 165, 205-219, 222, 223, 229-245, 269, 270, 284, 286, 297, 309, 312, 313, 320, 321
E-Learning 163, 174-177, 185-187, 199-204, 228, 241
Electronic Health Records (EHR) 44-48, 58-73, 80-86, 127, 214, 224, 227, 233, 234, 240, 245-248, 251, 260-263, 269, 270, 283, 290
End-User 44-49, 52-61, 73-81, 86, 298, 308, 309
End-User Involvement 45, 49, 54, 57, 58, 61, 73-77, 81, 86
End-User Participation 44-47, 52, 57, 61, 73, 78, 80, 86
E-Prescriptions 225, 245
Evaluation Method 44-46, 49-54, 57-63, 67, 73-78

F

Formative Evaluation 44, 45, 48, 49, 61, 65, 76, 78
Frequency 19, 20, 27, 42, 131, 210, 218, 236, 245, 306

G

Georeferencing 231, 245
Gestational Diabetes Mellitus (GDM) 14-19, 24-32, 35-42

H

Healthcare Information Systems (HIS) 82, 89, 103, 108, 171, 202, 267-271, 275-280, 284, 286, 294, 298-307, 310, 314, 320, 322
Healthcare Services 3, 27, 96, 102, 107, 111, 112, 143, 205-207, 210-213, 219, 220, 223-226, 230, 231, 235, 241, 269, 283, 286, 288, 291, 295, 307
Healthcare Telephone System 87-90, 93, 104, 108, 110, 131
Health Information Technology 61, 80, 81, 161, 164, 211, 236-243, 284, 312, 320
Healthy 3.0 287, 308, 309, 322
Heterogeneity 246-253, 263, 265
Higher Education 173, 174, 204
HIS integration 269, 280, 286
HIS Interoperability 286
HIS Measurement 322
Hospitals 17, 21, 32, 33, 40, 41, 48, 60, 63, 67, 84, 89, 103, 104, 121, 132-155, 160-168, 171, 211, 213, 218, 224, 226, 232, 239, 251, 269, 281, 312, 316

I

ICT acceptance 287, 293, 307, 319, 322
ICT Induce Benefits 322
ICT Performance 322
ICT ROI 322
ICT Support 25, 322
Information Requirements Definition (IRD) 141, 142, 150, 153, 172
Information Technology (IT) 47, 133, 172, 270
Information Technology Outsourcing 156, 161, 172
Interactive Voice Response System (IVRS) 95, 101-103, 113, 118-124, 131
Internet-Based Technologies 205, 206, 219-221, 225, 229, 235, 236
Internet of Things 115, 240, 244, 245
Interoperability 5, 9, 33, 40, 212, 246-254, 260-271, 277, 284-286, 292, 293, 297, 300, 302, 305, 306, 309, 310
IT evaluation 132-136, 139, 153
IT Investment Evaluation Methodologies 136, 172

J

Japan 120, 166, 173-179, 197-204

L

Learning Management System (LMS) 173, 178, 186, 191, 192
Lifelong Education 173, 174, 200

M

Machine to Machine (M2M) Communication 231, 239, 245
Mobile Health 3, 6-14, 97, 112, 115
Monitoring Diabetes 17, 28, 29, 35, 36

N

New Economy 158

O

On-Call Physician 87, 103, 104, 131
Ontology 248, 249, 253-257, 261-265
Organizational Factors 129, 163, 233
Outsourcing Projects 132, 135, 146, 148, 151, 154

P

Participation 18, 44-47, 52, 54, 57, 61-64, 73, 74, 78-82, 85, 86, 135, 139, 145, 146, 152-155, 158, 159, 167, 218, 234, 294
Patient Centered E-Health (PCEH) 270, 286
Pervasive Technology Solution 42
Platform Independent 42

R

Radio Frequency Identification (RFID) 245

S

Semantic Web Services 246, 263
Service Oriented Architecture (SOA) 266-286
Service Oriented Architecture (SOA) Governance 266-286
Social Carriers of Technology 52, 86

T

Task Complexity 19, 42
Technological Lifecycle 48, 52-54, 60, 65, 78
Tele-Diagnosis 87, 95, 98, 99, 111, 131
Tele-Health 87-91, 96, 99, 105, 107, 110-112, 129, 131
Telemedicine 9, 12, 19, 29, 31, 36-38, 46, 89, 91, 106, 107, 112-118, 121-129, 210, 214-217, 236-244, 282-284, 312, 315, 320, 321
Telephone-Triage 131
Top Management Support 135, 139, 140, 145-147, 152, 166, 169, 172
Transaction Cost Economics (TCE) Theory 14, 17, 19, 33, 40, 43
Transaction Costs 14

U

Underreferral 87, 98, 110, 119, 131
User Involvement 32, 39, 48, 81, 85, 146, 156, 166

W

Wearable Technology 245
Workload Reduction 47, 58, 66-70, 86

www.ingramcontent.com/pod-product-compliance
Lightning Source LLC
LaVergne TN
LVHW062109200926
848484LV00007B/1627
* 9 7 8 1 4 6 6 6 9 8 7 0 3 *